ASTHMA

PHYSIOLOGY, IMMUNOPHARMACOLOGY, AND TREATMENT

THIRD INTERNATIONAL SYMPOSIUM

Proceedings of the Third International Conference on Asthma,
Nuneham Park, Nuneham Courtenay, Oxford, U.K., May 16–18, 1983

ASTHMA

PHYSIOLOGY, IMMUNOPHARMACOLOGY, AND TREATMENT

THIRD INTERNATIONAL SYMPOSIUM

Edited by

A. BARRY KAY, Ph.D., F.R.C.P.

Cardiothoracic Institute, Brompton Hospital
London, United Kingdom

K. FRANK AUSTEN, M.D.

Harvard Medical School
Boston, Massachusetts

LAWRENCE M. LICHTENSTEIN, M.D., Ph.D.

The Johns Hopkins University School of Medicine
Baltimore, Maryland

ACADEMIC PRESS *(Harcourt Brace Jovanovich, Publishers)* 1984
London   Orlando   San Diego   New York
Toronto   Montreal   Sydney   Tokyo

ACADEMIC PRESS, INC. (LONDON) LTD.
24-28 Oval Road,
London NW1 7DX

United States Edition published by
ACADEMIC PRESS, INC.
Orlando, Florida 32887

LIBRARY OF CONGRESS CATALOG CARD NUMBER: 84-45454

ISBN 0-12-402750-4

PRINTED IN THE UNITED STATES OF AMERICA

84 85 86 87   9 8 7 6 5 4 3 2 1

Contents

Chapter 1   *In Vitro* **and** *in Vivo* **Studies of Mediator Release from Human Mast Cells**

Lawrence M. Lichtenstein, Robert P. Schleimer, Donald W. MacGlashan, Jr., Stephen P. Peters, Edward S. Schulman, David Proud, Peter S. Creticos, Robert M. Naclerio, and Anne Kagey-Sobotka

Chapter 2   **Tryptase from Human Pulmonary Mast Cells**

Lawrence B. Schwartz

Chapter 15 An Animal Model of the Late Asthmatic Response to Antigen Challenge

Gary L. Larsen, Mark P. Shampain, William R. Marsh, and B. Lyn Behrens

Chapter 16 Bronchial Responsiveness and Late Asthmatic Response

Frederick E. Hargreave and Jerry Dolovich

Chapter 17 Mediators in Exercise-Induced Asthma

T. H. Lee, O. Cromwell, T. Nagakura, and A. B. Kay

Chapter 18   **Airborne Allergen Exposure, Allergen Avoidance, and Bronchial Hyperreactivity**

Thomas A. E. Platts-Mills, E. Bruce Mitchell, Euan R. Tovey, Martin D. Chapman, and Susan R. Wilkins

Chapter 19   **Respiratory Heat Exchange and the Asthmatic Response**

E. R. McFadden, Jr., B. M. Pichurko, N. A. Soter, E. W. Ringel, and I. M. Mefford

Chapter 20   **The Effect of Mucosal Inflammation on Airways Reactivity**

J. C. Hogg, W. C. Hulbert, C. Armour, and P. D. Pare

Chapter 21   **β-Adrenoceptors in Asthma and Their Response to Agonists**

Peter J. Barnes, Philip W. Ind, and Colin T. Dollery

Chapter 22   **Corticosteroid Resistance in Chronic Asthma**

I. W. B. Grant, A. H. Wyllie, M. C. Poznansky, A. C. H. Gordon, and J. G. Douglas

Chapter 23   **Physiological and Pharmacological Control of the Respiratory Drive in Asthma**

D. C. Flenley

Contributors

Numbers in parentheses indicate the pages on which the authors' contributions begin.

G. KENNETH ADAMS III (101), Clinical Immunology Division, The Johns Hopkins University School of Medicine at the Good Samaritan Hospital, Baltimore, Maryland 21239, U.S.A.

C. ARMOUR* (327), Pulmonary Research Laboratory, St. Paul's Hospital, University of British Columbia, Vancouver, British Columbia V6Z 1Y6, Canada

PHILIP W. ASKENASE (157), Section of Clinical Immunology and Allergy, Department of Medicine, Yale University School of Medicine, New Haven, Connecticut 06510, U.S.A.

K. FRANK AUSTEN (63), Department of Medicine, Harvard Medical School, Robert B. Brigham Division, Brigham and Women's Hospital, Boston, Massachusetts 02115, U.S.A.

PETER J. BARNES (339), Department of Medicine, Royal Postgraduate Medical School, Hammersmith Hospital, London W12 OHS, U.K.

B. LYN BEHRENS† (245), Department of Pediatrics, National Jewish Hospital and Research Center, National Asthma Center, Denver, Colorado 80206, U.S.A.

MARY CARROLL‡ (211), Department of Allergy and Clinical Immunology, Cardiothoracic Institute, Brompton Hospital, London SW3 6HP, U.K.

*Present address: National Health and Medical Research Council, Department of Pharmacology, University of Sydney, Sydney, N.S.W. 2227, Australia.
†Present address: Department of Pediatrics, Loma Linda University Medical Center, Loma Linda, California 92354, U.S.A.
‡Present address: St. Helier Hospital, Carshalton, Surrey SM5 1AA, U.K.

MARTIN D. CHAPMAN (297), Division of Allergy and Clinical Immunology, Department of Internal Medicine, University of Virginia, Charlottesville, Virginia 22908, U.S.A.

P. K. CHIANG (173), Walter Reed Army Institute of Research, Washington, D.C. 20012, U.S.A.

MARTIN K. CHURCH (391), Department of Clinical Pharmacology, University of Southampton, Southampton General Hospital, Southampton SO9 4XY, U.K.

PETER S. CRETICOS (1), Clinical Immunology Division, The Johns Hopkins University School of Medicine at the Good Samaritan Hospital, Baltimore, Maryland 21239, U.S.A.

O. CROMWELL (211, 279), Department of Allergy and Clinical Immunology, Cardiothoracic Institute, Brompton Hospital, London SW3 6HP, U.K.

MICHAEL J. CUSHLEY (391), Faculty of Medicine, University of Southampton, Southampton General Hospital, Southampton SO9 4XY, U.K.

COLIN T. DOLLERY (339), Department of Clinical Pharmacology, Royal Postgraduate Medical School, Hammersmith Hospital, London W12 OHS, U.K.

JERRY DOLOVICH (263), Department of Pediatrics, McMaster University Medical Centre and McMaster University, Hamilton, Ontario H5C 3V47, Canada

J. G. DOUGLAS (359), Department of General Medicine, Royal Infirmary of Edinburgh, Edinburgh EH3 9YW, U.K.

JEFFREY M. DRAZEN (85), Respiratory Disease Division, Brigham and Women's Hospital, Harvard Medical School, Boston, Massachusetts 02115, U.S.A.

S. R. DURHAM (211), Department of Allergy and Clinical Immunology, Cardiothoracic Institute, Brompton Hospital, London SW3 6HP, U.K.

W. V. FILLEY* (195), Allergic Diseases Research Laboratory, Mayo Clinic, Rochester, Minnesota 55905, U.S.A.

D. C. FLENLEY (375), Department of Respiratory Medicine, City Hospital, Edinburgh EH10 5SB, U.K.

E. FRIGAS (195), Consultant Internal Medicine and Allergic Diseases, Mayo Clinic, Rochester, Minnesota 55905, U.S.A.

I. GARCIA-CASTRO (173), Walter Reed Army Institute of Research, Washington, D.C. 20012, U.S.A.

*Present address: Oklahoma Allergy Clinic, Oklahoma City, Oklahoma 73126.

V. GEETHA (173), National Institute of Dental Research, National Institutes of Health, Bethesda, Maryland 20205, U.S.A.

G. J. GLEICH (195), Allergic Diseases Research Laboratory, Mayo Clinic, Rochester, Minnesota 55905, U.S.A.

A. C. H. GORDON (359), Department of Medical Neurology, Northern General Hospital, Edinburgh EH5 2DQ, U.K.

I. W. B. GRANT (359), Respiratory Unit, Northern General Hospital, Edinburgh EH5 2DQ, U.K.

FREDERICK E. HARGREAVE (263), Firestone Regional Chest and Allergy Unit, Department of Medicine, St. Joseph's Hospital, Hamilton, Ontario L8N 4A6, Canada

J. C. HOGG (327), Pulmonary Research Laboratory, St. Paul's Hospital, University of British Columbia, Vancouver, British Columbia V6Z 1Y6, Canada

STEPHEN T. HOLGATE (391), Faculty of Medicine, University of Southampton, Southampton General Hospital, Southampton SO9 4XY, U.K.

MICHAEL J. HOLTZMAN (129), Cardiovascular Research Institute, and Department of Medicine, University of California, San Francisco, California 94143, U.S.A.

PETER H. HOWARTH (391), Faculty of Medicine, University of Southampton, Southampton General Hospital, Southampton SO9 4XY, U.K.

W. C. HULBERT* (327), Pulmonary Research Laboratory, St. Paul's Hospital, University of British Columbia, Vancouver, British Columbia V6Z 1Y6, Canada

PHILIP W. IND (339), Respiratory Unit, Royal Postgraduate Medical School, Hammersmith Hospital, London W12 OHS, U.K.

TERUKO ISHIZAKA (39), Subdepartment of Immunology, The Johns Hopkins University School of Medicine at the Good Samaritan Hospital, Baltimore, Maryland 21239, U.S.A.

ANNE KAGEY-SOBOTKA (1), Clinical Immunology Division, The Johns Hopkins University School of Medicine at the Good Samaritan Hospital, Baltimore, Maryland 21239, U.S.A.

*Present address: Department of Medicine, University of Alberta, Edmonton, Alberta T6G 2G3, Canada.

MICHAEL KALINER (229), Laboratory of Clinical Investigation, National Institute of Allergy and Infectious Diseases, National Institutes of Health, Bethesda, Maryland 20205, U.S.A.

A. B. KAY (211, 279), Department of Allergy and Clinical Immunology, Cardiothoracic Institute, Brompton Hospital, London SW3 6HP, U.K.

GARY L. LARSEN (245), Department of Pediatrics, National Jewish Hospital and Research Center, National Asthma Center, Denver, Colorado 80206, U.S.A.

CHONG W. LEE* (63), Department of Medicine, Harvard Medical School, Boston, Massachusetts 02115, U.S.A.

T. H. LEE† (211, 279), Department of Allergy and Clinical Immunology, Cardiothoracic Institute, Brompton Hospital, London SW3 6HP, U.K.

A. G. LEITCH (85), City Hospital, and Department of Respiratory Medicine, University of Edinburgh, Edinburgh EH10 5SB, U.K.

ROBERT LEMANSKE, JR. (229), Departments of Medicine and Pediatrics, University of Wisconsin Medical School, Madison, Wisconsin 53792, U.S.A.

L. G. LETTS (113), Merck Frosst Laboratories, Pointe Claire-Dorval, Quebec H9R 4P8, Canada

ROBERT A. LEWIS (63), Department of Rheumatology and Immunology, Brigham and Women's Hospital, Boston, Massachusetts 02115, U.S.A.

LAWRENCE M. LICHTENSTEIN (1, 101), Clinical Immunology Division, The Johns Hopkins University School of Medicine at the Good Samaritan Hospital, Baltimore, Maryland 21239, U.S.A.

D. A. LOEGERING (195), Allergic Diseases Research Laboratory, Mayo Clinic, Rochester, Minnesota 55905, U.S.A.

E. R. MCFADDEN, JR. (315), Shipley Institute of Medicine, Brigham and Women's Hospital, Harvard Medical School, Boston, Massachusetts 02115, U.S.A.

DONALD W. MACGLASHAN, JR. (1), Clinical Immunology Division, The Johns Hopkins University School of Medicine at the Good Samaritan Hospital, Baltimore, Maryland 21239, U.S.A.

*Present address: Pulmonary Unit, Massachussetts General Hospital, Boston, Massachusetts 02114, U.S.A.
†Present address: Department of Medicine, Harvard Medical School, Boston, Massachusetts 02115, U.S.A.

R. MANJUNATH* (173), National Institute of Child Health and Human Development, National Institutes of Health, Bethesda, Maryland 20205, U.S.A.

JONATHAN S. MANN (391), Faculty of Medicine, University of Southampton, Southampton General Hospital, Southampton SO9 4XY, U.K.

WILLIAM R. MARSH (245), Department of Pediatrics, National Jewish Hospital and Research Center, National Asthma Center, Denver, Colorado 80206, U.S.A.

J. MATO (173), National Institute of Dental Research, National Institutes of Health, Bethesda, Maryland 20205, U.S.A.

I. M. MEFFORD (315), Department of Chemistry, Boston College, Chestnut Hill, Massachusetts 02167, U.S.A.

JEAN-MICHEL MENCIA-HUERTA† (63), Department of Medicine, Harvard Medical School, Boston, Massachusetts 02115, U.S.A.

E. BRUCE MITCHELL (297), Division of Immunology, Clinical Research Centre, Harrow HA1 3UJ, U.K.

A. MUKHERJEE (173), National Institute of Child Health and Human Development, National Institutes of Health, Bethesda, Maryland 20205, U.S.A.

ROBERT M. NACLERIO (1), Clinical Immunology Division, The Johns Hopkins University School of Medicine at the Good Samaritan Hospital, Baltimore, Maryland 21239, U.S.A.

JAY A. NADEL (129), Section of Pulmonary Diseases, Cardiovascular Research Institute, and Departments of Medicine and Physiology, University of California, San Francisco, California 94143, U.S.A.

T. NAGAKURA‡ (211, 279), Department of Allergy and Clinical Immunology, Cardiothoracic Institute, Brompton Hospital, London SW3 6HP, U.K.

JOHN A. OATES (55), Departments of Medicine and Pharmacology, Vanderbilt University School of Medicine, Nashville, Tennessee 37232, U.S.A.

NIKI PAPAGEORGIOU§ (211), Department of Allergy and Clinical Immunology, Cardiothoracic Institute, Brompton Hospital, London SW3 6HP, U.K.

*Present address: Department of Microbiology, Dartmouth Medical School, Hanover, New Hampshire 03756, U.S.A.
†Present address: INSERM U200, 92140 Clamart, France.
‡Present address: Department of Allergy, National Children's Hospital, 3-35-31 Taishido, Setagaya-ku, Tokyo, Japan.
§Present address: Hospital for Thoracic Diseases, Athens, Greece.

P. D. PARE (327), Pulmonary Research Laboratory, St. Paul's Hospital, University of British Columbia, Vancouver, British Columbia V6Z 1Y6, Canada

D. PENCEV (173), National Institute of Dental Research, National Institutes of Health, Bethesda, Maryland 20205, U.S.A.

STEPHEN P. PETERS (1, 101), Clinical Immunology Division, The Johns Hopkins University School of Medicine at the Good Samaritan Hospital, Baltimore, Maryland 21239, U.S.A.

B. M. PICHURKO (315), Respiratory Disease Division, Brigham and Women's Hospital, Harvard Medical School, Boston, Massachusetts 02115, U.S.A.

PRISCILLA J. PIPER (113), Department of Pharmacology, Institute of Basic Medical Sciences, Royal College of Surgeons of England, London WC2A 3PN, U.K.

THOMAS A. E. PLATTS-MILLS (297), Division of Allergy and Clinical Immunology, Department of Internal Medicine, University of Virginia, Charlottesville, Virginia 22908, U.S.A.

M. C. POZNANSKY (359), Department of Pathology, University of Edinburgh Medical School, Edinburgh EH8 9AG, U.K.

DAVID PROUD (1), Clinical Immunology Division, The Johns Hopkins University School of Medicine at the Good Samaritan Hospital, Baltimore, Maryland 21239, U.S.A.

JOHN A. RANKIN (157), Pulmonary Disease Section, Department of Medicine, Yale University School of Medicine, New Haven, Connecticut 06510, U.S.A.

P. S. RICHARDSON (113), Department of Physiology, St. George's Hospital Medical School, London SW17 ORE, U.K.

E. W. RINGEL (315), Respiratory Disease Division, Brigham and Women's Hospital, Harvard Medical School, Boston, Massachusetts 02115, U.S.A.

L. JACKSON ROBERTS II (55), Departments of Medicine and Pharmacology, Vanderbilt University School of Medicine, Nashville, Tennessee 37232, U.S.A.

CLIVE ROBINSON (391), Department of Clinical Pharmacology, Southampton General Hospital, Southampton SO9 4XY, U.K.

ELLIOTT SCHIFFMANN (173), Laboratory of Developmental Biology and Anomalies, National Institute of Dental Research, National Institutes of Health, Bethesda, Maryland 20205, U.S.A.

ROBERT P. SCHLEIMER (1), Clinical Immunology Division, The Johns Hopkins University School of Medicine at the Good Samaritan Hospital, Baltimore, Maryland 21239, U.S.A.

EDWARD S. SCHULMAN (1), Clinical Immunology Division, The Johns Hopkins University School of Medicine at the Good Samaritan Hospital, Baltimore, Maryland 21239, U.S.A.

LAWRENCE B. SCHWARTZ (19), Department of Internal Medicine, Medical College of Virginia, Virginia Commonwealth University, Richmond, Virginia 23298, U.S.A.

MARK P. SHAMPAIN* (245), Department of Pediatrics, National Jewish Hospital and Research Center, National Asthma Center, Denver, Colorado 80206, U.S.A.

R. J. SHAW (211), Department of Allergy and Clinical Immunology, Cardiothoracic Institute, Brompton Hospital, London SW3 6HP, U.K.

N. A. SOTER† (315), Shipley Institute of Medicine, Brigham and Women's Hospital, Harvard Medical School, Boston, Massachusetts 02115, U.S.A.

BRIAN J. SWEETMAN (55), Departments of Medicine and Pharmacology, Vanderbilt University School of Medicine, Nashville, Tennessee 37232, U.S.A.

EUAN R. TOVEY‡ (297), Division of Allergy and Clinical Immunology, Department of Internal Medicine, University of Virginia, Charlottesville, Virginia 22908, U.S.A.

MARGARET TURNER-WARWICK (417), Department of Medicine (Thoracic Medicine), Cardiothoracic Institute, Brompton Hospital, London SW3 6HP, U.K.

SUSAN R. WILKINS (297), Division of Allergy and Clinical Immunology, Department of Internal Medicine, University of Virginia, Charlottesville, Virginia 22908, U.S.A.

A. H. WYLLIE (359), Department of Pathology, University of Edinburgh Medical School, Edinburgh EH8 9AG, U.K.

---

*Present address: 3131 College Heights Boulevard, Allentown, Pennsylvania 18104, U.S.A.
†Present address: Department of Dermatology, New York University Medical Center, New York, New York 10016, U.S.A.
‡Present address: Kolling Institute, Royal North Shore Hospital, St. Leonards NSW 2065, Australia.

Participants

G. KENNETH ADAMS III, Clinical Immunology Division, The Johns Hopkins University School of Medicine at the Good Samaritan Hospital, Baltimore, Maryland 21239, U.S.A.

PHILIP W. ASKENASE, Section of Clinical Immunology, Department of Internal Medicine, Yale University School of Medicine, New Haven, Connecticut 06510, U.S.A.

K. FRANK AUSTEN, Department of Medicine, Harvard Medical School, Robert B. Brigham Division, Brigham and Women's Hospital, Boston, Massachusetts 02115, U.S.A.

MICHAEL K. BACH, Hypersensitivity Diseases Research, The Upjohn Company, Kalamazoo, Michigan 49001, U.S.A.

PETER J. BARNES, Department of Medicine, Royal Postgraduate Medical School, Hammersmith Hospital, London W12 OHS, U.K.

T. J. H. CLARK, Guy's Hospital Medical and Dental Schools, London SE1 9RT, U.K.

COLIN T. DOLLERY, Department of Clinical Pharmacology, Royal Postgraduate Medical School, Hammersmith Hospital, London W12 OHS, U.K.

D. C. FLENLEY, Department of Respiratory Medicine, City Hospital, Edinburgh EH10 5SB, U.K.

G. J. GLEICH, Allergic Diseases Research Laboratory, Mayo Clinic, Rochester, Minnesota 55905, U.S.A.

I. W. B. GRANT, Respiratory Unit, Northern General Hospital, Edinburgh EH5 2DQ, U.K.

FREDERICK E. HARGREAVE, Firestone Regional Chest and Allergy Unit, Department of Medicine, St. Joseph's Hospital, Hamilton, Ontario L8N 4A6, Canada

J. C. HOGG, Pulmonary Research Laboratory, St. Paul's Hospital, University of British Columbia, Vancouver, British Columbia V6Z 1Y6, Canada

STEPHEN T. HOLGATE, Faculty of Medicine, University of Southampton, Southampton General Hospital, Southampton SO9 4XY, U.K.

TERUKO ISHIZAKA, Subdepartment of Immunology, The Johns Hopkins University School of Medicine at the Good Samaritan Hospital, Baltimore, Maryland 21239, U.S.A.

S. G. O. JOHANSSON, Department of Clinical Immunology, Karolinska sjukhuset, Stockholm S-104 01, Sweden.

ANNE KAGEY-SOBOTKA, Clinical Immunology Division, The Johns Hopkins University School of Medicine at the Good Samaritan Hospital, Baltimore, Maryland 21239, U.S.A.

MICHAEL KALINER, Laboratory of Clinical Investigation, National Institute of Allergy and Infectious Diseases, National Institutes of Health, Bethesda, Maryland 20205, U.S.A.

ALLEN P. KAPLAN, Division of Allergy, Rheumatology and Clinical Immunology, Health Sciences Center, State University of New York at Stony Brook, Stony Brook, New York 11794, U.S.A.

A. B. KAY, Department of Allergy and Clinical Immunology, Cardiothoracic Institute, Brompton Hospital, London SW3 6HP, U.K.

JAMES W. KERR, Department of Respiratory Medicine, Western Infirmary, Glasgow G11 6NT, U.K.

GARY L. LARSEN, Department of Pediatrics, National Jewish Hospital and Research Center, National Asthma Center, Denver, Colorado 80206, U.S.A.

T. H. LEE, Department of Allergy and Clinical Immunology, Cardiothoracic Institute, Brompton Hospital, London SW3 6HP, U.K.

A. G. LEITCH, City Hospital, and Department of Respiratory Medicine, University of Edinburgh, Edinburgh EH10 5SB, U.K.

M. H. LESSOF, Department of Medicine, Guy's Hospital Medical School, London SE1 9RT, U.K.

ROBERT A. LEWIS, Department of Rheumatology and Immunology, Brigham and Women's Hospital, Boston, Massachusetts 02115, U.S.A.

LAWRENCE M. LICHTENSTEIN, Clinical Immunology Division, The Johns Hopkins University School of Medicine at the Good Samaritan Hospital, Baltimore, Maryland 21239, U.S.A.

E. R. McFADDEN, JR., Shipley Institute of Medicine, Brigham and Women's Hospital, Harvard Medical School, Boston, Massachusetts 02115, U.S.A.

JOHN MORLEY, Department of Clinical Pharmacology, Cardiothoracic Institute, Brompton Hospital, London SW3 6HP, U.K.

JAY A. NADEL, Section of Pulmonary Diseases, Cardiovascular Research Institute, and Departments of Medicine and Physiology, University of California, San Francisco, California 94143, U.S.A.

A. J. NEWMAN TAYLOR, Department of Occupational Medicine, Brompton Hospital, London SW3 6HP, U.K.

JOHN A. OATES, Departments of Medicine and Pharmacology, Vanderbilt University School of Medicine, Nashville, Tennessee 37232, U.S.A.

PRISCILLA J. PIPER, Department of Pharmacology, Institute of Basic Medical Sciences, Royal College of Surgeons of England, London WC2A 3PN, U.K.

THOMAS A. E. PLATTS-MILLS, Division of Allergy and Clinical Immunology, Department of Internal Medicine, University of Virginia, Charlottesville, Virginia 22908, U.S.A.

NEIL PRIDE, Department of Medicine (Respiratory Division), Royal Postgraduate Medical School, Hammersmith Hospital, London W12 OHS, U.K.

ELLIOTT SCHIFFMANN, Laboratory of Developmental Biology and Anomalics, National Institute of Dental Research, National Institutes of Health, Bethesda, Maryland 20205, U.S.A.

ROBERT P. SCHLEIMER, Clinical Immunology Division, The Johns Hopkins University School of Medicine at the Good Samaritan Hospital, Baltimore, Maryland 21239, U.S.A.

LAWRENCE B. SCHWARTZ, Department of Internal Medicine, Medical College of Virginia, Virginia Commonwealth University, Richmond, Virginia 23298, U.S.A.

ANNE E. TATTERSFIELD, Faculty of Medicine, University of Southampton, Southampton General Hospital, Southampton SO9 4XY, U.K.

MARGARET TURNER-WARWICK, Department of Medicine (Thoracic Medicine), Cardiothoracic Institute, Brompton Hospital, London SW3 6HP, U.K.

J. O. WARNER, Department of Paediatrics, Brompton Hospital, London SW3 6HP, U.K.

STEPHEN I. WASSERMAN, Division of Rheumatic Diseases, School of Medicine, University Hospital, San Diego, California 92103, U.S.A.

A. H. WYLLIE, Department of Pathology, University of Edinburgh Medical School, Edinburgh EH8 9AG, U.K.

Preface

The study of the pathobiology of bronchial asthma occupies investigators in increasing numbers in various laboratories throughout the world. Their reports are dispersed in journals devoted to allergy, biochemistry, immunology, pharmacology, pathology, and physiology. The need for a multidisciplinary analysis of the current knowledge of pathobiological mechanisms in asthma prompted the initial symposia in 1972 and 1976. It was for the same reason that the Third International Symposium was held in 1983; the proceedings of that symposium are recorded in this volume.

The Third International Symposium, affectionately referred to as "Asthma III," took place in the Palladian surroundings of Nuneham Park, Oxford. During those three days in May 1983 a number of issues were raised which were in essence a continuation of the discussions initiated during the First and Second International Symposia. In addition participants addressed themselves to areas in which there had been remarkable progress in both fundamental and applied knowledge. The vigour of the discussion reflected the excellence of the presentations, the particular timeliness of the subject, and the astuteness of the session chairmen. We owe a particular debt of gratitude to Professor Margaret Turner-Warwick for her scholarly and thoughtful summing up and for the clarity with which she identified those issues that remain unsolved.

We are most grateful to our sponsors, Roussel, for making this event possible. In addition we would like to thank the manager and staff of Nuneham Park, Mr. Marcus Summersfield and his team of conference organizers, Miss Margaret Jolly (Roussel), and most especially, Miss Jennifer Mitchell for the untiring and skilful manner in which she guided the editorial aspects of this volume.

A. B. KAY
K. FRANK AUSTEN
LAWRENCE M. LICHTENSTEIN

ASTHMA

PHYSIOLOGY, IMMUNOPHARMACOLOGY, AND TREATMENT

THIRD INTERNATIONAL SYMPOSIUM

CHAPTER 1

In Vitro and in Vivo Studies of Mediator Release from Human Mast Cells*,†

LAWRENCE M. LICHTENSTEIN, ROBERT P. SCHLEIMER, DONALD W.
MACGLASHAN, JR., STEPHEN P. PETERS, EDWARD S. SCHULMAN,
DAVID PROUD, PETER S. CRETICOS, ROBERT M. NACLERIO, and
ANNE KAGEY-SOBOTKA

*Clinical Immunology Division,
The Johns Hopkins University School of Medicine
at The Good Samaritan Hospital
Baltimore, Maryland, U.S.A.*

INTRODUCTION

In the decade since the initiation of this series of conferences, research concerning the pathogenesis of asthma has entered a new and exciting phase. There has been a congenial marriage between those who previously approached the problem from a physiologic point of view and those whose training was in immunology, biochemistry, or pharmacology. Remarkable progress has occurred, most notably in the identification of what we suppose to be major mediators of asthma. Slow-reacting substance has been identified as several arachidonic acid metabolites, leukotrienes C_4, D_4, and E_4, and platelet-activating factor has been characterized as acetylglyceryl ether–phosphorylcholine (AGEPC) (1,2). The availability of purified, human mediator-containing cells has led to the solution of puzzling questions about origins of these mediators and now

* Supported by Grants AI-07290 and HL-23586 from the National Institutes of Health, Bethesda, Maryland 21205.
 † In addition to the collaborators listed as coauthors, I would like to acknowledge the collaboration of my more senior colleagues, Drs. Philip S. Norman, N. Franklin Adkinson, Jr., R. Neal Pinckard, and Edward Hayes.

ASTHMA: Physiology,
Immunopharmacology,
and Treatment
THIRD INTERNATIONAL SYMPOSIUM

1

allows us to pose a series of important biochemical and pharmacologic questions (3,4). Perhaps the most unifying development has been the general recognition that the mast cell and its products are of central importance in the pathogenesis of asthma. At the first meeting this was viewed quite skeptically by some, but it now appears clear that not only are antigen-induced asthmatic episodes related to the mast cell but also that such nonspecific stimuli as exercise can cause mediator release (5). Finally, because clinical asthma resembles the late phase reaction more than the acute response, the recognition that mast cells are capable of generating mediators that cause such late reactions has reinforced its importance (6). This presentation will focus on recent *in vitro* studies with human mast cells, contrasting them with human basophils, and examining the *in vivo* relevance of some of these findings.

IN VITRO STUDIES

Which Mediators Are in Mast Cells and Basophils?

The purification of human basophils and mast cells has allowed us to characterize the mediators contained in these cells. There was, for example, some uncertainty about whether slow-reacting substance (SRS) was derived from human mast cells. We found, however, that 3 and 98% human mast cells from the same lung preparation generated approximately equivalent amounts of SRS, as determined by bioassay or radioimmunoassay (RIA) ($\sim$320 $pM/10^6$ cells) (7). Preliminary HPLC studies combined with an RIA suggest that the predominant mast cell product is leukotriene C_4 (LTC_4) with purified cells generating little or no leukotriene D_4 (LTD_4) or leukotriene E_4 (LTE_4) (8). Human mast cells also produce a material which cochromatographs on HPLC with leukotriene B_4 (LTB_4) and is recognized by an RIA for LTB_4. The major monohydroxy arachidonate derivative of the mast cell is 5-monohydroxyeicosatetraenoic acid (5-HETE), an observation that is important in the context of certain pharmacologic studies to be discussed below.

The primary cyclooxygenase product of the mast cell, as previously demonstrated by others, is prostaglandin D_2 (PGD_2), and there can now be no uncertainty that this is the cell source, because PGD_2 generation has been observed with mast cells purified to essential homogeneity (9,10). Mast cells also produce a small amount of thromboxane A_2 (measured as B_2) and perhaps $PGF_{2\alpha}$ but none of the other cyclooxygenase products (e.g., PGE_2 and PGI_2) have been identified by HPLC or specific RIAs.

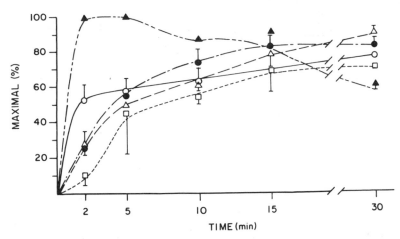

Fig. 1.   Release of mediators from purified human lung mast cells ($n = 4$). Data are from a single experiment in the case of AGEPC. Cells were challenged with 2 µg/ml anti-IgE. AGEPC (▲) was assayed in cell pellets; the release of histamine (○), prostaglandin D_2 (●), thromboxane B_2 (△), and leukotriene C_4 (□) was monitored by assay of cell-free supernatants.

Another important lipid mediator, platelet-activating factor, cannot be obtained from unstimulated mast cells; after stimulation however, these cells produce 10–30 times as much AGEPC as, for example, human polymorphonuclear cells (1.6 ng/10^6 cells). It is curious that under the conditions we used that little or none of the generated AGEPC was released into the fluid phase.

In terms of chemotactic mediators, the mast cells release factors that attract both neutrophils and eosinophils. The neutrophil chemotactic factor has been characterized by S. I. Wasserman as being of relatively high molecular weight (personal communication). The mast cell also secretes other preformed mediators, specifically several proteolytic enzymes that interact with the Hageman factor-dependent pathways. Of particular interest is a kininogenase that interacts with both low and high molecular weight kininogen to generate biologically active kinin, quantitated by a highly specific RIA. Additionally, the cells contain an enzyme that activates prekallikrein and another that cleaves Hageman Factor.

The mast cells generate and/or release these several mediators at differing rates. A summation of several experiments is shown in Fig. 1. AGEPC is generated very rapidly and is significantly degraded with time. Histamine is the first mediator to be released, followed by the cyclooxygenase products, and LTC_4 is released into the fluid phase at the slowest rate.

While the human basophil generates SRS-A, the proteolytic enzymes,

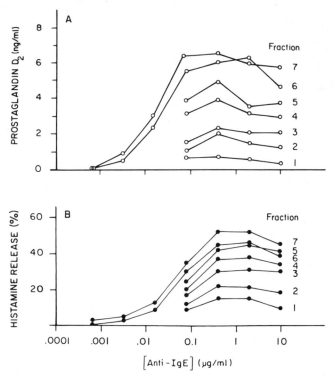

Fig. 2. Dose–response curves of anti-IgE-induced release of (A) the nonpreformed mast cell mediator, PGD$_2$, and (B) the preformed mediator, histamine, from mast cells of different sizes. The seven fractions were obtained by countercurrent elutriation, with the smallest cells in Fraction 1. Each point represents the mean of replicates in which 20,000 mast cells were challenged.

and tentatively, AGEPC, we are not able to detect any basophil-derived PGD$_2$ or other cyclooxygenase products. It is clear that in terms of arachidonate metabolism the basophil is far less active than the mast cell.

Mast Cell Heterogeneity

The mast cell purification technique involves countercurrent elutriation, which yields mast cells of varying sizes. These cells differ in their histamine content, ranging from <2 pg/cell in the smallest to >15 pg/cell in the largest cells. They also differ in terms of the percentage (and therefore absolute amount) of histamine released, with the small cells releasing poorly relative to the larger cells (Fig. 2). This differential ability to respond to IgE-mediated signals carries over to the nonpreformed mediator PGD$_2$: again, the small cells release relatively poorly while the large cells are more effective (11). The surface density of IgE antibodies on mast cells is greatest in the poorly releasing, smaller cells; the large cells contain about one-fifth as many IgE receptors per square micrometer of cell surface (11). This inverse relationship between IgE antibody and release reinforces the concept of releasability, the nonimmunologic parameter which, in basophils, correlates with the asthmatic diathesis (12).

One of the interesting, and troubling, new pieces of information is that mast cells from different locations (e.g., peritoneal versus intestinal, skin versus lung) appear to have different characteristics (13). Perhaps some or all of these differences may be attributed to differences in cell size and/or maturity, rather than being fundamental attributes.

Pharmacologic Studies

Agonists that increase the intracellular level of cyclic AMP, such as isoproterenol and E prostaglandins, inhibit mast cell histamine release; as suggested by Kaliner, the mast cell is unlike the basophil in that it lacks a histamine-2 receptor (14,15). Another difference is that PGD_2, which potentiates basophil histamine release, fails to affect the mast cell (16).

Based on experiments with basophils, we have hypothesized that the lipoxygenase pathways are important not only in generating inflammatory mediators but that they are also intimately involved in the mechanism of mediator release (17). By and large, these were indirect pharmacologic studies utilizing putative inhibitors of these pathways (18). Studies in the mast cell have not yet reached the biochemical stage, but the same inhibitors of arachidonic acid generation (bromphenacetyl bromide; mepacrine) and lipoxygenase activity (ETYA; ETI; nordihydroguiaretic acid; phenidone) also inhibit the mast cell (19). In the basophil, we feel that it is the 5-lipoxygenase pathway that is involved in the release reaction, based on the fact that only this mono-HETE enhances IgE-mediated histamine release and causes direct noncytotoxic release in the presence of cytochalasin B (20,21). The mast cell, which generates significant quantities of leukotriene C_4, certainly has this pathway, and as noted the predominant mono-HETE generated is the 5-product. Exogenous 5-HETE, however, has little or no effect on the mast cell.

The corticosteroids, which are of central importance in the treatment of asthma, have been the subject of much investigation because of the suggestion that they act by causing the synthesis of a polypeptide that blocks phospholipase A_2 and thereby impairs the release of arachidonic acid (22–24). When basophils were incubated for 12 to 24 hr with pharmacologic levels ($\sim 10^{-9}$ M) of dexamethasone or other steroids, histamine release was inhibited (25). Our studies suggested, however, that this inhibition was not caused by impaired phospholipase A_2 activity (26). Human mast cells, unlike murine mast cells, were singularly unaffected by the same or higher concentrations of corticosteroids: As shown in Fig. 3A, the steroids affected neither histamine release nor the generation of PGD_2 and SRS (10). This is not surprising because steroids have no *in vivo* effect on acute, IgE-mediated reactions such as occur during bronchoprovocation (27). The pharmacologic potency of the steroids in asthma may be related in part to the observations shown in Fig. 3B. While steroid treatment of whole human lung tissue followed by challenge with anti-IgE does not affect the release of mast cell mediators, it significantly inhibits the release of proinflammatory cyclooxygenase products from other lung cell types (10). Preliminary studies suggest that steroid treatment of chopped human lung tissue also inhibits the release of nonmast cell lipoxygenase products. It is interesting that the time course of the action of steroids on the basophils and its therapeutic effects in man are quite similar; the fact that steroids block late phase bronchoprovocation is compatible with mast cell-induced basophil activation as a part of this phenomenon.

Biochemical Studies

The major advantage in having purified human mediator-containing cells is the ability to pose biochemical questions. Since our last meeting, there has been remarkable progress in defining the biochemical concomitants of IgE stimulation, based primarily on studies with purified murine mast cells. The ability to examine the relevance of these studies in human cells cannot be overemphasized, although as yet only preliminary work has been performed.

The role of cAMP in IgE-mediated release mechanisms has had a long and complex history since its involvement was suggested, based on pharmacologic studies in basophils (28). In the murine system, early studies showed that stimulation of the mast cells induced a fall in cAMP levels, but more recent studies demonstrated an early and transient increase in the cAMP concentration (29,30). Elegant studies by Austen and his colleagues, with ribose and purine (R and P) site adenosine analogs, have shown that an increase in the cAMP level is associated with increased mediator release and vice versa (31), although PGD_2, which increases cAMP in the rat mast cell, did not affect release (32). In terms of human cells, some years ago we reported, using the basophils of a patient with chronic myelogenous leukemia, that there was an early increase in cAMP (and a subsequent fall) after anti-IgE stimulation (33). In our studies with human mast cells, however, we have found no significant change in cAMP

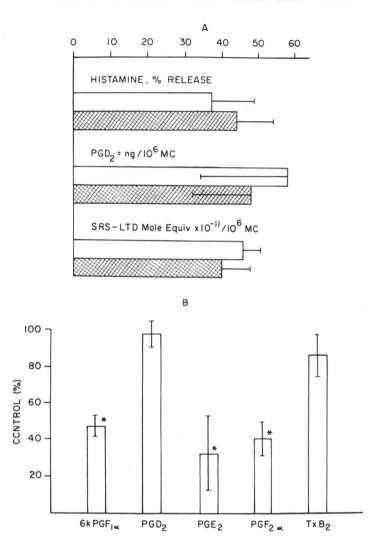

Fig. 3. Effect of dexamethasone on mediator release from purified human lung mast cells and human lung fragments. (A) Anti-IgE-induced release of histamine, PGD_2, and SRS from control and dexamethasone-treated (24 hr, 10^{-6} M drug) mast cells (MC purity = 92 ± 2.3%, N = 5). Open bars, control; hatched bars, dexamethasone added. (B) Anti-IgE-induced net release of arachidonate cycloxygenase metabolites from human lung fragments. Data are normalized to show the release of each metabolite from dexamethasone-treated fragments (10^{-6} M, 24 hr) expressed as percentage of release from control fragments (n = 3). In the same experiments, dexamethasone did not inhibit histamine release from the lung fragments (not shown). Asterisks indicate $p < .05$ versus control.

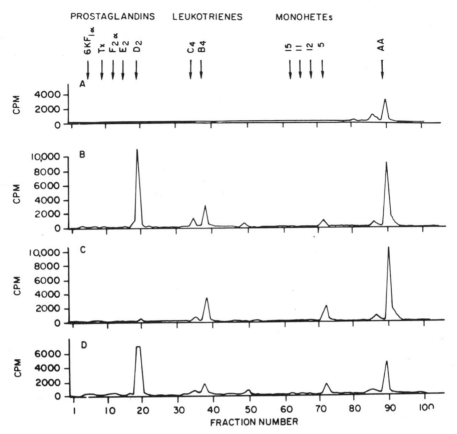

Fig. 4. The release of arachidonic acid metabolites from purified human lung mast cells prelabeled with [³H]arachidonic acid. Human lung mast cells were prepared and cultured overnight in the presence of [³H]arachidonic acid. After washing, they were challenged with the indicated stimulus (600,000 mast cells of 96% purity in a volume of 0.5 ml). (A) Normal goat serum (NGS, at 2 μg/ml); (B) anti-IgE (a-IgE, at 2 μg/ml); (C) preincubated with indomethacin (Indo, 3 μM); (D) ionophore A23187. Histamine release was (A) 1%, (B) 29%, (C) 34%, and (D) 69%. Standards elute as shown on the top of the figure.

levels after anti-IgE stimulation; in the same experiments, the positive control, fenoterol, caused a 50–150% increase. Using somewhat different conditions, Dr. T. Ishizaka found an increase in cAMP levels. Thus, there may be an increase in the cAMP level under certain circumstances but this does not necessarily occur, suggesting that in the human mast cell these changes are unrelated to the mechanisms of release.

Indeed, this discrepancy focuses upon a fundamental caveat that must be considered with respect to all biochemical studies. Biochemical changes that are temporally associated with mediator release need not be mechanistically related to the process; efforts to alter conditions or studies with pharmacologic agonists to disassociate the release process and the biochemical parameter under study are required. Insofar as these remain associated, a causal relationship is supported, but when they are disassociated, causality must be questioned.

Our major biochemical interest in the mast cell has involved gaining an understanding of this cell's pathways of arachidonic acid metabolism, in preparation for a parallel analysis of the effects of lipoxygenase inhibitors on arachidonate metabolism and mediator release. We would like to prove or disprove a role for the 5-lipoxygenase pathway in the release reaction. An HPLC technique has been developed that allows us to determine, in a single chromatographic procedure, the generation and release of the major cyclooxygenase products, leukotrienes, and mono-HETEs (8). A typical experiment (98% mast cells) is shown in Fig. 4: anti-IgE or ionophore stimulation leads to the production of metabolites that coelute with PGD_2, LTC_4, LTB_4, 5-HETE, and arachidonic acid. These peaks can be quantitated by calibration with standards; PGD_2, leukotriene C_4, and leukotriene B_4 have also been identified in the appropriate elution fractions by RIAs. In preliminary experiments we found that ionophore and anti-IgE induce the same pattern and quantity of metabolites; indomethacin blocks PGD_2 production without a marked effect on leukotriene production; and, in a single experiment, ETI decreases the release of arachidonic acid and its metabolites at the same concentration that it blocks histamine release.

IN VIVO STUDIES

The intensity of the recent *in vitro* work has led to an increased desire to validate these studies by examining mediator release *in vivo*. Most attempts to do so have centered around antigen- or exercise-induced bronchospasm and the results have been somewhat conflicting. Some investigators have been able to measure increased serum levels of histamine and neutrophil chemotactic factors (NCF) after various types of provocation, but others have not (5,34). To the readers of these papers, the recent demonstration that the *in vivo* measurement of mediators is fraught with difficulties suggests caution (35). It does appear that antigen-induced bronchospasm is accompanied by increased levels of histamine and NCF in the blood, and that the same mediators appear to be generated in the appropriate patients by exercise (5,36). As noted, the release of a mast cell mediator after a nonantigenically induced asthmatic episode is of critical importance to the thesis that the mast cell plays a central role in asthma.

In our own studies, antigen bronchoprovocation was found to cause an increase in the plasma level of a platelet factor (PF_4); one scenario suggests a mechanism involving activation of platelets by mast cell-derived AGEPC or TxA_2 (10,37). Wasserman, challenging the skin with antigen or cold (in patients with cold urticaria), also demonstrated PF_4 in venous blood; Kaplan, in an elegant series of experiments, demonstrated histamine release after physical stimulation of the skin of appropriate patients (38,39).

We have utilized a simpler *in vivo* system to assess mediator release after antigen stimulation. This involves nasal challenge of ragweed-sensitive individuals with either ragweed pollen grains or ragweed extract (40). In sensitive individuals, as few as 10 grains of ragweed pollen induced sneezing (by which we "quantitate" the clinical response) and mediator release into the nasal fluids, which are then washed from the nose and assayed. The question posed first was whether the mediators that we find to be derived from mast cells *in vitro* are also found *in vivo*. This question is examined in Fig. 5. There is a clear relationship between pollen instillation, the clinical response, and the release into the nasal airways of histamine, PGD_2, SRS, TAMe-esterase, and kinin. We can be certain that the histamine is derived from the mast cell (or from basophils); it also seems highly probable that the PGD_2 and SRS are similarly derived. The TAMe-esterase has the same characteristics (inhibition profile) as does the esterase derived from mast cells; these characteristics differ from those of serum or glandular-derived TAMe-esterases. The mechanism by which kinin is generated is not clear, but certainly the mast cell kininogenase is a reasonable candidate (41).

This *in vivo* system appears to be an excellent vehicle for pharmacologic studies. The most fundamental question is whether drugs that stop the release of all mediators *in vitro* have this effect *in vivo* as well. Some years ago, we showed that tricyclic antihistamines, including azatadine, blocked the release of histamine and SRS from human basophils and chopped primate lung (42). Since azatadine has none of the smooth muscle or vascular effects of most of other inhibitors, we selected it for our first trial of "antirelease" agents. The protocol called for three repetitive antigen challenges on day 1, recording sneezing and the release of TAMe-esterase. On the drug day the first antigen challenge was repeated to ascertain that reactivity was qualitatively the same. The drug was then administered intranasally and the patient subjected to the next two anti-

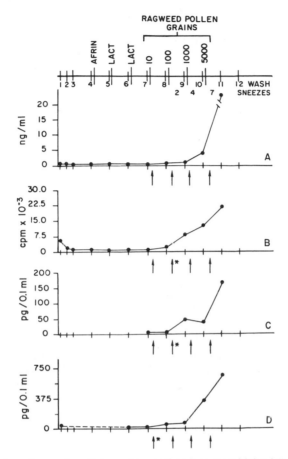

Fig. 5. *In vivo* release of mediators of immediate hypersensitivity following intranasal challenge with antigen. The protocol for challenge is shown at the top of the figure. Measurement of the release of four mediators into the nasal wash fluids is shown. Note that the appearance of (A) histamine, (B) TAMe-esterase activity, (C) PGD$_2$, and (D) leukotrienes occurred in a dose-related fashion after nasal antigen challenge, and that the detection of these mediators correlates with the clinical response of sneezing.

gen challenges. The results were clearcut inhibition of both sneezing and mediator release (Fig. 6).

The other therapeutic modality we examined was immunotherapy, which is widely employed in the treatment of allergic asthmatics although its efficacy has not been clearly established. Immunotherapy has, in some hands, been shown to decrease a patient's sensitivity to inhaled antigen, as judged by measurements of bronchospasm. In other studies no change

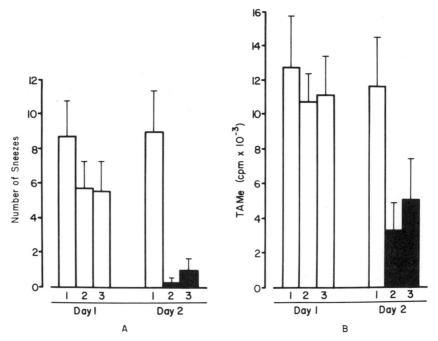

Fig. 6. Inhibition of the clinical response (A) of sneezing and (B) mediator release (TAMe-esterase) by topical azatadine base, 0.08 ml of a 2% solution. The amount of allergen used was the same for each challenge and had previously been shown to elicit a clinical response and mediator release. Thirty-four minutes were allowed to elapse between each challenge. Means ± SEM of seven subjects are shown. Shaded bars, with drug; open bars, without drug.

has been noted. Our results suggest that after immunotherapy there is both lessened sneezing and a marked reduction in the release of histamine, TAMe-esterase, PGD_2, and bradykinin on nasal challenge.

CONCLUSION

Immediate hypersensitivity has been under investigation since the turn of the century, with excellent work extending back at least 50 years. While it does not seem inappropriate to feel a particular pride in the quality of the current work, we cannot yet claim that it has led to the introduction of new modalities for the therapy of asthma. Whatever its ultimate value, cromolyn was developed empirically; inhaled β-adrenergic agonists and steroids were simply technological advances. It is our perception, however, that the field is on the brink of remarkable pharmacologic progress which will lead to drugs that materially alleviate the clinical severity of asthma. It is to be hoped and anticipated that these will provide the focus of our next meeting.

REFERENCES

1. Samuelsson, B., Borgeat, P., Hammarström, S., and Murphy, R. C. Introduction of a nomenclature; leukotrienes. *Prostaglandins* **17:**785–787, 1979.
2. Demopoulos, C. A., Pinckard, R. N., and Hanahan, D. J. Platelet activating factor. Evidence for 1-O-alkyl-2-acetyl-*sn*-glyceryl-3-phosphorylcholine as the active component (a new class of lipid chemical mediators). *J. Biol. Chem.* **254:**9355–9358, 1979.
3. MacGlashan, D. W., Jr., and Lichtenstein, L. M. The purification of human basophils. *J. Immunol.* **124:**2519–2521, 1980.
4. Schulman, E. S., MacGlashan, D. W., Jr., Peters, S. P., Schleimer, R. P., Newball, H. H., and Lichtenstein, L. M. Human lung mast cells: Purification and characterization. *J. Immunol.* **129:**2662–2667, 1982.
5. Lee, T. H., Nagy, T., Nagakura, T., Walport, M. J., and Kay, A. B. Identification and partial purification of an exercise-induced neutrophil chemotactic factor in bronchial asthma. *J. Clin. Invest.* **69:**889–899, 1982.
6. Oertel, H. L., and Kaliner, M. The biological activity of mast cell granules. III. Purification of inflammatory factors of anaphylaxis (IF-A) responsible for causing late-phase reactions. *J. Immunol.* **127:**1398–1402, 1981.
7. MacGlashan, D. W., Jr., Schleimer, R. P., Peters, S. P., Schulman, E. S., Adams, G. K., III, Newball, H. H., and Lichtenstein, L. M. Generation of leukotrienes by purified human lung mast cells. *J. Clin. Invest.* **70:**747–751, 1982.
8. Peters, S. P., MacGlashan, D. W., Jr., Schulman, E. S., Schleimer, R. P., and Lichtenstein, L. M. The production of arachidonic acid metabolites by purified human lung mast cells. *Fed. Proc., Fed. Am. Soc. Exp. Biol.* **42:**1375, 1983.
9. Lewis, R. A., Holgate, S. T., Roberts, L. J., Oates, J. A., and Austen, K. F. Preferential generation of prostaglandin D$_2$ by rat and human mast cells. *In* "Biochemistry of the Acute Allergic Reactions" (E. L. Becker, A. S. Simon, and K. F. Austen, eds.), pp. 239–254. A. R. Liss, Inc., New York, 1981.
10. Schleimer, R. P., Schulman, E. S., MacGlashan, D. W., Jr., Peters, S. P., Adams, G. K., III, Lichtenstein, L. M., and Adkinson, N. F., Jr. Effects of dexamethasone on mediator release from human lung fragments, and purified human lung mast cells. *J. Clin. Invest.* **71:**1830–1835, 1983.
11. Schulman, E. S., Kagey-Sobotka, A., MacGlashan, D. W., Jr., Adkinson, N. F., Jr., Peters, S. P., Schleimer, R. P., and Lichtenstein, L. M. Heterogeneity of human lung mast cells. *J. Immunol.* **131:**1936–1941, 1983.
12. Tung, R., and Lichtenstein, L. M. *In vitro* histamine release from basophils of asthmatic and atopic individuals in D$_2$O. *J. Immunol.* **128:**2067–2072, 1982.
13. Befus, A. D., Pierce, F. L., Gauldie, J., Holswood, P., and Bienenstock, J. Mucosal mast cells. I. Isolation and functional characteristics of rat intestinal mast cells. *J. Immunol.* **128:**2475, 1982.
14. Peters, S. P., Schulman, E. S., Schleimer, R. P., MacGlashan, D. W., Jr., Newball, H.

H., and Lichtenstein, L. M. Dispersed human lung mast cells: Pharmacology and comparison with human lung tissue fragments. *Am. Rev. Respir. Dis.* **126:**1034–1039, 1982.

15. Kaliner, M. Human lung tissue and anaphylaxis: The effects of histamine on the immunologic release of mediators. *Am. Rev. Respir. Dis.* **118:**1015–1022, 1978.

16. Peters, S. P., Schleimer, R. P., Kagey-Sobotka, A., Naclerio, R. M., MacGlashan, D. W., Jr., Schulman, E. S., Adkinson, N. F., Jr., and Lichtenstein, L. M. The role of prostaglandin D_2 in IgE-mediated reactions in man. *Trans. Assoc. Am. Physicians* **95:**221–228, 1982.

17. Marone, G., Sobotka, A. K., and Lichtenstein, L. M. Effects of arachidonic acid and its metabolites on antigen induced histamine release from human basophils *in vitro. J. Immunol.* **123:**1669–1677, 1979.

18. Marone, G., Kagey-Sobotka, A., and Lichtenstein, L. M. Possible role of phospholipase A_2 in triggering histamine secretion from human basophils *in vitro. Clin. Immunol. Immunopathol.* **20:**231–239, 1981.

19. MacGlashan, D. W., Jr., Schleimer, R. P., Peters, S. P., Schulman, E. S., Adams, G. K., III, Sobotka, A. K., Newball, H. H., and Lichtenstein, L. M. Comparative studies of human basophils and mast cells. *Fed. Proc., Fed. Am. Soc. Exp. Biol.* **42:**2662–2667, 1983.

20. Peters, S. P., Kagey-Sobotka, A., MacGlashan, D. W., Jr., Siegel, M. I., and Lichtenstein, L. M. The modulation of human basophil histamine release by products of the 5-lipoxygenase pathway. *J. Immunol.* **129:**797–803, 1982.

21. Kagey-Sobotka, A., Schleimer, R. P., Peters, S. P., and Lichtenstein, L. M. Lipoxygenase (LO) products release histamine from human basophils. *Fed. Proc., Fed. Am. Soc. Exp. Biol.* **42:**1342, 1983.

22. Danon, A., and Assouline, G. Inhibition of prostaglandin biosynthesis by corticosteroids requires RNA and protein synthesis. *Nature (London)* **273:**552–554, 1978.

23. Flower, R. J., and Blackwell, G. J. Anti-inflammatory steroids induce biosynthesis of a phospholipase A_2 inhibitor which prevents prostaglandin generation. *Nature (London)* **278:**456–459, 1979.

24. Hirata, F., Schiffmann, E., Venkatasubramanian, K., Salomon, D., and Axelrod, J. A phospholipase A_2 inhibitory protein in rabbit neutrophils induced by glucocorticoids. *Proc. Natl. Acad. Sci. U.S.A.* **77:**2533–2536, 1980.

25. Schleimer, R. P., Lichtenstein, L. M., and Gillespie, E. Inhibition of basophil histamine release by anti-inflammatory steroids. *Nature (London)* **292:**454–455, 1981.

26. Schleimer, R. P., MacGlashan, D. W., Jr., Gillespie, E., and Lichtenstein, L. M. Inhibition of basophil histamine release by anti-inflammatory steroids. II. Studies on the mechanism of action. *J. Immunol.* **129:**1632–1636, 1982.

27. Pepys, J., Davies, R. J., Breslin, A. B. X., Hendrick, D. J., and Hutchcroft, B. J. The effects of inhaled beclomethasone dipropionate (Becotide) and sodium cromoglycate on asthmatic reactions to provocation tests. *Clin. Allergy* **4:**13–24, 1974.

28. Lichtenstein, L. M., and Margolis, S. Histamine release *in vitro:* Inhibition by catecholamines and methylxanthines. *Science* **161:**902–903, 1968.

29. Kaliner, M., and Austen, K. F. Cyclic AMP, ATP, and reversed anaphylactic histamine release from rat mast cells. *J. Immunol.* **112:**664–674, 1974.

30. Sullivan, T. J., Parker, K. L., Kulczychi, A., and Parker, C. W. Modulation of cyclic AMP in purified rat mast cells. III. Studies on the effect of Concanavalin A and anti-IgE on cyclic AMP concentration during histamine release. *J. Immunol.* **117:**713–716, 1976.

31. Holgate, S. T., Lewis, R. A., and Austen, K. F. Role of adenylate cyclase in immunologic release of mediators from rat mast cells: Agonist and antagonist effects of purine and ribose modified adenosine analogs. *Proc. Natl. Acad. Sci. U.S.A.* **77:**6800–6806, 1980.

32. Holgate, S. T., Winslow, C. M., Lewis, R. A., and Austen, K. F. Effects of prostaglandin D_2 and theophylline on rat serosal mast cells: Discordance between increased cellular levels of cyclic AMP and activation of cyclic AMP-dependent protein kinase. *J. Immunol.* **127**:1530–1533, 1981.
33. Lichtenstein, L. M., Kagey-Sobotka, A., Malveaux, F. J., and Gillespie, E. IgE-induced changes in human basophil cyclic AMP levels. *Int. Arch. Allergy Appl. Immunol.* **56**:473–478, 1978.
34. Deal, E. C., Jr., Wasserman, S. I., Soter, N. A., Ingram, R. H., Jr., and McFadden, E. R., Jr. Evaluation of the role played by mediators of immediate hypersensitivity in exercise-induced asthma. *J. Clin. Invest.* **65**:659–665, 1980.
35. Gleich, G. J., and Hall, W. M. Measurement of histamine: A quality control study. *J. Allergy Clin. Immunol.* **66**:295–298, 1980.
36. Lee, T. H., Brown, M. J., Nagy, L., Causon, R., Walport, M. J., and Kay, A. B. Exercise-induced release of histamine and neutrophil chemotactic factor in atopic asthmatics. *J. Allergy Clin. Immunol.* **70**:73–81, 1982.
37. Knauer, K. A., Lichtenstein, L. M., Adkinson, N. F., Jr., and Fish, J. Platelet activation during antigen-induced airway reactions in asthmatic subjects. *N. Engl. J. Med.* **304**:1404–1407, 1981.
38. Wasserman, S. I. Personal communication, 1983.
39. Kaplan, A. P., Gray, L., Shaff, R. C., Horakova, Z., and Beaven, M. A. *In vivo* studies of mediator release in cold and cholinergic urticaria. *J. Allergy Clin. Immunol.* **55**:394, 1975.
40. Naclerio, R. M., Meier, H. L., Kagey-Sobotka, A., Adkinson, N. F., Jr., Meyers, D. A., Norman, P. S., and Lichtenstein, L. M. Mediator release after nasal airway challenge with allergen. *Am. Rev. Respir. Dis.* **128**:597–602.
41. Proud, D., Togias, A., Naclerio, R. M., Crush, S. A., Norman, P. S., and Lichtenstein, L. M. Kinins in allergic rhinitis. *Fed. Proc., Fed. Am. Soc. Exp. Biol.* **42**:250, 1983.
42. Lichtenstein, L. M., and Gillespie, E. The effects of the H1 and H2 antihistamines on "allergic" histamine release and its inhibition by histamine. *J. Pharmacol. Exp. Ther.* **192**:441–450, 1975.

DISCUSSION

Austen: Is there any technical reason for the poor ability of human basophils to generate and use arachidonic acid; that is, is it due to technical factors in cell isolation? How was 5-HETE quantitated? If you use exogenous arachidonate, the profile of products may not reflect actual quantitative product profile.

Lichtenstein: The basophils have about one-fourth as much histamine and only ~5% as much LTC_4/D_4 as the mast cell. If our data with AGEPC hold up, the basophil will have a similarly small amount of this mediator. We have not been able to measure PGD_2 in the basophil. Yet, I don't agree that it is a "crippled" cell. It is not clear whether these cells require large concentrations of mediators, such as those contained in the mast cell, to produce their effects. The quantitation of 5-HETE is simply in terms of the percentage of the total AA products it represents. After overnight incubation with exogenous arachidonate, it was but a few percent. These were experiments of Dr. S. Peters and they are subject to the usual caveats that attend the use of exogenous reagents.

Lewis: Was there a discrepancy between measurements of bradykinin (BK) and lysyl bradykinin (LBK) by RIA and by absorbance after HPLC?

Lichtenstein: The data shown on kinins in the nasal fluids after ragweed pollen challenge were as follows: Dr. D. Proud ran BK and LBK standards on HPLC and these were localized by UV absorption. He then performed a RIA on the HPLC fractions of the standards. Finally, he subjected the nasal solutions to HPLC and determined the antigenicity of the material that coeluted with BK and LBK. There were no discrepancies.

Oates: When purifying rat serosal mast cells, the concentrations of both histamine and PGD_2 (ng/number of total cells) increases as the relative content of mast cells increases. Do you see such an enrichment of LTC_4 in parallel with that of histamine as the human pulmonary cell mixtures are purified to yield progressively higher percentages of mast cells?

Lichtenstein: The human lung mast cell produces both PGD_2 and LTC_4 (D. W. MacGlashan, R. P. Schleimer, S. P. Peters, E. S. Schulman, G. K. Adams, H. H. Newball, and L. M. Lichtenstein, *J. Clin. Invest.* **70:**747, 1982). The quantity of LTC_4 per mast cell is the same in 3% as in 98% mast cells. Thus, the LTC_4 concentration per total cell number in a preparation does, of course, increase as the mast cells are purified.

We suspect that most or all of the LTC_4/D_4 produced by human lung following challenge with anti-IgE is derived from the mast cell. Recently Bob Murphy in Colorado undertook immunofluorescence with anti-LTD_4/C_4 in guinea pig lung after antigen challenge. Only the mast cells produced leukotrienes [R. C. Murphy, B. Hoffer, M. Palmer, L. Olson, E. C. Hayes, A. Rosenthal, R. N. Young, and J. Rokach, *in* "Leukotrienes and Other Lipoxygenase Products" (P. J. Piper, ed.). Research Studies Press, Chichester, New York, p. 70, 1983].

Wassserman: Glucocorticoids inhibit mouse and rat mast cell mediator release as well as human basophil mediator release. The failure to inhibit human lung mast cell mediator release after *in vitro* glucocorticoid administration may reflect the source and history of lung mast cells; that is, they are obtained from patients undergoing surgical procedures and general anesthesia, events associated with steroid release. It is possible that lung mast cells have already responded fully to steroids. For this reason it is important to consider the methods of cell purification and the clinical history in interpreting *in vitro* studies.

Lichtenstein: It is possible that the source of the mast cell precludes seeing a steroid effect if, as you suggest, the stress of surgery had "desensitized" the cells to steroids.

The steroids also fail to block mediator release from chopped human lung, so the failure to see an effect is not due to the enzyme treatment.

Schleimer: We cannot eliminate the possibility that mast cells obtained from human lung have already been exposed to steroids *in vivo*. However, the lack of effect of steroids on the acute *in vivo* response to experimental challenge with antigen in human lung, skin, or nasal mucosa fits in well with our observation of a lack of mast cell response to steroids *in vitro*. Furthermore, the fact that we do see a steroid inhibition of the release of arachidonate metabolites from other cells in the lung makes an *in vivo* desensitization seem less likely. We also want to test human peritoneal mast cells to determine whether these cells are steroid sensitive, as is the case with murine peritoneal mast cells.

Schiffmann: Is mast cell activation inhibited by inhibiting an esterase? Or is the desensitization reaction alone specifically inhibited by the inhibition of esterase?

Lichtenstein: Like others, we have also found that DFP inhibits histamine release at high concentrations, that is, at about 5 mM. The effect I cited was at 0.1 to 0.5 mM, where DFP blocks an antigen-activated enzyme that appears to *cause* desensitization. This suggests that desensitization is an active process. At those concentrations DFP enhances the percentage basophil histamine release, and there is good correlation between the degree of enhancement and the inhibition of desensitization, suggesting that the latter process controls release.

Askenase: Regarding the mediator content of basophils versus mast cells, it is clear that mast cells have a much larger content of the mediators that we think are important in allergic reactions. However, it must be remembered that the mast cell content in tissues is relatively static, but can increase in chronic lesions or in specialized situations such as the gut response to worms. Basophils, on the other hand, are clearly infiltrating cells that can be continually delivered to and accumulate in a tissue site. They can be 10^4–10^5 times more frequent than mast cells. Thus, I regard the basophil as a "cheap" mast cell, but a deliverable and renewable (they regranulate) mediator-containing cell.

With regard to reactions to radio-contrast media and the possible cell type involved (basophil versus mast cell), do you know if steroids regulate release from human lung mast cells under hyperosmolar conditions?

Lichtenstein: We have not studied the effect of steroids on hyperosmolar histamine release from human mast cells.

Schwartz: Can one definitively distinguish the cell of origin of the mediators released into nasal secretions?

Lichtenstein: No. We assume that the histamine comes from mast cells or basophils. The TAMe-esterase has the inhibition profile of a mast cell enzyme rather than the serum enzyme. We view the mast cell or basophil as the most probable origin of PGD_2 and LTC_4/D_4. How the kinins are generated remains to be seen, although the mast cell has enzymes that can generate it.

Platts-Mills: In view of your comments about a different effect of steroids on basophils and mast cells, how do you think beclomethasone acts in hayfever? Does it act on basophils present in the mucus?

Lichtenstein: I don't, of course, know how steroids work in hayfever. I have given you two effects: they block basophil histamine release and they inhibit the release of cyclooxygenase products from other cells that are driven by a mast cell product. I suspect that the basophil is involved in allergic rhinitis and that this is one of the ways that steroids act.

Holgate: Rat mast cells respond to a variety of nonimmunological secretagogs for mediator release—do human lung mast cells respond to similar stimuli?

Lichtenstein: We have not examined a whole host of releasing agents. The anaphylatoxins cause some release and the ionophore is an excellent releaser. Dr. Eggleston has shown that the mast cell is even more sensitive to hyperosmolar stimuli than is the basophil. This stimulus may well have relevance for exercise-induced asthma, because it can cause a few percent release at ~50 mOsmol above normal. Further, a mast cell that has been exposed to antigen is exquisitely sensitive to increased osmolarity.

Morley: With reference to your comments on the parallel between a lack of efficacy of steroids on human mast cells *in vitro* and the failure of steroids to affect the acute response to allergen inhalation *in vivo,* what is the effect of disodium cromoglycate (DSCG) on mediator release by isolated human mast cells?

Lichtenstein: We can observe some inhibition, by DSCG, of histamine release from human lung fragments. It has been reported that in about 100 human chopped lung preparations, inhibition varied from 0 to 100%; the inhibition was obtained at variable concentrations. We noted no dose relationship. With isolated mast cells we failed to see an effect of DSCG even at very high concentrations.

Nadel: Your observation is that DSCG inhibits (variably) mediator release from chopped lung but not from isolated mast cells. Please comment on the three following possibilities and how one might determine which is correct: (1) the mast cells are different; (2) cell isolation techniques have affected differently their abilities to respond; or (3) chopped lung contains other cells, such as epithelial cells, macrophages, neutrophils, whose actions are inhibited by cromolyn?

Lichtenstein: I agree. The failure of DSCG to inhibit mast cell release could result from the isolation of the mast cell (i.e., the inhibition would be mediated by other cells) or to the enzymatic treatment.

Bach: Inhibition of mediator release by cromolyn-like drugs is inversely related to the extent of the uninhibited mediator release in any given experiment. Therefore, has this observation been considered in drawing your conclusions about the failure of DSCG to inhibit mediator release from purified mast cells?

Lichtenstein: We have reported that many agonists are more effective at low levels of release (R. S. Tung and L. M. Lichtenstein, *J. Pharmacol. Exp. Ther.* **218:**642, 1981) but we have not studied in detail the amount of individual release as it relates to DSCG.

Ishizaka: We have unpublished data that demonstrate dissociation in the effect of cromolyn *in vivo* and *in vitro*. When monkey lung fragments sensitized with human IgE antibody were incubated with varying concentrations of cromolyn and challenged with antigen, no significant inhibition of histamine or SRS-A release was observed. However, the same concentrations of cromolyn inhibited IgE-mediated skin reaction in the monkeys. We speculated that skin mast cells and lung mast cells may have different sensitivity for cromolyn, or that other types of the cells in the skin may play an essential role in the inhibition of histamine release from skin mast cells.

CHAPTER 2

Tryptase from Human Pulmonary Mast Cells

LAWRENCE B. SCHWARTZ

Division of Immunology and Connective Tissue Diseases
Section of Allergy and Clinical Immunology
Department of Internal Medicine
Medical College of Virginia, Virginia Commonwealth University
Richmond, Virginia, U.S.A.

INTRODUCTION

Human mast cells mediate immediate hypersensitivity reactions by release of mediators that are stored preformed in mast cell secretory granules and by secretion of newly generated mediators (reviewed in ref. 1). The former include predominantly the biogenic amine histamine (2); a highly sulfated proteoglycan, heparin proteoglycan (3); and a neutral protease, tryptase (4), along with the less abundant acid hydrolases, β-hexosaminidase, β-glucuronidase, and arylsulfatase (4). The latter include, most notably, prostaglandin D_2 (PGD_2) (5), sulfidopeptide leukotrienes (slow-reacting substances) (6,7), and platelet-activating factor (8). Tryptase, the dominant protein component and neutral protease in human mast cells, will be the major focus of this chapter.

HISTOCHEMICAL STUDIES OF NEUTRAL PROTEASES

The presence of neutral protease activity in mast cells was initially demonstrated by histochemical techniques. In studies of the evolution of mast cells in five vertebrate classes, detectable levels of heparin-like proteoglycan were present in mast cells of fish, amphibians, reptiles, birds, and mammals; histamine appeared only in the latter three groups, and

ASTHMA: Physiology,
Immunopharmacology,
and treatment
THIRD INTERNATIONAL SYMPOSIUM

19

neutral proteases appeared primarily in mammals and reptiles (9). Although the presence of neutral proteases in mast cell secretory granules may be a late evolutionary development, compared with proteoglycan and biogenic amines, in rodent and human mast cells neutral proteases are the major component of secretory granules on the basis of weight. Furthermore, the detection of neutral proteases and proteoglycan during mast cell maturation in embryonic and fetal rodent tissues (10), and perhaps during reformation of secretory granules in the mature rat peritoneal mast cell after degranulation (11,12), is an early event relative to the appearance of histamine. Thus, structural organization of the secretory granule matrix may occur prior to the presence of histamine (13).

Mast cells in different taxa contain distinct neutral proteases. Trypsin-like activity is characteristic of human, monkey, and turtle mast cells, whereas a chymotrypsin-like activity is found in rat connective tissue mast cells (9). Neutral protease activity in rat mast cells was first indicated in 1953, when these cells were stained with the histochemical substrate, 3-chloracetoxy-2-naphthoic acid anilide (14), and was characterized in 1959 as having a substrate specificity similar to that of chymotrypsin and not trypsin by cleavage of the acetyl ethyl esters of aromatic and not basic amino acids (15). Human cutaneous and gingival mast cells express esterase activity comparable to that of trypsin, as ascertained by cleavage of histochemical substrates such as N-α-benzoyl-DL-arginine-β-naphthylamide hydrochloride (16). Kinetic analysis of this trypsin-like enzyme by histochemical techniques showed Michaelis–Menton kinetics and suggested that a single enzyme was responsible for this activity (17).

SOLUBILIZATION AND SUBCELLULAR LOCALIZATION OF TRYPTASE

The subcellular localization of mast cell enzymes to cytoplasmic granules has been based upon histochemical techniques, subcellular fractionation, and noncytotoxic immunologic secretion in parallel with histamine. Only the latter technique discriminates between components of secretory and nonsecretory granules and permits quantification of mediator levels in each granule subtype. Tryptase was shown to be released in parallel with histamine from human pulmonary mast cells by an IgE-dependent mechanism and was thereby localized to the secretory granules (4).

Tryptase can be solubilized from dispersed mast cell preparations by sonication in 1 M NaCl. The enzyme is a neutral endopeptidase that, like bovine trypsin, cleaves peptide and ester bonds on the carboxyl side of basic amino acids and can be quantified by hydrolysis of tosyl-L-arginine methyl ester (TAMe) (4) and p-nitroanilide derivatives of synthetic peptides (18). The pH optimum for esterase activity is ~8.0 and for peptidase activity ~7.4. Its inhibition by diisopropylfluorophosphate and N-α-p-tosyl-L-lysine chloromethyl ketone and not by L-1-tosylamide-2-phenylethyl chloromethyl ketone indicates that the active site contains serine and histidine and is similar to the active site of trypsin, but the absence of inhibition by α-1 trypsin inhibitor, aprotinin, and lima bean, soybean, and ovomucoid trypsin inhibitors clearly distinguishes tryptase from bovine trypsin (4). Like the neutral endopeptidase and exopeptidase enzymes, chymase and carboxypeptidase A from rat mast cells (19), tryptase binds tightly to heparin in physiologic buffers *in vitro* and may reside as a complex with heparin proteoglycan *in vivo*.

PURIFICATION AND SUBUNIT STRUCTURE

Tryptase has been purified to apparent homogeneity from dispersed and partially purified human pulmonary mast cells by sequential chromatography on Dowex 1-X2, DEAE-Sephadex, and heparin-agarose (20). Selected biochemical characteristics of the enzyme are summarized in Table I. Purified enzyme yields a single stained band of protein after electrophoresis in a 7.5% polyacrylamide gel containing 4 M urea at pH 4.5. Less dissociative conditions in buffers lacking urea at acid or alkaline pH fail to permit entry of tryptase into 5% polyacrylamide gels, possibly because of

TABLE I
Biochemical Characteristics of Tryptase

Subunit composition	A_2B_2
	where A = 37,000 MW
	B = 36,000 MW
Standard assay	One unit cleaves 1 μmol of tosyl-L-arginine
	methylester per minute at 37°C;
	specific activity = 100 units/mg
Inhibitors	Diisopropylfluorophosphate
	Tosyl-L-lysine chloromethyl ketone
Heparin affinity	Elution from heparin-agarose at 0.75 M NaCl
Quantity per pulmonary mast cell	12 pg (~23% of total cell protein)

TABLE II
The Major Components of Human Mast Cell
Secretory Granules

Component	fmol/cell	pg/cell
Histamine (2)	15.3	1.7
Heparin proteoglycan (3)	0.07	4
Tryptase (20)	0.08	12

aggregation of the protein at low ionic strength. Analysis of the subunit structure of purified tryptase by SDS polyacrylamide gel electrophoresis revealed equal amounts of two stained protein bands with apparent MW of 37,000 and 35,000 with and without reduction and alkylation. Because of its apparent MW of 120,000 to 140,000 by gel filtration, the holoenzyme is considered to be a tetramer with a MW calculated to be 144,000 and composed of two subunits of 37,000 MW and two subunits of 35,000 MW. Autodegradation of purified holoenzyme was observed by analysis in SDS polyacrylamide gels to occur after incubation at room temperature, and this may account for the minor peak of TAMe-esterase activity eluted from heparin-agarose columns at 0.08 M NaCl. Both subunits bind [^{3}H]diisopropylfluorophosphate and therefore each subunit may contain an active catalytic site. The mast cell content of tryptase is about 12 pg, establishing it as the major component in human lung mast cell secretory granules on a weight basis (Table II). Tryptase may account for about 23% of total mast cell protein, a similar percentage of protein to that accounted for by the two neutral proteases in rat serosal mast cells, chymase and carboxypeptidase A (19,21,22), and the neutral protease in rat mucosal mast cells, rat mast cell protease II (23,24). Levels of TAMe-esterase in human lung mast cells are more than 100-fold higher than those in human neutrophils, eosinophils, and monocytes (20). Furthermore, levels of tryptase on a weight basis are at least one order of magnitude higher than the levels of the neutral proteases characteristically found in other cell types, such as elastase and cathepsin G in human neutrophils (25,26). From mast cell concentrations found in normal human skin ($\sim$10,000/mm^3) (27,28) and from the assumption that pulmonary and cutaneous mast cells have equivalent amounts of tryptase, a concentration of tryptase in cutaneous tissue of about 150 μg/cm^3 would be expected. A dominant tryptic activity with an apparent MW of $\sim$120,000 that is not inhibited by α-1 trypsin inhibitor or serum has been reported in human skin and may correspond to mast cell tryptase (29).

INTERACTION OF TRYPTASE WITH C3

An action of tryptase on plasma proteins is possible, because of the influx of plasma known to occur at tissue sites of mast cell activation as a result of the actions of other mediators derived from human mast cells such as histamine (2,30), sulfidopeptide leukotrienes (6,7), prostaglandin D_2 (5,7), and possibly platelet-activating factor (8) to increase venular permeability as illustrated in Fig. 1. The complement factor, C3, is present in plasma at concentrations between 1 and 2 mg/ml and is composed of two subunits, a 110,000 MW α chain and a 70,000 MW β chain (31). Physiologic activation of C3 to C3b (170,000 MW) and the anaphylatoxic fragment designated C3a (9,000 MW) occurs by a selective proteolytic cleavage of the α chain (32) by either the classical C3 convertase (C4b, 2a) (33) or the alternative pathway amplification C3 convertase (C3b, Bb) (34,35). C3 can also be cleaved by bovine trypsin to yield the C3a fragment (36). The biology of C3a anaphylatoxin can be summarized as follows:

1. smooth muscle spasmogen,
2. venular permeability, and
3. activation of rat serosal mast cells.

C3a enhances cutaneous vascular permeability and contracts ileal smooth muscle of guinea pigs (37), directly initiates histamine release from rat mast cells (38), and causes wheal and flare formation when injected into human skin (39,40).

Purified tryptase (0.2 μg) from human pulmonary mast cells catalyzed cleavage of the α chain of native human C3 (15 μg), whereas the β chain remained intact (41), as shown schematically in Fig. 2. Major cleavage fragments of 105,000 (α'), 39,500, 34,000, 29,000, and 9,000 MW were detected by electrophoresis in polyacrylamide gels with reduction; only

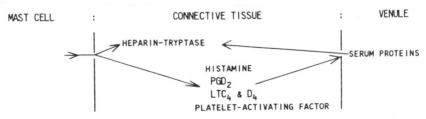

Fig. 1. Activation of mast cells at the interface between connective tissue and the postcapillary venule.

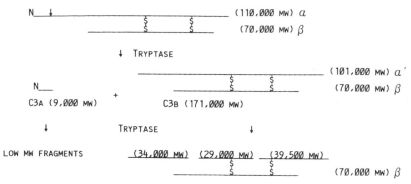

Fig. 2. Metabolism of human C3 by purified tryptase.

the 34,000 and 9,000 MW fragments were detected without reduction. By 9 hr, the α' fragment was almost completely degraded to the final products. Molar ratios of the 39,500, 34,000, 29,000, and 9,000 MW end-stage fragments to β subunit all approached unity. Because the 39,500 and 29,000 MW fragments were observed only after reduction, it is likely that they were linked to the β chain by disulfide bonds and presumably were related, at least in part, to the α^c and α^b fragments described by Harrison and Lachmann (42). The fragment of 34,000 MW may contain C3^d or C3^{de} sections of the α chain.

The C3 fragment generated by tryptase at 9,000 MW was observed to comigrate with purified C3a and with trypsin-generated C3a in SDS polyacrylamide gels, and therefore it corresponds in size to authentic C3a (41). A portion of this material was antigenically and functionally identified as C3a by radioimmunoassay and by bioactivity on the guinea pig ileum, respectively. That a fraction of the material detected at 9,000 MW might not be C3a was indicated by the lower amounts of C3a detected by bioassay and radioimmunoassay as compared to densitometric scanning of the 9,000 MW fragment. This inactive material may represent fragments from regions of the α chain other than C3a, as well as degradation fragments of C3a. The latter may account for much of this material, because the electrophoretic mobility of authentic C3a was not noticeably altered by incubation with tryptase although C3a antigenic and contractile activities were ultimately lost.

The effect of porcine heparin on the interaction of tryptase with C3 was examined because of the probable association of tryptase and heparin proteoglycan in the extracellular milieu after degranulation (20). Under conditions of relative heparin excess over a 9-hr time course, no appreciable differences in the rates of appearance and the MW of the major tryptase-cleavage fragments of C3 were found, with the single exception that no C3a-like material was detected by radioimmunoassay, bioassay, or in a stained polyacrylamide gel. Heparin selectively enhanced the rate of catabolism of C3a by more than 100-fold, which resulted in a concomitant loss of contractile activity. A similar enhancement of bovine trypsin-catalyzed degradation of C3a was not observed. Human heparin proteoglycan resides in the complex milieu of mast cell secretory granules in a weight ratio to tryptase of 1:3 (3,20), whereas porcine heparin was employed *in vitro* at ratios of heparin to tryptase ranging from 4 to 10:1. This may be of biologic relevance because of the similar biologic and chemical properties of porcine and human heparins (3). Whether heparin acts on C3a *in vitro* to increase its susceptibility to tryptase or on tryptase to selectively enhance its activity against C3a is not known. One favored possibility is that through a binding interaction between heparin and C3a, destabilization of the α-helical structure of C3a (43) may occur, thereby exposing otherwise protected internal peptide regions to attack by tryptase.

Anaphylatoxin C3a has biologic activities that include smooth muscle contraction of the guinea pig ileum at levels of 6–9 nM and enhancement of vascular permeability in human skin at levels of 1 to 100 pmol/0.1 ml injection (40,44). Histamine release *in vitro* from rat mast cells occurs at 1,000 to 10,000 nM C3a, concentrations that seem unlikely to be achieved *in vivo*. However, histologic studies of cutaneous tissues after intradermal challenge of humans with C3a (5 pmol in 0.1 ml) have shown mast cell degranulation (40). With guinea pig trachea (45) and pulmonary parenchyma (46,47) target tissues, the smooth muscle response to porcine C3a and C5a appears to be primarily histamine independent, whereas guinea pig ileum contractility may be primarily histamine dependent (38). In guinea pig lung tissue, C5a and C5a$_{des\ Arg}$ act in part through the secondary generation of sulfidopeptide leukotrienes C$_4$, D$_4$, and E$_4$ (48), the biologically and chemically defined slow-reacting substances of anaphylaxis (49). Analogous studies with C3a are not available. Biological concentrations of tryptase possible in human skin can be estimated at ~830 nM on the basis of mast cell concentrations in normal human skin of about 10,000/mm^3 (50,51) and a content of 12 pg tryptase/mast cell (20). A C3 concentration of 3,300 nM and a tryptase concentration of 70 nM were employed in the *in vitro* experiments summarized above. C3, which has a plasma concentration of about 8,000 nM, could reach sites of mast cell activation at a concentration that is sufficient for the generation of effective levels of C3a.

THE INTERACTION OF TRYPTASE WITH HIGH MOLECULAR WEIGHT KININOGEN

In systemic reactions of anaphylaxis consumption of high molecular weight kininogen (HMWK), fibrinogen, and coagulation Factors V and VIII has been reported to occur without evidence for activation of coagulation Factor XII and prekallikrein, two proenzymes of the contact activation phase of intrinsic coagulation and kinin generation (52). The participation of proteases that are distinct from those normally associated with utilization of HMWK and activation of the intrinsic coagulation pathway was therefore postulated. The plasma protein, HMWK as noted for C3, could be made available to tryptase *in vivo* because of the capacity of other mediators derived from activated human mast cells to augment venular permeability. Anaphylactic release of kinin-generating, prekallikrein-activating, and Hageman factor-activating activities from human lung fragments have also been observed (53), although a cell source for these activities, the physicochemical characterization of the enzymes involved, and their relationship to tryptase have not been reported as yet.

HMWK, as outlined in Table III, is required as a cofactor for the Hageman factor- (Factor XIIa-) dependent activation of Factor XI of the intrinsic coagulation pathway (reviewed in ref. 54). Patients lacking HMWK (Fitzgerald trait) have a prolonged partial thromboplastin time (intrinsic coagulation pathway), a normal prothrombin time (extrinsic coagulation pathway), and no clinically significant abnormalities of blood coagulation (54). The vasoactive bradykinin and lysyl-bradykinin peptide sequences are located internally in HMWK and low molecular weight kininogen (55) but can be selectively released by the limited proteolytic action of kallikrein (kininogenase) enzymes (56). HMWK circulates in plasma as a complex with Factor XI or prekallikrein, a precursor of plasma kallikrein (54). HMWK directs deposition of these complexes

TABLE III
The Biology of High Molecular Weight Kininogen (Fitzgerald Factor)

1. Resides as a complex in plasma with Factor XI or with prekallikrein
2. Amplifies the initial contact phase reactions for kinin generation and for the intrinsic coagulation pathway
   a. XIIa-dependent activation of Factor XI and of prekallikrein
   b. Kallikrein-dependent activation of Factor XII
3. Source of bradykinin (BK)

onto surfaces with a negative charge (57,58), where Factor XII may also reside (54,58). HMWK facilitates the reciprocal activation of prekallikrein by Factor XIIa and of Factor XII by kallikrein (54,58,59), leading to amplification of the initial contact phase step for kinin generation and for the intrinsic coagulation pathway.

Although bovine trypsin can release bradykinin from HMWK with retention of residual procoagulant activity, human lung mast cell tryptase catalyzes the destruction of human HMWK as a kallikrein-dependent source of kinin activity and as a procoagulant factor of the intrinsic coagulation system without concomitant generation of kinin activity (60). HMWK (5,600 nM) was 50% destroyed as a source of kallikrein-generated kinin after a 5-min incubation with tryptase (31 nM). Tryptase, when incubated with bradykinin or human pancreatic and urinary kallikreins, had no direct effect on their biologic activities, and reciprocally, human urinary kallikrein had no effect on the TAMe-esterase activity of tryptase. Destruction of bradykinin does not occur with tryptase or kallikrein enzymes, but is attributed primarily to the actions of a dipeptide hydrolase (kininase II, angiotensin I converting enzyme) (61) or a C-terminal protease, carboxypeptidase N (62), that is also the complement anaphylatoxin inactivator (63).

Human mast cell tryptase was reported to inactivate the HMWK-dependent procoagulant activity of both native HMWK and the purified procoagulant chain that is derived from HMWK (60). Incubation of HMWK (51 nM) or procoagulant chain (40 nM) with tryptase (0.04 and 0.02 nM, respectively) resulted in a 72% loss of HMWK procoagulant activity by 7 min. In contrast, human urinary and pancreatic kallikreins did not alter the procoagulant activity of HMWK under conditions where the substrate was cleaved to generate kinin (64).

Structural changes in HMWK caused by tryptase were analyzed by electrophoresis under denaturing conditions in SDS polyacrylamide gels and are illustrated in Fig. 3. Native HMWK (4600 nM) was completely cleaved by tryptase (69 nM) between 2 and 10 min. The native chain was sequentially converted to forms that, when not reduced, had apparent MW of 100,000 and 95,000 by 2 min and of 74,000 and 67,000 by 10 to 30 min. With reduction, two major fragments at 67,000 and 66,000 apparent MW that stained with about equal intensity were found at preincubation times from 0.17 to 30 min. These two products could have originated from regions on opposite ends of HMWK or from the same end. When HMWK is cleaved by kallikreins to release kinin, the residual kinin-free substrate consists of two disulfide linked chains, each ~65,000 MW (64,65). Studies with plasma kallikrein have shown that the carboxy-terminal chain quantitatively retains procoagulant activity, even after further limited cleavage

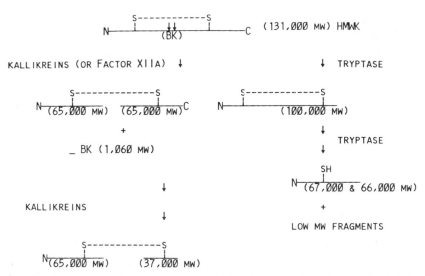

Fig. 3. Comparison of the metabolism of high molecular weight kininogen by kallikrein enzymes and purified tryptase.

to forms as small as 54,000 (65), 44,000 (66), or 37,000 (67) MW. Thus, the time-dependent accumulation of very low MW products in both the reduced and nonreduced samples together with the rapid loss of procoagulant activity from native HMWK and its isolated procoagulant chain suggest that tryptase extensively degrades this region of HMWK. Consequently, the 66,000 and 67,000 MW reduced products observed at 30 min most likely represent portions of the amino-terminal region of the native substrate. Inactivation of tryptase-treated HMWK as a source of kinin could result from a conformational change that makes the usual site of cleavage by kallikrein unavailable or from direct cleavage within the kinin peptide segment of the protein substrate.

The average concentration of tryptase in human skin, as noted before, can be estimated at ~830 nM. The normal plasma concentration of HMWK is ~600 nM (66). Thus, concentrations of tryptase possible in connective tissue at sites of mast cell activation are sufficient for the rapid inactivation of any HMWK that might diffuse into these locations. During a limited and localized mast cell response, catabolism of an insignificant portion of total plasma HMWK may occur, whereas a larger systemic activation of mast cells may result in depletion of an appreciable amount of HMWK. Consistent with the latter circumstance is the report mentioned previously that during systemic anaphylactic reactions to bee venom, plasma HMWK, as assessed by procoagulant activity, is depleted in the absence of consumption of Factor XII (Hageman Factor) or of prekallikrein (52).

CONCLUDING REMARKS

Mast cells occupy sentinel positions in and around venules and at cutaneous, mucosal, and serosal surfaces of connective tissue (68). Mediators released and generated at these sites may be expected to exert much of their activity at the interface between connective tissue and the corresponding surface. Indeed, the pathobiologic alterations at vascular, gastrointestinal, cutaneous, ocular, and bronchial surfaces known to occur with allergic disorders confirm this expectation, whereas the physiologic functions of mast cells are not generally understood.

A window of communication between the connective tissue and plasma compartments is opened by release of histamine, PGD_2, sulfidopeptide leukotrienes, and possibly platelet-activating factor from human pulmonary mast cells, all of which enhance vascular permeability and concomitant diffusion of plasma proteins into tissues (Fig. 1). Human pulmonary, rat serosal, and rat mucosal mast cells release neutral proteases that in the first two cell types exist as an insoluble macromolecular complex with heparin proteoglycan. This complex may serve to restrict the diffusion and possibly the substrate specificity of these enzymes.

Human pulmonary mast cell secretory granules, like those in rat mast cells, contain neutral proteases that appear to be qualitatively distinct from components in granules of basophils and other cell types. Measurements of these cell-specific mediators in biologic fluids may be helpful in distinguishing the relative activity of each cell type in a given situation *in vivo* in which both mast cells and basophils are present. The presence of chymase and heparin proteoglycan in the rat serosal (connective tissue) mast cell, and of rat mast cell protease II along with chondroitin sulfate in the mucosal (bone marrow derived, T lymphocyte dependent) mast cells, serves to distinguish these two mast cell subtypes from one another as well as from other cell types (22,24,69). The presence of analogous mast cell subtypes in human tissues remains to be documented. Whether the different compositions of secretory granules in different mast cell subtypes represent different stages of mast cell maturation or depends upon the ultimate tissue destination of the mast cell, and whether these mast cell subtypes originate from distinct stem cells, need further clarification.

Coagulation and fibrin deposition in areas of mast cell activation may not occur because of mast cell-derived mediators such as heparin proteoglycan, an anticoagulant that combines with antithrombin III to inhibit thrombin and coagulation Factors Xa, XIa, and XIIa (reviewed in ref. 70); prostaglandin D_2, an inhibitor of platelet aggregation (71); and potentially fibrinogenolytic proteases. The capacity of tryptase from human lung mast cells to inactivate human HMWK is consistent with the ability of other mast cell-derived mediators to suppress blood coagulation and thrombosis, whereas inactivation of HMWK as a precursor for kinin production involves a different biologic pathway. These factors may explain why the hive that results from a local influx of plasma remains soft and painless and resolves in less than 24 hr, as opposed to the cutaneous lesion of delayed-type or cutaneous basophil hypersensitivity that is indurated, persistent, and characterized in part by deposition of fibrin. In human basophils none of the anticoagulant mediators present in mast cells has been detected. In fact, activated basophils have been reported to secrete bradykinin activator and a Hageman factor activator that may actually promote coagulation and generate kinins (72,73).

A histamine-independent role for mast cell involvement in human bronchial asthma can now be postulated based on the *in vitro* capacity of mast cell tryptase to generate anaphylatoxin from serum complement, in addition to the generation by mast cells of other smooth muscle spasmogens, such as the sulfidopeptide leukotrienes. Generation of peptides with chemotactic activity by mast cells through protease action on available proteins is also a likely possibility and may be of particular significance in late onset cutaneous, pulmonary, and nasal reactions that involve an influx of polymorphonuclear and mononuclear cells.

A role for mast cells in defense against parasitic disease has been suspected based upon the increased numbers of mast cells found in gastrointestinal tissues of animals infected with helminths (74), the decreased resistance to infection when IgE synthesis is suppressed (75), and the ability of mast cell mediators to mobilize eosinophils *in vitro* and to enhance eosinophil-mediated killing of these helminths (76). The rat mucosal mast cell neutral protease, RMCP II, is the dominant soluble protein component of intestinal mucus (23), and may impart a protective effect to this biologic fluid against parasitic infestation. That neutral protease activities are important in cell-mediated cytotoxicity by murine T lymphocytes (77) and activated murine peritoneal macrophages (78,79), and in the inhibition of leukocyte migration by the lymphokine termed leukocyte inhibitory factor (80), suggests a broader potential role for mast cell proteases in policing the connective tissue and mucosal environments. The role of mast cell enzymes in wound healing (81) and in growth of solid tumors (82) also needs clarification because of the implication of mast cells and proteases in these tissue processes. The capabilities of mast cells and mast cell subtypes to play a role in diverse biologic events will be better understood as their special neutral proteases are further characterized.

REFERENCES

1. Schwartz, L. B., and Austen, K. F. Mast cells and mediators. *In* "Clinical Aspects of Immunology" (P. J. Lachmann and D. K. Peters, eds.), pp. 130–157. Blackwell, Oxford, 1982.
2. Patterson, N. A. M., Wasserman, S. I., Said, J. W., and Austen, K. F. Release of chemical mediators from partially purified human lung mast cells. *J. Immunol.* **117:**1356–1362, 1976.
3. Metcalfe, D. D., Lewis, R. A., Silbert, J. E., Rosenberg, R. D., Wasserman, S. I., and Austen, K. F. Isolation and characterization of heparin from human lung. *J. Clin. Invest.* **64:**1537–1543, 1979.
4. Schwartz, L. B., Lewis, R. A., Seldin, D., and Austen, K. F. Acid hydrolases and tryptase from secretory granules of dispersed human lung mast cells. *J. Immunol.* **126:**1290–1294, 1981.
5. Lewis, R. A., Soter, N. A., Diamond, P. T., Austen, K. F., Oates, J. A., and Roberts, L. J., II. Prostaglandin D_2 generation after activation of rat and human mast cells with anti-IgE. *J. Immunol.* **129:**1627–1631, 1982.
6. MacGlashan, D. W., Jr., Schleimer, R. P., Peters, S. P., Schulman, E. S., Adams, G. K., III, Newball, H. H., and Lichtenstein, L. M. Generation of leukotrienes by purified human lung mast cells. *J. Clin. Invest.* **70:**747–751, 1982.
7. Soter, N. A., Lewis, R. A., Corey, E. J., and Austen, K. F. Local effects of synthetic LTs (C4, D4, E4, and B4) in human skin. *J. Invest. Dermatol.* **80:**115–119, 1983.
8. Pinckard, R. N. "Platelet Activating Factor: Is it a Mediator of Anaphylaxis? pp. 1–8. "The American Academy of Allergy Postgraduate Syllabus, Montreal, 1982.
9. Chiu, H., and Lagunoff, D. Histochemical comparison of vertebrate mast cells. *Histochem. J.* **4:**135–144, 1972.
10. Combs, J. W., Lagunoff, D., and Benditt, E. P. Differentiation and proliferation of embryonic mast cells of the rat. *J. Cell Biol.* **25:**577–592, 1965.
11. Czarnetzki, B. M., and Behrendt, H. Studies on the *in vitro* development of rat peritoneal mast cells. *Immunobiology* **159:**256–268, 1981.
12. Krüger, P. G., and Lagunoff, D. Mast cell restoration: A study of the rat peritoneal mast cells after depletion with polymyxin B. *Int. Arch. Allergy Appl. Immunol.* **65:**278–290, 1981.
13. Combs, J. W. Maturation of rat mast cells: An electron microscope study. *J. Cell Biol.* **31:**563–575, 1966.
14. Gomori, G. Chloracetyl esters as histochemical substrates. *J. Histochem. Cytochem.* **1:**469–470, 1953.
15. Benditt, E. P., and Arase, M. An enzyme in mast cells with properties like chymotrypsin. *J. Exp. Med.* **110:**451–460, 1959.
16. Glenner, C. G., and Cohen, L. A. Histochemical demonstration of a species-specific trypsin-like enzyme in mast cells. *Nature (London)* **185:**846–847, 1960.
17. Hopsu-Havu, V. K., and Glenner, G. G. A histochemical enzyme kinetic system applied to the trypsin-like amidase and esterase activity in human mast cells. *J. Cell Biol.* **17:**503–520, 1963.
18. Schwartz, L. B., Schratz, J. J., Vik, D., Fearon, D. T., and Austen, K. F. Cleavage of

human C3 by human mast cell tryptase. *Fed. Proc., Fed. Am. Soc. Exp. Biol.* **41**:487, 1982.

19. Schwartz, L. B., Riedel, C., Schratz, J. J., and Austen, K. F. Localization of carboxypeptidase A to the macromolecular heparin proteoglycan–protein complex in secretory granules of rat serosal mast cells. *J. Immunol.* **128**:1128–1133, 1982.

20. Schwartz, L. B., Lewis, R. A., and Austen, K. F. Tryptase from human pulmonary mast cells: purification and characterization. *J. Biol. Chem.* **256**:11939–11943, 1981.

21. DuBuske, L., Schwartz, L. B., and Austen, K. F. Carboxypeptidase A (CPA) from rat serosal mast cells (RSMC). *J. Allergy Clin. Immunol.* (abstr.) **71**:135, 1983.

22. Schwartz, L. B., Riedel, C., Caulfield, J. P., Wasserman, S. I., and Austen, K. F. Cell association of complexes of chymase, heparin proteoglycan, and protein after degranulation by rat mast cells. *J. Immunol.* **126**:2071–2078, 1981.

23. Woodbury, R. G., and Miller, H. R. P. Quantitative analysis of mucosal mast cell protease in the intestines of *Nippostrongylus*-infected rats. *Immunology* **46**:487–495, 1982.

24. Haig, D. M., McKee, T. A., Jarrett, E. E., Woodbury, R., and Miller, H. R. Generation of mucosal mast cells is stimulated *in vitro* by factors derived from T cells of helminth-infected rats. *Nature (London)* **300**:188–190, 1982.

25. Plow, E. F. The major fibrinolytic proteases of human leukocytes. *Biochim. Biophys. Acta* **630**:46–47, 1980.

26. Feinstein, G., and Janoff, A. A rapid method for purification of human granulocyte cationic neutral proteases: Purification and characterization of human granulocyte chymotrypsin-like enzyme. *Biochim. Biophys. Acta* **403**:477–492, 1975.

27. Mikhail, G. R., and Miller-Milinska, A. Mast cell population in human skin. *J. Invest. Dermatol.* **43**:249–254, 1964.

28. Soter, N. A., Mihm, M. C., Jr., Dvorak, H. F., and Austen, K. F. Cutaneous necrotizing venulitis: a sequential analysis of the morphological alterations occurring after mast cell degranulation in a patient with a unique syndrome. *Clin. Exp. Immunol.* **32**:46–58, 1978.

29. Fräki, J. E., and Hopsu-Havu, V. K. Human skin proteases. Separation and characterization of two alkaline proteases, one splitting trypsin and the other chymotrypsin substrates. *Arch. Dermatol. Res.* **253**:261–276, 1975.

30. Robertson, I., and Greaves, M. W. Responses of human skin blood vessels to synthetic histamine analogues. *Br. J. Clin. Pharmacol.* **5**:319, 1978.

31. Tack, B. F., and Prahl, J. W. Third component of human complement: Purification from plasma and physicochemical characteristics. *Biochemistry* **15**:4513–4521, 1976.

32. Müller-Eberhard, H. J., Dalmasso, A. P., and Calcott, M. A. The reaction mechanism of β1c-globulin (C'3) in immune hemolysis. *J. Exp. Med.* **123**:33–54, 1966.

33. Müller-Eberhard, H. J., Polley, M. J., and Calcott, M. A. Formation and functional significance of a molecular complex derived from the second and the fourth component of human complement. *J. Exp. Med.* **125**:359–380, 1967.

34. Götze, O., and Müller-Eberhard, H. J. The C3-activator system: An alternate pathway of complement activation. *J. Exp. Med.* **134**:90s, 1971.

35. Fearon, D. T., Austen, K. F., and Ruddy, S. Formation of a hemolytically active cellular intermediate by the interaction between properdin factors B and D and the activated third component of complement. *J. Exp. Med.* **138**:1305–1313, 1973.

36. Bokisch, V. A., Müller-Eberhard, H. J., and Cochrane, C. G. Isolation of a fragment (C3a) of the third component of human complement containing anaphylatoxin and chemotactic activity and description of an anaphylatoxin inactivator of human serum. *J. Exp. Med.* **129**:1109–1130, 1969.

37. Dias da Silva, W., Eisele, J. W., and Lepow, I. H. Complement as a mediator of inflammation. III. Purification of the activity with anaphylatoxin properties generated by interaction of the first four components of complement and its identification as a cleavage product of C'3. *J. Exp. Med.* **126:**1027–1048, 1967.

38. Cochrane, C. G., and Müller-Eberhard, H. J. The derivation of two distinct anaphylatoxin activities from the third and fifth components of human complement. *J. Exp. Med.* **127:**371–386, 1968.

39. Hugli, T. E. Complement anaphylatoxins as plasma mediators, spasmogens and chemotaxins. *In* "The Chemistry and Physiology of Human Plasma Proteins" (D. H. Bing, ed.), pp. 255–280. Pergamon, Oxford, 1979.

40. Lepow, I. H., Willms-Kretschmer, K., Patrick, R. A., and Rosen, F. S. Observations on lesions produced by intradermal injection of human C3a in man. *Am. J. Pathol.* **61:**13–24, 1970.

41. Schwartz, L. B., Kawahara, M. S., Hugli, T. E., Vik, D., Fearon, D. T., and Austen, K. F. Generation of C3a anaphylatoxin from human C3 by human mast cell tryptase. *J. Immunol.* **130:**1891–1895, 1983.

42. Harrison, R. A., and Lachmann, P. J. The physiological breakdown of the third component of human complement. *Mol. Immunol.* **17:**9–20, 1980.

43. Huber, R., Scholze, H., Paques, E. P., and Deisenhofer, J. Crystal structure analysis and molecular model of human C3a anaphylatoxin. *Hoppe-Seyler's Z. Physiol. Chem.* **361:**1389–1399, 1980.

44. Hugli, T. E., Vallota, E. H., and Müller-Eberhard, H. J. Purification and partial characterization of human and porcine C3a anaphylatoxin. *J. Biol. Chem.* **250:**1472–1478, 1975.

45. Regal, J. F., Eastman, A. Y., and Pickering, R. J. C5a-induced tracheal contraction: A histamine independent mechanism. *J. Immunol.* **124:**2876–2878, 1980.

46. Stimler, N. P., Hugli, T. E., and Bloor, C. M. Pulmonary injury induced by C3a and C5a anaphylatoxins. *Am. J. Pathol.* **100:**327–348, 1980.

47. Stimler, N. P., Brocklehurst, W. E., Bloor, C. M., and Hugli, T. E. Anaphylatoxin-mediated contraction of guinea pig lung strips: A nonhistamine tissue response. *J. Immunol.* **126:**2258–2261, 1981.

48. Stimler, N. P., Bach, M. K., Bloor, C. M., and Hugli, T. E. Release of leukotrienes from guinea pig lung stimulated by C5a$_{\text{des Arg}}$ anaphylatoxin. *J. Immunol.* **128:**2247–2252, 1982.

49. Lewis, R. A., and Austen, K. F. Mediation of local homeostasis and inflammation by leukotrienes and other mast cell-dependent compounds. *Nature (London)* **293:**103–108, 1982.

50. Mikhail, G. R., and Miller-Milinska, A. Mast cell population in human skin. *J. Invest. Dermatol.* **43:**249–254, 1964.

51. Soter, N. A., Mihm, M. C., Jr., Dvorak, H. F., and Austen, K. F. Cutaneous necrotizing venulitis: A sequential analysis of the morphologic alterations occurring after mast cell degranulation in a patient with a unique syndrom. *Clin Exp. Immunol.* **32:**46–58, 1978.

52. Smith, P. L., Sobotka, A. K., Bleecker, E. R., Traystman, R., Kaplan, A. P., Gralnick, H., Valentine, M. D., Permutt, S., and Lichtenstein, L. M. Physiologic manifestations of human anaphylaxis. *J. Clin. Invest.* **66:**1072–1080, 1980.

53. Meier, H. L., Revak, S. D., Kaplan, A. P., Berninger, R. W., Cochrane, C. G., Lichtenstein, L. M., and Newball, H. H. Inflammatory proteases of anaphylaxis. *In* "Advances in Allergy and Applied Immunology" (A. Oehling, I. Glazer, E. Mathov, and C. Arbesman, eds.), p. 652. Pergamon, Oxford, 1980.

54. Saito, H. The 'contact system' in health and disease. *Adv. Intern. Med.* **30:**217–238, 1980.

55. Nagasawa, S., and Nakayasu, T. Enzymatic and chemical cleavages of human kininogens. *DHEW Publ. (NIH) (U.S.)* **NIH 76-791:**139, 1976.

56. Habal, F. M., Movat, H. Z., and Burrowes, C. E. Isolation of two functionally different kininogens from human plasma—separation from proteinase inhibitors and interaction with plasma kallikrein. *Biochem. Pharmacol.* **23:**2291–2303, 1974.

57. Wiggins, R. C., Bouma, B. N., Cochrane, C. G., and Griffin, J. H. Role of high molecular weight kininogen in surface-binding and activation of coagulation factor XI and prekallikrein. *Proc. Natl. Acad. Sci. U.S.A.* **74:**4636–4640, 1977.

58. Silverberg, M., Nicoll, J. E., and Kaplan, A. P. The mechanism by which light chain of cleaved HMW-kininogen augments the activation of prekallikrein, Factor XI and Hageman Factor. *Thromb. Res.* **20:**173–189, 1980.

59. Cochrane, C. G., and Revak, S. D. Dissemination of contact activation in plasma by plasma kallikrein. *J. Exp. Med.* **152:**608–619, 1980.

60. Maier, M., Spragg, J., and Schwartz, L. B. Inactivation of human high molecular weight kininogen by human mast cell tryptase. *J. Immunol.* **130:**2352–2356, 1983.

61. Yang, H. Y. T., Erdös, E. G., and Levin, Y. Characterization of a dipeptide hydrolase (kininase II: angiotensin I converting enzyme). *J. Pharmacol. Exp. Ther.* **177:**291–300, 1971.

62. Erdös, E. G., Sloane, E. M., and Wohler, I. M. Carboxypeptidase in blood and other fluids. I. Properties, distribution, and partial purification of the enzyme. *Biochem. Pharmacol.* **13:**893–905, 1964.

63. Bokisch, V. A., and Müller-Eberhard, H. J. Anaphylatoxin inactivator of human plasma: Its isolation and characterization as a carboxypeptidase. *J. Clin. Invest.* **49:**2427–2436, 1970.

64. Maier, M., Austen, K. F., and Spagg, J. Characterization of the procoagulant chain derived from human high molecular weight kininogen (Fitzgerald factor) by human tissue kallikrein. *Blood* **62:**457–463, 1983.

65. Schiffman, S., Mannhalter, C., and Tyner, K. D. Human high molecular weight kininogen. Effects of cleavage by kallikrein on protein structure and procoagulant activity. *J. Biol. Chem.* **255:**6433–6438, 1980.

66. Kerbiriou, D. M., and Griffin, J. H. Human high molecular weight kininogen. Studies of structure–function relationships and of proteolysis of the molecule occurring during contact activation of plasma. *J. Biol. Chem.* **254:**12020–12027, 1979.

67. Thompson, R. E., Mandle, R., Jr., and Kaplan, A. P. Characterization of human high molecular weight kininogen. Procoagulant activity associated with the light chain of kinin-free high molecular weight kininogen. *J. Exp. Med.* **147:**488–499, 1978.

68. Selye, H. "The Mast Cells." Butterworth, London, 1965.

69. Woodbury, R. G., Gruzenski, G. M., and Lagunoff, D. Immunofluorescent localization of a serine protease in rat small intestine. *Proc. Natl. Acad. Sci. U.S.A.* **75:**2785–2789, 1978.

70. Harpel, P. C., and Rosenberg, R. D. α2-macroglobulin and antithrombin-heparin cofactor: Modulators of hemostatic and inflammatory reactions. *Proc. Hemostasis Thromb.* **3:**145–189, 1976.

71. Mills, D. C., and MacFarlane, D. E. Stimulation of human platelet adenyl cyclase by prostaglandin D_2. *Thromb. Res.* **5:**401–412, 1974.

72. Newball, H. H., Berninger, R. W., Talamo, R. C., and Lichtenstein, L. M. Anaphylactic release of a basophil kallikrein-like activity. I. Purification and characterization. *J. Clin. Invest.* **64:**457–465, 1979.

73. Newball, H. H., Talamo, R. C., and Lichtenstein, L. M. Anaphylactic release of a basophil kallikrein-like activity. II. A mediator of immediate hypersensitivity reaction. *J. Clin. Invest.* **64:**466–475, 1979.
74. Miller, H. R. P., and Jarrett, W. F. H. Immune reactions in mucous membranes. I. Intestinal mast cell response during helminth expulsion in the rat. *Immunology* **20:**277–288, 1971.
75. Dessein, A. J., Parker, W. L., James, S. L., and David, J. R. IgE antibody and resistance to infection. I. Selective suppression of the IgE antibody response in rats diminishes the resistance and the eosinophil response to *Trichinella spiralis* infection. *J. Exp. Med.* **153:**423–436, 1981.
76. Anwar, A. R. E., McKean, J. R., Smithers, S. R., and Kay, A. B. Human eosinophil- and neutrophil-mediated killing of schistosomula of Schistosoma mansoni *in vitro*. I. Enhancement of complement-dependent damage by mast cell-derived mediators and formyl methionyl peptides. *J. Immunol.* **124:**1122–1129, 1980.
77. Redelman, D., and Hudig, D. The mechanism of cell-mediated cytotoxicity. I. Killing by murine cytotoxic T lymphocytes requires cell surface thiols and activated proteases. *J. Immunol.* **124:**870–878, 1980.
78. Adams, D. O. Effector mechanisms of cytolytically activated macrophages. I. Secretion of neutral proteases and effect of protease inhibitors. *J. Immunol.* **124:**286–292, 1980.
79. Adams, D. O., Kao, K., Farb, R., and Pizzo, S. V. Effector mechanisms of cytolytically activated macrophages. II. Secretion of a cytolytic factor by activated macrophages and its relationship to secreted neutral proteases. *J. Immunol.* **124:**293–300, 1980.
80. Bendtzen, K., and Rocklin, R. E. Use of benzoyl-L-phenylalanyl-L-valyl-L-arginine [³H]methyl ester as a sensitive and selective substrate for the human lymphokine, leukocyte migration inhibitory factor (LIF). *J. Immunol.* **125:**1775–1781, 1980.
81. Matsuda, H., and Kitamura, Y. Migration of stromal cells supporting mast-cell differentiation into open wound produced in the skin of mice. *Exp. Hematol.* **9:**38–43, 1981.
82. Azizkhan, R. G., Azizkhan, J. C., Zetter, B. R., and Folkman, J. Mast cell heparin stimulates migration of capillary endothelial cells *in vitro*. *J. Exp. Med.* **152:**931–944, 1980.

DISCUSSION

Austen: Could Drs. Schwartz and Lichtenstein discuss more fully the possible range of proteases in human mast cells as revealed by different assays?

Schwartz: Approximately 90 to 95% of the TAMe-esterase activity in human lung mast cells can be ascribed to tryptase. A minor amount of TAMe-esterase has been observed that elutes from heparin-agarose at a lower ionic strength than tryptase.

Lichtenstein: The mast cells appear to have a prekallikrein activator, an enzyme that cleaves Hageman factor and a kininogenase. These enzymes have not been fully characterized. The kininogenase, however, is preformed and obtainable from mast cells of greater than 98% purity.

Schwartz: Although tryptase does not generate bradykinin from heat-inactivated plasma or from purified high molecular weight kininogen, it is still possible that other proteases exist in mast cells with these activities. By analogy to rat serosal mast cells, which contain two distinct proteases, chymase and carboxypeptidase A, it would not be surprising to find multiple proteases in the human mast cells.

Gleich: I have two questions and a comment. (1) Are inhibitors of tryptase present in body fluids? (2) Do you have antibody to the tryptase? The latter question is prompted by the need for specific histochemical markers for vasoactive amine containing cells. We have found that basophils contain many of the same molecules as do eosinophils. For example, basophils contain quantities of the Charcot-Leyden crystals, which are indistinguishable from the amounts present in eosinophils. Similarly, basophils contain the eosinophil granule major basic protein, albeit in quantities much less than in the eosinophil, namely 1/10 to 1/100. These observations point to immunochemical similarities between basophils and eosinophils and emphasize the need for cell-specific immunohistochemical markers for these cells.

Schwartz: Tryptase is clearly different from trypsin because of the lack of inhibition of tryptase by soybean, lima bean, and ovamucoid trypsin inhibitors, and by α-1-antitrypsin and trasylol. Furthermore, a trypsin-like enzyme of apparent 120,000 MW from human cutaneous tissue that might be tryptase was not inhibited by human serum (J. E. Fräki and V. K. Hapsu-Havu, *Arch. Dermatol. Res.*, **253:**261, 1975).

Antibodies specific for tryptase are being developed and will be of great value for conformation of the cellular and subcellular localization of tryptase, for definition of the antigenic relationship of the two different tryptase subunits, and for development of a radioimmunoassay with specificity and sensitivity to measure the enzyme in complex biologic fluids and tissues.

The levels of esterase activity in basophils as shown by histochemical techniques are much less than in mast cells. Proteases that have been associated with basophils and cleave TAMe as described (H. H. Newball, R. W. Berninger, R. C. Talamo, and L. M. Lichtenstein, *J. Clin. Invest.* **64:**457, 1979) appear to be of different molecular weight than tryptase. Nevertheless, vigorous exclusion of tryptase in basophils must await development of sensitive immunoassays specific for tryptase.

Hogg: How does the enzyme compare with the neutral proteases of the PMN described by Janoff and others?

Schwartz: The two enzymes have different physicochemical characteristics and substrate specificities. Elastase is a small molecular weight enzyme, whereas tryptase is a tetramer of MW 144,000. Tryptase also does not cleave the elastase synthetic substrate succinyl-ala-ala-ala-*p*-nitroanalide.

Wasserman: In light of altered tryptase specificity for C3a in the presence of heparin, have you data regarding tryptase–high-MW kininogen interaction in the presence of heparin? Also a comment: as human heparin proteoglycan has a molecular weight of 60,000 it is unlikely it will alter the diffusability of tryptase to any great degree.

Schwartz: The effect of commercial heparin glycosaminoglycan to selectively enhance tryptase-catalysed degradation of C3a could result either from an action on tryptase or C3a. The latter possibility is favored because of the known binding of C3a to heparin, an event that may cause conformational changes in C3a that increases its susceptibility to protease action. The use of excess heparin *in vitro*, however, may not accurately reflect what actually happens *in vivo* where heparin may be completely saturated with protein such that its binding to C3a would be prevented.

Schleimer: Work in Dr. Austen's lab has shown that rat mast cell chymase stimulates histamine release from the rat serosal mast cells. Does tryptase have any such activity on the human mast cells?

Neutral proteases have recently been discovered that activate the calcium-dependent protein kinase by cleavage. This is exciting to those who study early events in cell activation since protein phosphorylation is likely to be an important modulator of cell responses. It might be interesting to study the effects of neutral proteases such as the ones you are working with on the calcium-dependent protein kinase.

Schwartz: It is true that chymase from rat serosal mast cells, like chymotrypsin, activates the secretory process in these cells (B. Schick, K. F. Austen, and L. B. Schwartz, *Fed. Proc., Fed. Am. Soc. Exp. Biol.* **42:**2454, 1983). Trypsin works less well (D. Lagunoff, E. Y. Chi, and H. Wan, *Biochem. Pharmacol.* **24:**1573, 1975). I have no data on the activation of human mast cells by proteases.

Compartmentalization of tryptase in the secretory granules and protein kinases in the cytoplasm may restrict any action of granule proteases on these kinases.

Larsen: C5 fragments, specifically C5a and $C5a_{des\ Arg}$, are also phlogistic agents with activities similar to those described for C3a. In addition, these C5 fragments are chemotactic for neutrophils by direct and/or indirect mechanisms. Will tryptase also cleave C5a and/or $C5a_{des\ Arg}$ from C5?

Schwartz: An action of tryptase on C5 to yield the anaphylatoxin C5a with its potent spasmogenic and chemotactic activities, would be of great interest and will be examined in detail over the next year.

Platts-Mills: Do you think your results on repeat application suggest a role for antigen persistence in the LAR?

Schwartz: Mast cell neutral protease in general, or tryptase in particular, may play a role in late-phase reactions in skin and pulmonary tissues that cannot be accounted for by histamine. Of possibly greater importance is the role these proteases may have in the physiologic actions of mast cells that have yet to be defined.

Schiffmann: Is heparin degraded upon release from mast cells? If so this might be a control mechanism for the relative persistence of C3a after its generation by tryptase.

Schwartz: There are no data in the human system for degradation of heparin proteoglycan by the protease, sulphatase, or glycosidases known to reside in mast cell secretory granules. In the rat mast cell the $(Ser-Gly-)_n$ sequence of the heparin protein core is very resistant to digestion by trypsin and chymotrypsin-like enzymes because of the lack of internal basic and aromatic amino acid residues and the dense distribution of glycosaminoglycan side chains attached to the protein core.

Austen: Neither the heparin proteoglycan of rat mast cells nor the chondroitin sulphate E proteoglycan of mouse bone marrow-derived mast cells are reduced in size during activation secretion responses.

CHAPTER 3

IgE-Mediated Triggering Signals for Mediator Release from Human Mast Cells and Basophils*

TERUKO ISHIZAKA

Subdepartment of Immunology
The Johns Hopkins University School of Medicine
at the Good Samaritan Hospital
Baltimore, Maryland, U.S.A.

In IgE-mediated hypersensitivity reactions, IgE molecules bind to specific receptors on mast cells and basophils with high affinity (1,2), and the reaction of cell-bound IgE molecules with multivalent ligand initiates the release of a variety of preformed and newly generated mediators (reviewed in ref. 3). Our previous studies on rat mast cells revealed that bridging of IgE receptors on rat mast cells, either directly by divalent antireceptor antibodies or indirectly through cell-bound IgE and anti-IgE, induced a marked increase in phospholipid methylation and a monophasic rise in cyclic AMP (cAMP), which were followed by an increase in ^{45}Ca uptake and histamine release (4–6). Since inhibition of phospholipid methylation by specific inhibitors resulted in the inhibition of ^{45}Ca uptake and histamine release, we concluded that phospholipid methylation is involved in transduction of IgE-mediated triggering signals for histamine release. Our results also showed that inhibitors of chymotrypsin and trypsin inhibited both phospholipid methylation and cAMP rise induced by receptor bridging, suggesting that membrane-associated proteolytic enzyme(s) is activated by receptor bridging prior to the activation of methyltransferases and adenylate cyclase (7).

A question was raised as to whether the early biochemical events following the bridging of IgE receptors are common in rat mast cells and

* This work was supported by research grant AI-10060 from the U.S. Public Health Service, and from Lillia Babbitt Hyde Foundation. This article is publication No. 515 from the O'Neill Laboratories at the Good Samaritan Hospital.

ASTHMA:
Physiology, Immunopharmacology,
and Treatment
THIRD INTERNATIONAL SYMPOSIUM

human mast cells. Using human mast cells isolated from lung tissues and cultured human basophils, which have become available in our laboratory, we analyzed early membrane events involved in IgE-mediated histamine release from human mast cells and basophils.

BIOCHEMICAL EVENTS INVOLVED IN IgE-MEDIATED HISTAMINE RELEASE FROM HUMAN LUNG MAST CELLS

Mast cells in a single-cell suspension were prepared by digestion of lung fragments with proteolytic enzymes (8,9) and were partially purified by countercurrent centrifugation and elutriation (10). In our experiments, partially purified mast cells were cultured overnight with 10 μg/ml of human IgE to saturate IgE receptors. Cells recovered from the culture were further purified by flotation through discontinuous Percoll layers. Approximately 10^7 cells suspended in 90% Percoll solution were placed at the bottom of the tube, and different concentrations of Percoll were layered. The tubes were then centrifuged at 400 g for 12 min. In general, mast cells were found at the 60/70% and 50/60% Percoll interfaces. The purity of mast cells in the preparation recovered from these interfaces was in the range of 70 to 98% (11).

Using purified human lung mast cells, we examined possible changes in phospholipid methylation, intracellular cAMP level, and ^{45}Ca uptake following the bridging of IgE receptors (11). Purified mast cells sensitized with human IgE were challenged with anti-IgE, and the kinetics of the phospholipid methylation, cAMP rise, ^{45}Ca uptake, and histamine release were analyzed. As shown in Fig. 1, challenge of mast cells with anti-IgE resulted in a marked enhancement of phospholipid methylation and an increase in intracellular cAMP, followed by ^{45}Ca uptake and histamine release. Phospholipid methylation reached maximum at 30 sec after the challenge; cAMP level reached maximum at 1 min. Both phospholipid methylation and cAMP level declined to baseline within 3 to 5 min. In human mast cells, ^{45}Ca uptake reached plateau at 2 to 3 min, and the maximum histamine release was obtained within 5 to 8 min. Chromatographic analysis of methylated phospholipids on Silica G plates (12) revealed that the formation of monomethyl- and dimethylphosphatidylethanolamine and phosphatidylcholine in mast cells markedly enhanced upon challenge with anti-IgE. Lysophosphatidylcholine was also detectable at 30 sec after challenge with anti-IgE.

As demonstrated in rat mast cells by Lewis (13), 10 μM of indomethacin failed to inhibit the initial rise in cAMP induced by anti-IgE, indicating

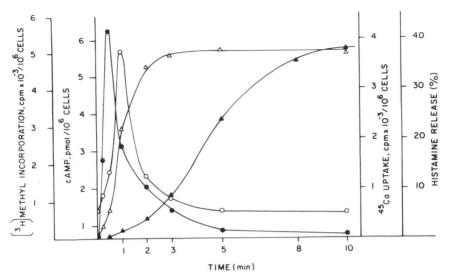

Fig. 1. Kinetics of [³H]methyl incorporation into phospholipids (●), cAMP rise (○), ⁴⁵Ca uptake (△), and histamine release (▲) induced by anti-IgE. Purified lung mast cells were incubated overnight with E myeloma protein to saturate IgE receptors and then challenged with 0.9 μg/ml of anti-IgE. The same mast cell preparation (purity, 90%) was employed in all measurements. Each point is an average of duplicated measurements. The original cAMP level in the unstimulated cells was 1.45 pmol/10^6 cells.

that the increase of cAMP is not the result of prostaglandin synthesis. Thus, it appears that initial biochemical events induced by receptor bridging are similar in both rat and human mast cells. The main difference between rat mast cells and human mast cells was that all of the biochemical events occur more slowly in human mast cell system (cf. 5,6).

In order to confirm that these biochemical events are indeed the results of bridging of IgE-receptors, human mast cells saturated with IgE were challenged by the F(ab′)₂ fragments or Fab′ monomer fragments of anti-IgE. It was found that F(ab′)₂ induced phospholipid methylation, cAMP rise, ⁴⁵Ca uptake, and histamine release. Kinetics of these reactions were identical to those induced by anti-IgE. By contrast, Fab′ monomer fragment of the antibody did not induce any of these reactions.

In order to prove that phospholipid methylation induced by receptor bridging is actually involved in opening Ca^{2+} channels, we studied the effect of inhibitors of phospholipid methylation on ⁴⁵Ca uptake and histamine release. Purified lung mast cells sensitized with IgE were preincubated with various concentrations of 3-deazaadenosine together with 100 μM L-homocysteine thiolactone at 37°C for 30 min, and the cells were challenged by an optimal concentration of anti-IgE. Incorporation of

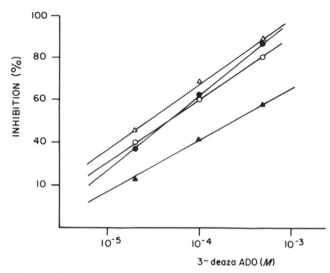

Fig. 2.   Inhibition of anti-IgE-induced [³H]methyl incorporation (○), cAMP rise (●), ⁴⁵Ca uptake (△), and histamine release (▲) by 3-deazaadenosine (3-deaza ADO) and L-homocysteine thiolactone. Aliquots of lung mast cells (93% pure) were preincubated at 37°C for 30 min with various concentrations of 3-deazaadenosine together with 100 μM L-homocysteine thiolactone, and the cells were challenged with 0.9 μg/ml anti-IgE. [³H]methyl incorporation into phospholipid, cAMP levels, ⁴⁵Ca uptake, and histamine release were measured in duplicate at 30 sec, 1 min, 3 min, and 15 min, respectively.

[³H]methyl groups into phospholipid, intracellular cAMP, ⁴⁵Ca uptake, and histamine release were determined at 30 sec, 1 min, 3 min, and 15 min after the challenge, respectively. Representative results are shown in Fig. 2. Preincubation of purified lung mast cells with 3-deazaadenosine with homocysteine thiolactone resulted in the inhibition of not only phospholipid methylation, but also cAMP rise, ⁴⁵Ca uptake, and histamine release in a dose–response fashion. Another inhibitor of phospholipid methylation, 3-deaza-SIBA, gave similar results. The results indicate that phospholipid methylation plays an important role in the IgE-mediated Ca²⁺ uptake and histamine release.

Our recent studies revealed that purified human lung mast cells preincubated with [¹⁴C]arachidonic acid (AA), released [¹⁴C]AA upon challenge with anti-IgE and that the kinetics of [¹⁴C]AA release was identical to that of histamine release. It was also found that inhibitors of phospholipid methylation inhibited both IgE-mediated histamine release and [¹⁴C]AA release in an identical dose–response fashion. These results are in agreement with previous observations on rat mast cells and demonstrated that phospholipid methylation induced by receptor bridging is an essential step in IgE-mediated release of histamine and arachidonates from human lung mast cells.

BIOCHEMICAL EVENTS INVOLVED IN MEDIATOR RELEASE FROM HUMAN CULTURED BASOPHILS

Quite recently, we have succeeded in selective growth of human mast cells/basophils in suspension culture of mononuclear cells from umbilical cord blood (14), in collaboration with Dr. Makio Ogawa in the University of South Carolina. The mononuclear cells of cord blood were cultured in the presence of a fraction of culture supernatant of PHA-stimulated human T cells, which was purchased from Associated Biomedic Systems (Buffalo, New York). When cord blood mononuclear cells were cultured in the presence of the culture supernatant, a significant number of mast cells/basophils were developed in the culture. However, the majority of the cells in the culture were T cells. Thus, we fractionated the culture supernatant following the method described by Yung and co-workers (15) for the purification of growth factors for mouse mast cells. The mononuclear cells of cord blood were then cultured in the presence of a fraction of culture supernatant of PHA-stimulated human T cells from which interleukin-2 was eliminated, and the cells developed in the culture were examined.

After 2 to 4 weeks, 50–90% of the nonadherent cells in the culture contained metachromatic granules characteristic for mast cells and basophils. We were not able to conclude from examination under a light microscope whether these cultured cells were mast cells or basophils. Some cells had an oval nucleus with a dispersed chromatin pattern, which is attributed to mast cells, while many others had a segmented nucleus and dense heterochromatin (14). However, preliminary studies by electron microscopy carried out by Dr. Ann Dvorak revealed that the majority of the cultured cells showed ultrastructural features characteristic for human basophils. Based on this information, these cells are tentatively named cultured human basophils in this chapter. In mouse mast cells, Razin *et al.* (16,17) established the existence of two distinct subclasses of mast cells that differ in the nature of their proteoglycan and in the character of their oxidative products of AA. Thus, the final classification of cultured cells should be decided after the information on the characteristics of AA products and the nature of proteoglycan in the cells is available.

Cultured human basophils are OKT-3$^-$, OKM-1$^-$, and Ia$^-$ cells and bear $1.2–3.8 \times 10^5$ IgE receptors per cell. They contain 0.5–2 μg hista-

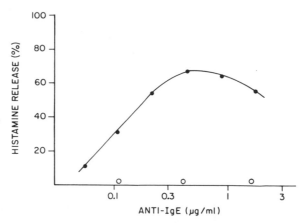

Fig. 3. Anti-IgE-induced histamine release from cultured human basophils. Aliquots of the cells sensitized with human IgE (●) and unsensitized cells (○) were incubated for 15 min at 37°C with various concentrations of anti-IgE. Each point represents mean of duplicate samples. Histamine content in the basophils was 0.96 μg/10^6 cells.

mine per 10^6 cells. As shown in Table I, IgE receptors on cultured basophils bind human IgE with high affinity. The kinetics of association and dissociation between E myeloma protein and receptors on the cultured basophils were determined by the methods described by Kulczycki and Metzger (18). The average forward rate constant k_1 and dissociation constant k_{-1}, calculated from three experiments, were $1.88 \times 10^5 M^{-1}$ sec^{-1} and 6.93×10^{-5} sec^{-1}, respectively. Average equilibrium constant of the binding between IgE and the receptors was $2.75 \times 10^9 M^{-1}$. These values are comparable to those of the binding of rodent IgE to rodent mast cells. The specific binding of human IgE to cultured cells with high affinity confirmed that the cells recovered from the suspension culture are indeed human basophils.

Histamine content in some of the cultured basophils was lower than that in basophils in human peripheral blood. However, cultured basophils sensitized with human IgE released a substantial amount of histamine upon exposure to anti-IgE, while unsensitized cells failed to do so (Fig. 3). Maximal histamine release from 11 different cell preparations was in the range of 22 to 81%. In all of the cell preparations sensitized with IgE, an optimal concentration of anti-IgE for maximal histamine release was 0.45 μg/ml, which was comparable to that of the same anti-IgE preparation to induce maximal histamine release from human peripheral blood basophils and human lung mast cells.

TABLE I
Histamine Content and IgE Receptors on Cultured Basophils

Culture		Basophils[a]				Binding characteristics		
No.	Days	Proportion (%)	Yield per flask ($\times 10^6$)[b]	Histamine per 10^6 cells (μg)	IgE[c] receptor per cell ($\times 10^5$)	$k_1 \times 10^{-5}$ ($M^{-1}\text{sec}^{-1}$)	$k_{-1} \times 10^5$ (sec^{-1})	$K_A \times 10^{-9}$ (M^{-1})
1	23	89	2.3	0.52	3.83	1.47	7.54	1.95
2	26	89	2.8	1.60				
3	29	70	1.2	0.96				
4	26	92	3.2	1.04	2.75	1.84	6.75	2.73
5	29	88	3.8	0.48	2.98	2.32	6.52	3.56
6	27	89	2.8	0.82	2.77			
7	29	74	2.4	0.68	1.20			
8	26	81	2.1	1.97				
Mean					2.71	1.88	6.93	2.75

[a] Metachromatic granules (+) cells by toluidine blue (pH 3.0) staining. From Ishizaka et al. (21).
[b] Six million mononuclear cells from cord blood were plated in each flask.
[c] Determined by direct binding assay using ^{125}I-labeled human IgE. From Kulczycki and Metzger (18).

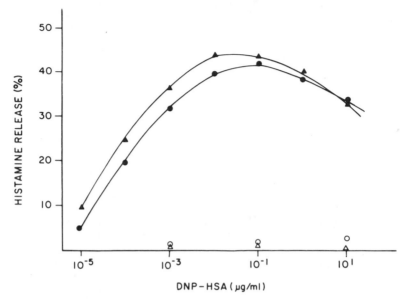

Fig. 4. Sensitization of purified lung mast cells and cultured basophils with monoclonal mouse anti-DNP IgE antibody. Aliquots of the mast cells (●) and the basophils (▲) sensitized with 10 μg/ml mouse anti-DNP IgE antibody, as well as unsensitized mast cells (○) and basophils (△), were challenged with various concentrations of $DNPL_{13}$-HSA for histamine release. Histamine content in the mast cells and cultured basophils was 8.76 and 1.51 μg/10^6 cells, respectively.

As demonstrated with peripheral blood basophils in our previous experiments (19), both human lung mast cells and cultured basophils could be sensitized with mouse IgE. As shown in Fig. 4, cultured basophils sensitized with monoclonal mouse anti-DNP IgE antibody (20) released histamine on challenge with DNP-HSA. The optimal concentration of DNP-HSA for maximal histamine release was 0.01–0.1 μg/ml in all of human mast cells, peripheral blood basophils, and cultured basophils. These results indicate that human basophils obtained in the culture are functionally mature cells.

Thus, we analyzed initial biochemical events involved in IgE-mediated histamine release from cultured basophils. The cells were incubated with 10 μg/ml of human IgE overnight for sensitization and were then challenged with either F(ab')₂ fragments or Fab' fragments of anti-IgE. As shown in Fig. 5, F(ab')₂ fragments of anti-IgE induced a marked enhancement in phospholipid methylation and an increase in cAMP, which were followed by ^{45}Ca uptake and histamine release. The kinetics of these responses were identical to those observed in human lung mast cells. As

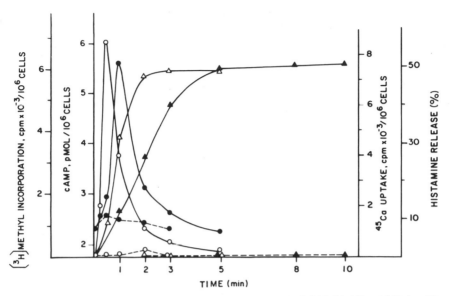

Fig. 5. Kinetics of [³H]methyl incorporation into phospholipid lipids (○), cAMP rise (●), ⁴⁵Ca uptake (△), and histamine release (▲) induced by F(ab′)₂ fragment of anti-IgE. Cultured basophils were incubated overnight with 10 μg/ml E myeloma protein and then challenged with an optimal concentration of F(ab′)₂ fragments (———) or Fab′ monomer (----) of anti-IgE. Purity of the basophils in the preparation was 91%. The cAMP level in the unstimulated cells was 1.54 pmol/10⁶ cells.

expected, the Fab′ fragments of the antibody failed to induce these responses.

Chromatographic analysis of methylated phospholipids in cultured basophils is shown in Table II. Sensitized cultured basophils were incubated with [³H]methyl methionine followed by the challenge with anti-IgE. At 30 sec after the challenge, phospholipids were extracted from the cells and analyzed by thin layer chromatography on Silica G plates. Formation of monomethyl- and dimethylphosphatidylethanolamine and phosphatidylcholine was markedly enhanced after the challenge with anti-IgE. The formation of lysophosphatidylcholine was also detectable at 30 sec after the challenge, indicating that phosphatidylcholine was cleaved by phospholipase A₂. When the cells were preincubated with 3-deazaadenosine and L-homocysteine thiolactone, and then challenged with anti-IgE, incorporation of [³H]methyl groups into the phospholipids was inhibited.

As demonstrated in human lung mast cells, sensitized cultured basophils preincubated with [¹⁴C]AA released [¹⁴C]AA upon challenge with anti-IgE. The kinetics of the [¹⁴C]AA release was identical to that of

TABLE II

Incorporation of [³H]Methyl into Phospholipids after Challenge with Anti-IgE[a]

Pretreatment with	Challenge with	Phospholipids (cpm/10⁶ cells)[b]				
		PE	PME	PDE	PC	LysoPC
None	Anti-IgE	144	10,415	1,466	10,882	990
3-Deaza-ADO[c] + Hcy	Anti-IgE	144	1,838	201	2,806	177
None	None	138	1,474	308	2,512	189

[a] Cultured basophils sensitized with human IgE were challenged with an optimal concentration of anti-IgE (0.45 μg/ml). At 30 sec after the challenge, phospholipids were extracted from the cells and analyzed by thin layer chromatography on Silica G plate. Numerals in the table represent mean values of two separate experiments. Variations between the two experiments (cpm) are 12% of the average.

[b] PE, phosphatidylethanolamine; PME, phosphatidyl-*N*-monomethyl-ethanolamine; PDE, phosphatidyl-*N,N*-dimethylethanolamine; PC, phosphatylcholine; LysoPC, lysophosphatidylcholine.

[c] A portion of the sensitized cells was preincubated with 1 m*M* 3-deaza-ADO and 100 μ*M* L-homocysteine thiolactone (Hcy) at 37°C for 30 min and then challenged with anti-IgE.

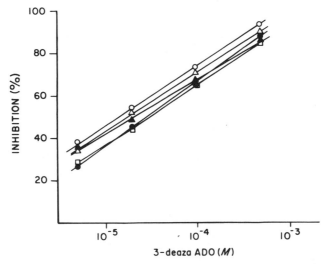

Fig. 6. Inhibition of anti-IgE-induced [³H]methyl incorporation into phospholipids (○), cAMP rise (●), ⁴⁵Ca uptake (△), histamine release (▲), and [¹⁴C]AA (□) release by 3-deaza-ADO and L-homocysteine thiolactone. Cultured basophils sensitized with human IgE were preincubated with various concentrations of 3-deaza-ADO together with 100 μM L-homocysteine thiolactone at 37°C for 30 min, and the cells were challenged with 0.45 μg/ml anti-IgE. [³H]methyl incorporation, cAMP level, ⁴⁵Ca uptake, and histamine, and [¹⁴C]AA release were determined in duplicate at 30 sec, 1 min, 3 min, and 15 min, respectively.

histamine release from the same cells. It was also found that inhibitors of phospholipid methylation, such as 3-deaza-ADO along with L-homocysteine thiolactone, inhibited not only phospholipid methylation but also all of subsequent biochemical events, that is, cAMP rise, ^{45}Ca uptake, and histamine and [^{14}C]AA release in a similar dose–response fashion (Fig. 6). Experiments were then carried out to exclude the possibility that inhibitors of phospholipid methylation might have affected other enzymes involved in mediator release. Because the inhibition of methyltransferases by 3-deazaadenosine must result from accumulation of S-adenosyl-L-homocysteine and its analogs, we examined whether the inhibition of histamine and [^{14}C]AA release by 3-deaza-ADO or 3-deaza-SIBA could be reversed by the addition of S-adenosyl-L-methionine (SAM). Cultured basophils sensitized with mouse monoclonal anti-DNP IgE antibody were preincubated with 3-deaza-SIBA or 3-deaza-ADO together with L-homocysteine thiolactone and then challenged with DNP-HSA in the presence or absence of 5 mM SAM. The results showed that the inhibition of histamine and [^{14}C]AA release by 3-deaza-ADO or 3-deaza-SIBA was reversed by the addition of SAM, indicating that accumulation of S-adenosyl-L-homocysteine was responsible for the inhibition of histamine and arachidonate release. Thus, it appears that phospholipid methylation is essential for the transduction of IgE-mediated triggering signals for mediator release.

SUMMARY

We succeeded in developing human basophils by culture of mononuclear cells of cord blood in the presence of conditioned medium of PHA-stimulated human T cells, from which IL-2 had been eliminated. Approximately 50–90% of cells recovered after 2 to 4 weeks culture were basophil granulocytes that bear receptors with high affinity for human IgE. Sensitization of the cells with human IgE followed by challenge with anti-IgE resulted in the release of histamine and arachidonic acid.

In both the cultured basophils and human lung mast cells, bridging of cell-bound IgE with anti-IgE induced a transient increase in phospholipid methylation and intracellular cAMP, and these processes were followed by Ca^{2+} uptake and both histamine and arachidonate release.

Evidence was obtained that phospholipid methylation induced by the bridging of IgE receptors is involved in subsequent increase in cAMP and is an essential step for transduction of triggering signals for mediator release.

ACKNOWLEDGMENTS

I would like to express my gratitude to Drs. K. Ishizaka, D. H. Conrad, E. S. Schulman, and M. Iwata, the Johns Hopkins University School of Medicine; Dr. Makio Ogawa, the VA Medical Center, Medical University of South Carolina; and Dr. Ann M. Dvorak, Beth Israel Hospital and Harvard Medical School, for their collaboration; and to Mr. A. R. Sterk and Mrs. Chiew G. L. Ko for their excellent technical assistance. I would also like to express my special appreciation to Drs. J. F. Burdick, J. R. Niebyl, and G. P. Marquette, The Johns Hopkins University, for supplying us with human lung tissues and umbilical cord blood on a regular basis. Their persistent efforts made it possible for me to carry on this series of studies.

REFERENCES

1. Ishizaka, K., Tomioka, H., and Ishizaka, T. Mechanisms of passive sensitization. I. Presence of IgE and IgG molecules on human leukocytes. *J. Immunol.* **105:**1459–1467, 1970.
2. Ishizaka, T., Ishizaka, K., and Tomioka, H. Release of histamine and slow reacting substance of anaphylaxis (SRS-A) by IgE–anti-IgE reaction on monkey mast cells. *J. Immunol.* **108:**513–520, 1972.
3. Austen, K. F., Wasserman, S. I., and Goetzl, E. J. Mast cell-derived mediators: Structural and functional diversity and regulation of expression. *In* "Molecular and Biological Aspects of the Acute Allergic Reactions" (S. G. O. Johansson, K. Strandberg, and B. Uvnas, eds.), pp. 293–318. Plenum, New York, 1976.
4. Ishizaka, T., Foreman, J. C., Sterk, A. R., and Ishizaka, K. Induction of calcium flux across the rat mast cell membrane by bridging IgE receptors. *Proc. Natl. Acad. Sci. U.S.A.* **76:**5858–5862, 1979.
5. Ishizaka, T., Hirata, F. Ishizaka, K., and Axelrod, J. Stimulation of phospholipid methylation, Ca^{2+} influx and histamine release by bridging of IgE receptors on rat mast cells. *Proc. Natl. Acad. Sci. U.S.A.* **77:**1903–1906, 1980.
6. Ishizaka, T., Hirata, F., Sterk, A. R., Ishizaka, K., and Axelrod, J. Bridging of IgE receptors activates phospholipid methylation and adenylate cyclase in mast cell plasma membranes. *Proc. Natl. Acad. Sci. U.S.A.* **78:**6812–6816, 1981.
7. Ishizaka, T. Analysis of triggering events in mast cells for immunoglobulin E-mediated histamine release. *J. Allergy Clin. Immunol.* **67:**90–96, 1981.
8. Gould, K. G., Clements, J. A., Jones, A. L., and Fells, F. M. Dispersal of rabbit lung into individual viable cells: A new method for the study of lung metabolism. *Science* **178:**1209–1211, 1972.
9. Lewis, R. A., Wasserman, S. I., Goetzl, E. J., and Austen, K. F. Formation of slow-reacting substance of anaphylaxis in human lung tissue and cells before release. *J. Exp. Med.* **140:**1133–1146, 1974.
10. Schulman, E. S., MacGlashan, D. W., Peters, S. P., Schleimer, R. P., Newball, H. H., and Lichtenstein, L. M. Human lung mast cells, purification and characterization. *J. Immunol.* **129:**2662–2667, 1982.
11. Ishizaka, T., Conrad, D. H., Schulman, E. S., Sterk, A. R., and Ishizaka, K. Biochemical analysis of initial triggering events of IgE-mediated histamine release from human lung mast cells. *J. Immunol.* (in press).

12. Hirata, F., Viveros, O. H., Diliberto, E. J., Jr., and Axelrod, J. Identification and properties of two methyltransferases in conversion of phosphatidylethanolamine to phosphatidylcholine. *Proc. Natl. Acad. Sci. U.S.A.* **75:**1718–1721, 1978.
13. Lewis, R. A., Holgate, S. T., Roberts, J. J., II, Maguire, J. F., Oates, J. A., and Austen K. F. Effects of indomethacine on cyclic nucleotide levels and histamine release from rat serosal mast cells. *J. Immunol.* **123:**1663–1668, 1979.
14. Ogawa, M., Nakahata, T., Leary, A. G., Sterk, A. R., Ishizaka, K., and Ishizaka, T. Suspension culture of human mast cells/basophils from umbilical cord blood mononuclear cells. *Proc. Natl. Acad. Sci. U.S.A.* (in press).
15. Yung, Y. P., Eger, R., Tertian, G., and Moore, M. A. S. Long-term *in vitro* culture of murine mast cells. II. Purification of a mast cell growth factor and its dissociation from TCGF. *J. Immunol.* **127:**794–799, 1981.
16. Razin, E., Stevens, R. I., Akiyama, F., Schmid, K., and Austen, K. F. Culture from mouse bone marrow of a subclass of mast cells possessing a distinct chondroitin sulfate proteoglycan with glycosaminoglycan rich in *N*-acetylgalactosamine-4,6-disulfate. *J. Biol. Chem.* **257:**7229–7235, 1982.
17. Razin, E., Mencia-Huerta, J. M., Stevens, R. L., Lewis, R. A., Liu, F. T., Corey, E. J., and Austen, K. F. IgE-mediated release of leukotriene C_4, chondroitin sulfate E proteoglycan, β-hexosaminidase and histamine from cultured bone marrow-derived mouse mast cells. *J. Exp. Med.* **157:**189–201, 1983.
18. Kulczycki, A., Jr., and Metzger, H. The interaction of IgE with rat basophilic leukemia cells. II. Quantitative aspects of the binding reaction. *J. Exp. Med.* **140:**1676–1695, 1974.
19. Conrad, D. H., Wingard, J. R., and Ishizaka, T. The interaction of human and rodent IgE with the human basophils. *J. Immunol.* **130:**327–333, 1983.
20. Liu, F. T., Bohn, J. W., Ferry, E. L., Yamamoto, H., Molinar, C. A., Sherman, L. A., Klinman, N. R., and Katz, D. H. Monoclonal dinitrophenyl specific murine IgE antibody. Preparation, isolation and characterization. *J. Immunol.* **124:**2728–2737, 1980.
21. Ishizaka, T., Soto, C. S., and Ishizaka, K. Mechanisms of passive sensitization III. Number of IgE molecules and their receptor sites on human basophil granulocytes. *J. Immunol.* **111:**500–511, 1973.

DISCUSSION

Holgate: Dr. Lichtenstein has reported that activation of highly purified human lung mast cells with anti-human IgE for mediator release is not associated with an early rise in cyclic AMP. Have you any explanation for the differences between your and Dr. Lichtenstein's findings?

Ishizaka: I would like to take this opportunity to explain in some detail the discrepancy between the results of Dr. Lichtenstein's group and my own findings on early changes in cAMP in human lung mast cells. First of all, we have run parallel experiments using the same purified human lung mast cells. The cells released over 83% of histamine upon challenge with an optimal concentration of anti-IgE, while normal rabbit serum of the same concentration induced only 4.5% histamine release. We both assayed time-dependent levels of cAMP on the same day. In my hands, at 1 min after challenge of mast cells with an optimal concentration of anti-IgE, there was a marked increase in intracellular cAMP, as compared to normal rabbit serum control. No cAMP rise by anti-IgE was detected by their assay. Response to PGE_2 was detected by both groups. However, the cAMP increase detected by our assay was approximately twofold higher than that obtained in their assay. Using the same method, they were also unable to detect a cAMP rise induced by anti-IgE in rat mast cells. We have confirmed the occurrence of the cAMP rise in human lung mast cells using several different anti-IgE preparations (both goat anti-IgE and rabbit anti-IgE). Thus it appears that the discrepancy is due to a methodologic problem in their assay system.

In their previous publication (L. M. Lichtenstein, A. K. Sobotka, H. J. Malveaux, and E. Gillespie, *Int. Arch. Allergy Appl. Immunol.* **56:**473, 1978), they reported an early rise in cAMP in basophils of a patient with chronic myelogenous leukemia upon stimulation with anti-IgE, and the kinetics of the rise they observed is similar to that observed in human lung mast cells and in cultured human basophils in our present experiments. The method used in their previous experiments was established by Dr. Elizabeth Gillespie and was different from their present assay. The sensitivity of her assay was confirmed to be comparable to that of ours. If they had used her original method, I wonder if they might have been able to detect an increase in cAMP by anti-IgE in both rat and human mast cells.

Thus, although IgE-mediated increase in cAMP in mast cells cannot be detected in their assay conditions, this does not necessarily mean that no cAMP change occurred, and this should not lead to the conclusion that cAMP changes are unrelated to the mechanisms of mediator release.

Lichtenstein: When I state our cAMP results I am not offering an opinion but citing our data. Of course I believe Teri's data. However, in a dozen experiments anti-IgE caused histamine release but did not induce a change in cAMP, while in the same cells an agonist caused a clear cut increase. It is not clear to me how a technical problem could lead to that result. I would certainly like to resolve the issue.

Schleimer: It is not yet clear what is responsible for the differences between our results and those of Dr. Ishizaka. We have validated our cAMP assay according to the methods described by Harper and Brooker (G. Brooker, J. F. Harper, W. L. Terasaki, and R. D. Moylan, *Adv. Cyclic Nucleotide Res.* **10:**1, 1979), and indeed the purified mast cells respond to the β-agonist fenoterol, and PGE_2 with elevations of cAMP up to three- or fourfold. In the single cAMP experiment which we have undertaken in parallel with Dr. Ishizaka, the following results were obtained:

	Picomoles cAMP/10^6 mast cells	
	Ishizaka	Schleimer
Anti-IgE ($\times 2000$)		
0 min	1.05	3.00
1 min	13.15	3.74
Normal rabbit serum ($\times 2000$)		
0 min	1.14	3.00
1 min	2.49	10.60
PGE_2 ($5 \times 10^{-5}\ M$)		
3 min	5.00	7.57

Neither laboratory was able to collect meaningful results when samples were exchanged and run in the other's assay. The buffer system that we have used (PIPES-buffered saline) differs from the HEPES/MES phosphatidylserine buffer that Dr. Ishizaka has used. The assay that we use (acetylation of samples prior to assay) cannot be used when phosphatidylserine is present in the buffer. Furthermore, the dose–response sensitivity of the mast cells to histamine release by anti-IgE differed in ours and Dr. Ishizaka's laboratories. Studies carried out by Dr. MacGlashan and others in our division have shown that ~30 times more of the goat anti-human IgE and the rabbit anti-human PS myeloma preparations are required to produce optimal release in the mast cell as compared to the basophil, while this shift in potency was not observed in Dr. Ishizaka's studies. It is our hope that the source of these divergent results will soon be clear.

Ishizaka: I would imagine that your observation may be the result of the anti-IgE preparation used in your experiments, rather than differences in human lung mast cells and basophils. I used four anti-IgE preparations for histamine release, one monospecific goat anti-IgE, one monospecific and one specifically purified rabbit anti-IgE, and a F(ab)$_2$ of rabbit anti-IgE. All anti-IgEs showed a broad optimal concentration range for maximum histamine release and the optimal concentration range was comparable for all of the human lung mast cell preparations, human peripheral blood basophils, and cultured human basophils.

Austen: In order to establish the IgE-Fc-initiated transmembrane activation of adenylate cyclase, we showed the resultant activation of cytoplasmic cAMP-dependent protein kinase in rat mast cells.

Gleich: I have two questions. First, are you describing a cell line or are these cells short lived? Second, do you see eosinophils along with basophils? The latter comment stems from observations that eosinophils and basophils may differentiate from a common precursor cell, as suggested by the findings of Denburg and his associates (J. A. Denburg, M. Richardson, S. Telizyo, G. J. Gleich, P. Dor, and J. Bienenstock, *Clin. Res.* **31:**163A, 1983), as well as our own findings that eosinophils and basophils share common molecules, for example, the Charcot–Leyden crystal protein (S. J. Ackerman, G. J. Weil, and G. J. Gleich, *J. Exp. Med.* **155:**1597, 1982) as well as the eosinophil granule major basic protein (S. J. Ackerman, G. M. Kephart, T. M. Habermann, P. R. Greipp, and G. J. Gleich, *J. Exp. Med.* **157:**1981, 1983).

Ishizaka: The major contaminant in the basophil culture is eosinophils. If human mast cell growth factors are similar to growth factors for mouse mast cells, our fractionated conditioned medium (10 mM phosphate buffer fraction) may contain granulocyte colony-stimulating factors as well as other cell colony-stimulating factors (Y. P. Yung, R. Eger, G. Tertian, and M. A. S. Moore, *J. Immunol.* **127:**794, 1981; I. Clark-Lewis and J. W. Schrader, *ibid.* p. 1941), in addition to mast cell growth factors, which may account for eosinophil growth in some cultures.

Schwartz: The kinetics of IgE-mediated histamine release from cultured basophils is similar to the release kinetics of pulmonary mast cells, not to peripheral blood basophils.

What are the morphologic features that define the cells cultured from umbilical cord as basophils rather than fetal or developing connective tissue mast cells or to the putative mucosal human mast cell equivalent that has been defined in rodent tissue?

Ishizaka: The cultured cells are now tentatively called cultured human basophils based on their ultrastructural features described by Dr. Ann Dvorak. Many of the cultured cells have a segmented nucleus and dense heterochromatin which is attributed to basophils.

Schiffmann: Does S-adenosyl-L-methionine (SAM) enter the cell or the cell membrane? If it does not, the mechanism of its effect on reversing the effect of deazaadenosine may be different from simply changing the ratio of SAM to S-adenosyl-L-homocysteine.

Ishizaka: We have not tested that possibility. It is a good suggestion and we shall test it in the near future.

Nadel: Will you describe the culture system? How much cord blood is used? How many basophils are derived per ml of cord blood? Over the 6-week period of culture, does cell function change?

Ishizaka: The yield of basophils in the culture is 20–60%. If 6×10^6 mononuclear cells of cord blood were plated per flask, 2 to 4×10^6 basophils can be recovered from nonadherent cells in the flask after 3–4 weeks culture. After 4 weeks culture, the histamine content in the cells does not increase and cells reach a mature state. As purity of the basophils reaches the highest value between 3 and 4 weeks, we usually use the cells for our experiments after 3 weeks culture.

Gleich: Have you identified conditions that direct the umbilical cord cells to differentiate into basophils? Have you tested interleukin 3, for example?

Ishizaka: Since no purified human IL-3 is available, we have not tested for it in our culture. However, mononuclear cells of cord blood cultured in the presence of the culture supernatant of a human T-cell hybridoma, maintained in Dr. C. S. Henney's lab, differentiated into basophils. Since the culture supernatant contains neither IL-1 nor IL-2, there is the possibility that growth factor(s) for human basophils (IL-3) may be characterized from the culture supernatant.

Austen: Homogenous interleukin 3 is available from mouse helper T cells, but has not yet been purified to homogeneity from human T-cell clones.

CHAPTER 4

The Release of Mediators of the Human Mast Cell: Investigations in Mastocytosis*

JOHN A. OATES, BRIAN J. SWEETMAN, and *L. JACKSON ROBERTS II*

Departments of Medicine and Pharmacology
Vanderbilt University
School of Medicine
Nashville, Tennessee, U.S.A.

The clinical syndrome of systemic mastocytosis has been investigated to better elucidate the mediators released from the superabundant mast cells, to examine their contributions to the clinical manifestations of the disease, and to assess the regulation of mediator release. Mastocytosis is characterized by an excessive proliferation of tissue mast cells that usually involves multiple organs in the body. As a consequence of the release of mediators from the mast cells, these patients may have a number of clinical manifestations including flushing, light-headedness, syncope, palpitations and tachycardia, dypsnea without wheezing, diarrhea and abdominal cramping, urticaria, and pruritis. Studies in mastocytosis have contributed substantially to the concept that prostaglandin D_2 is a major mediator of the human mastocyte.

In the rat serosal mast cell, prostaglandin D_2 (PGD_2) was found to be the principal cyclooxygenase metabolite of arachidonic acid, as determined by quantification of the prostaglandins and thromboxane B_2 with stable isotope dilution methods and further identification of the PGD_2 released by gas chromatography–mass spectrometry in a collaborative investigation with R. A. Lewis and K. F. Austen (1). The predominant production of PGD_2 by the mast cell was also demonstrated by studies in which radiolabeled arachidonic acid was added as a precursor. Activation of the rat serosal mast cells with either calcium ionophore (A23187) or

* This work was supported in part by NIH Grant GM #1543.

ASTHMA: Physiology,
Immunopharmacology,
and Treatment
THIRD INTERNATIONAL SYMPOSIUM

55

immunologically with anti-rat IgE or anti-rat $F(ab')_2$ causes release of PGD_2 in conjunction with histamine (2,3).

The first evidence that human mastocytosis produced PGD_2 was derived as a result of the observation that treatment with a combination of H_1- and H_2-histamine antagonists did not prevent the cardiovascular manifestations exhibited by patients with severe mastocytosis. This led to exploration of the possibility that these episodes, which previously had been termed "histamine shock," might be caused by some other mediator than histamine. This search was greatly aided by the previous elucidation of the metabolic fate of PGD_2 in the monkey (4). In the monkey, PGD_2 was found to be metabolized into a series of metabolites, the major proportion of which had a prostaglandin F-ring structure. Metabolites with both D- and F-ring structure had undergone metabolism by β-oxidation, 15-hydroxy-dehydrogenation, 13,14 reduction, and ω-oxidation singly or in combination. The biotransformation of PGD_2 to metabolites of $PGF_{2\alpha}$ is of importance in considering the interpretation of increased levels of $PGF_{2\alpha}$ metabolites in conditions such as asthma.

In the search for an additional mediator of the episodes of flushing and syncope in mastocytosis, the possibility that this might be a prostaglandin was examined. During the course of that investigation, an unknown compound was detected, which was found to have the structure of one of the urinary metabolites of PGD_2 that we previously had identified from the monkey. The structure of this compound was elucidated by analysis of the complete mass spectrum of the methyl ester, *O*-methyloxime, trimethylsilyl ether derivative. The spectrum proved to be identical with that previously determined for the PGD_2 metabolite 9α-hydroxy-11,15-dioxo-2,3,4,5-tetranorprostane-1,20-dioic acid (5). The large amount of this metabolite relative to that found in normal urine indicated marked overproduction of PGD_2 in mastocytosis. Subsequently, we have identified excessive quantities of 14 metabolites of PGD_2, including many with the F-ring structure, in the urine of patients with severe mastocytosis.

The production of PGD_2 by concentrated human lung tissue mast cells was then examined (2,3). It was found that PGD_2 was the overwhelmingly predominant cyclooxygenase product from these cells. Activation of the mast cell-enriched human pulmonary cells with anti-IgE led to release of PGD_2 in proportion to the extent of histamine release. Thus, evidence that PGD_2 is a mediator of human mast cells was derived both from the human pulmonary mast cell and from *in vivo* overproduction of PGD_2 in patients with mastocytosis.

In order to quantify the release of PGD_2 in mastocytosis, a method was developed for measuring the PGD_2 urinary metabolite 9α-hydroxy-11,15-dioxo-2,3,18,19-tetranorprost-5-ene-1,20-dioic acid (PGD-M) employing gas chromatography–mass spectrometry in the selected ion monitoring mode (6). The urinary excretion of PGD-M in normal individuals is 247 ± 150 ng/24 hr (mean ± 2 SD). Levels of this metabolite were measured in 18 patients with mastocytosis characterized by severe symptoms, including syncope, increased dermal proliferation of mast cells with 10 or more mast cells per high power field on skin biopsy, and increased urinary excretion of histamine to levels greater than 40 μg/24 hr (7). Thirteen of these patients had levels of PGD-M that were substantially elevated. In some patients with severe disease, the level of PGD-M was increased up to 150-fold above the normal range. It is of note that these measurements were made when the patients were not experiencing acute attacks.

Evidence for the release of PGD_2 during attacks of flushing was obtained by measuring the concentration of the metabolite in the urine collected during the first 4 hr after an attack. Increases of PGD-M excretion in the postattack urine of 9- and 80-fold were observed. These findings are interpreted as reflecting an increase in PGD_2 release in conjunction with the clinical attacks.

Based on the evidence for PGD_2 overproduction in patients with mastocytosis that is further increased during the flushing episodes, the effect of inhibiting the prostaglandin cyclooxygenase was evaluated in a group of patients with severe symptoms and recurrent episodes of syncope (7). Seven of eight patients treated with a combination of chlorpheniramine (32–48 mg/day) and cimetidine (1200 mg/day) continued to experience recurrent episodes of syncope in conjunction with severe symptoms associated with nonsyncopal attacks of flushing. In 13 patients it was possible to add treatment with high doses of aspirin to the combination of antihistamines. In 12 of these 13 there has been no recurrence of syncope, and their symptoms have been largely ameliorated. Aspirin was given in doses of 3.9 to 5.2 g/day with adjustment of the dose to achieve a plasma salicylate level between 20 and 30 mg/dl. Thus, in these patients the inhibition of PGD_2 biosynthesis was associated with alleviation of the episodes of syncope and attendant severe symptoms.

In a small subset of patients with mastocytosis (±5%), attacks are triggered by aspirin and other inhibitors of the fatty acid cyclooxygenase. In contrast to the therapeutic efficacy of administering aspirin in doses sufficient to inhibit PGD_2 biosynthesis in the usual patient with mastocytosis, the syndrome of aspirin-evoked mastocytosis (AEM) presents an apparent paradox and a challenge both clinically and scientifically.

In these susceptible patients, attacks provoked by aspirin and related nonsteroidal antiinflammatory drugs may be severe, resembling anaphylactic shock, and some have been fatal. Accordingly, this possibility requires intense diagnostic consideration, and it is essential that the initiation of aspirin treatment in patients with mastocytosis should be carefully dose ranged, beginning with doses of less than 50 mg, and conducted in a setting where emergency care is at hand.

The syndrome of AEM is a scientific puzzle in its own right, enhanced by the analogy to aspirin-evoked asthma. In aspirin-evoked asthma, removal of a prostaglandin bronchodilator has been proposed as a possible mechanism (8), but this could hardly be the explanation for AEM. Rather we considered that blockade of the cyclooxygenase is probably initiating an event that leads to mast cell activation. This concept would be consistent with the data demonstrating an increase in histamine levels in patients with aspirin-evoked asthma (9). Accordingly, we examined the possibility that the administration of aspirin led to mast cell activation in patients with AEM.

Evidence for mast cell activation was sought by measuring urinary histamine mass spectrometrically, employing negative ion chemical ionization. Two patients have been studied to date. In one, an attack of flushing, urticaria, and dyspnea was provoked by the administration of 150 mg of aspirin. This was associated with a more than threefold increase in the excretion of histamine during the attack. In a second patient, flushing, tachycardia, dyspnea, and bronchorrhea were provoked by the repeated administration of aspirin in doses of 10 to 20 mg given with the objective of producing tolerance to aspirin. This provoked a more protracted attack that was associated with an approximately fivefold increase in histamine excretion. Of note is that the doses of aspirin required to evoke these attacks are substantially less than those needed to effectively treat the usual patient with mastocytosis. The evidence from these two patients strongly supports the concept that inhibition of the fatty acid cyclooxygenase triggers mast cell activation.

Consideration of the mechanism of mast cell activation by cyclooxygenase inhibition should address two general possibilities: the critical site of cyclooxygenase inhibition leading to mast cell activation could take place within the mast cell itself, or it could occur within a different cell that participates in regulating mast cell mediator release. Inhibition of cyclooxygenase within the mast cell would lead to a decrease in PGD_2 biosynthesis and also reduce arachidonic acid disposition by the cyclooxygenase pathway, thus making the substrate available for biotransformation to other products that could influence mast cell function. Whereas other prostaglandins are capable of inhibiting mast cell activation, PGD_2 is at best a weak inhibitor in the rat serosal mast cell (10), and inhibition of its biosynthesis would not seem likely to evoke mediator release. To address more directly the possibility that inhibiting the cyclooxygenase within the human mast cell might be the critical event in mast cell activation in AEM, we have assessed the biosynthesis of PGD_2 during attacks provoked by aspirin.

In a patient with severe AEM and a 65-fold increase in PGD_2 production in the basal state, the effect of aspirin on PGD_2 metabolite excretion was assessed in two studies (11). In the first, a single dose of 40 mg of aspirin was found to evoke flushing and tachycardia after 2 hr. This led to an increase in the excretion of PGD-M from 11,564 ± 1,564 ng/g creatinine to a peak level of 20,973 ng/g 4 hr after the administration of aspirin. In a second study, repeated doses of 10 mg of aspirin over a 4-day period evoked multiple episodes of flushing and tachycardia, accompanied by a marked sustained increase in the urinary excretion of PGD-M to a peak of 29,499 ng/g creatinine on the fourth day. This occurred in conjunction with the increase in histamine excretion discussed above. These data indicate that the very small doses of aspirin required to evoke mast cell mediator release did not inhibit biosynthesis of PGD_2; rather, mast cell activation under these circumstances was associated with increased release of prostaglandin D_2. In addition, aspirin administration was continued in this patient in conjunction with the use of epinephrine infusion to attenuate the attacks, and when the aspirin dosage was increased to the higher doses sufficient to inhibit prostaglandin D_2 biosynthesis, the patient's spontaneous attacks of flushing, dyspnea, tachycardia, and hypotension were completely inhibited. Thus, all of the evidence obtained in the study of this patient indicates that the low doses of aspirin that trigger mast cell activation do not do so by inhibiting the cyclooxygenase within the mast cell itself. These findings strongly suggest that the critical site of cyclooxygenase inhibition that results in mast cell activation must be in a cell other than the mast cell that is exerting major control over the process that engenders mast cell activation.

REFERENCES

1. Roberts, L. J., Lewis, R. A., Oates, J. A., and Austen, K. F. Prostaglandins, thromboxane and 12-hydroxy-5,8,11,14-eicosatetraenoic acid production by ionophore-stimulated rat serosal mast cells. *Biochim. Biophys. Acta* **575**:185–192, 1979.
2. Lewis, R. A., Soter, N. A., Diamond, P. T., Austen, K. F., Oates, J. A., and Roberts, L. J., II Prostaglandin D_2 generation after activation of rat and human mast cells with anti-IgE. *J. Immunol.* **129**(4):1627–1631, 1982.
3. Lewis, R. A., Holgate, S. T., Roberts, L. J., Oates, J. A., and Austen, K. F. Preferential generation of prostaglandin D_2 by rat and human mast cells. *Kroc Found. Ser.* **14**:239–254, 1981.
4. Ellis, C. K., Smigel, M. D., Oates, J. A., Oelz, O., and Sweetman, B. J. Metabolism of prostaglandin D_2 in the monkey. *J. Biol. Chem.* **254**:4152–4163, 1979.

5. Roberts, L. J., II, Sweetman, B. J., Lewis, R. A., Austen, K. F., and Oates, J. A. Increased production of prostaglandin D_2 in patients with systemic mastocytosis. *N. Engl. J. Med.* **303**(24):f1400–1414, 1980.

6. Roberts, L. J., II Quantification of the PGD_2 urinary metabolite 9α-hydroxy-11,15-dioxo-2,3,18,19-tetranorprost-5-ene-1,20-dioic acid by stable isotope dilution–mass spectrometric assay. *In* "Methods in Enzymology" 86, p. 559. Academic Press, New York, 1982.

7. Roberts, L. J., Fields, J. P., and Oates, J. A. Mastocytosis without urticaria pigmentosa: A frequently unrecognized cause of recurrent syncope. *Trans. Assoc. Am. Physicians* **95**:36, 1982.

8. Szceklik, A., Gryglewski, R. J., and Czernawoska-Mysik, G. Clinical patterns of hypersensitivity to non-steroidal anti-inflammatory drugs and their pathogenesis. *J. Allergy Clin. Immunol.* **60**:264–284, 1977.

9. Szmit, M., Grzelewska-Rzymowska, I., Rozniecki, J., Kowalski, M. L., and Rychlika, I. Histaminemia after aspirin challenge in aspirin sensitive asthmatics. *Agents Actions* **11**:105–107, 1981.

10. Holgate, S. T., Lewis, R. A., MacGuire, J. F., Roberts, L. J., II, Oates, J. A., and Austen, K. F. Effects of prostaglandin D_2 on rat serosal mast cells. *J. Immunol.* **125**:1367–1373, 1980.

11. Roberts, L. J., II, and Oates, J. A. Evidence against a role of mast cell cyclooxygenase inhibition in aspirin hypersensitivity reactions. *Clin. Res.* **31**:165A, 1983.

DISCUSSION

Austen: What do you feel is the mechanism of aspirin activation?

Oates: Our data serve to place the critical inhibition of cyclooxygenase at some site outside the mast cell but do not define that site. It could be removal of an activation inhibitor such as PGE_2, or it could be removal of the endothelial prostaglandins that inhibit ingress of cells that have the capacity to activate mastocytes.

Gleich: Concerning the putative accessory cells needed to produce the syndrome of vasodepression, it would seem reasonable to implicate those cells in proximity to the mast cells. Therefore we need to know what cells are in the vicinity of the mast cells?

Kaliner: In collaborative investigations presented at the March 1983 American Academy of Allergy meetings and published in abstract form (R. Simon, W. Pleskow, M. Kaliner, S. Wasserman, J. Curd, and D. Stevenson, *J. Allergy Clin. Immunol.* **71**:146, 1983), we reported on plasma histamine, plasma neutrophil chemotactic activity, and urinary histamine levels in more than 20 ASA-sensitive asthmatics. In these subjects, followed serially after positive provocation, there was no detectable mediator release. Concurrently, we examined plasma histamines after bronchial antigen inhalation challenge (P. Atkins, B. Zweiman, J. Dyers, P. M. Bédard, and M. Kaliner, *J. Allergy Clin. Immunol.* **71**:151, 1983) and easily measured histamine release. Therefore, based upon these data, we have no evidence for mast cell mediator release in ASA-asthma. I would therefore stress caution in extrapolating your ASA-sensitive mastocytosis observations to the ASA-sensitive asthma subjects.

Oates: I would agree that the similarity is in the biochemical mechanism of activation, and clearly the ultimate reactions are different.

Austen: Patients with syncope and systemic mastocytosis have biopsy proven increased mast cells in various organs such as the liver.

Kaliner: We are also following a large population of mastocytosis patients and do not see spontaneous syncope in any. By contrast, we followed a population of subjects experiencing recurring idiopathic anaphylaxis (E. Bacal, R. Patterson, and C. R. Reiss, *Clin. Allergy* **8**:295, 1978; P. Lieberman and W. W. Taylor, *Arch. Intern. Med.* **139**:1032, 1979) who have the following characteristics: most are female; many are atopic; the syndromes experienced include flushing, syncope, asthma, abdominal distress, hypotension, and bronchomotor reactions. These subjects do not have urticaria pigmentosa and may have normal urine histamine (and plasma histamine) levels between attacks with elevations concurrent with attacks (G. Myers, M. Donlon, and M. Kaliner, *J. Allergy Clin. Immunol.* **67**:305, 1981). These subjects are distinct from the systemic mastocytosis patients in our experience, and I therefore wonder if your syncope group is a relatively distinct subgroup of your mastocytosis subjects that most closely resembles the idiopathic anaphylaxis category?

Oates: First, we have seen syncope in patients with the type of mastocytosis that is associated with urticaria pigmentosa. Second, many of our patients without visible skin lesions do have characteristics of the group called "idiopathic anaphylaxis"; some of these have increased histamine and/or PGD_2 metabolites between attacks whereas others do not. Importantly, the haemodynamic, respiratory, and intestinal manifestations seen in these patients can be markedly ameliorated by administration of aspirin in doses sufficient to inhibit PGD_2 biosynthesis. I would suggest that many of the groups of patients previously called idiopathic anaphylaxis have a form of mastocytosis, but I do not think the data base that currently exists will permit accurate subclassification of the broad categories of mastocytosis. Certainly, further evaluation of the histopathology and the biochemical markers should be expected to yield a sound basis for dividing mastocytosis into a number of subcategories, and I strongly concur with your overall suggestion that such subsets do exist.

Lessof: It is tempting to look for a common explanation for aspirin-sensitive reactions in mastocytosis and in other conditions, such as aspirin-evoked urticaria, as studied by Asad *et al.* (S. I. Asad, L. J. F. Youlten, and M. H. Lessof, *Clin. Allergy* **13**:459, 1983). In aspirin-evoked urticaria, before challenge venous levels of $PGF_{2\alpha}$ are about three times normal. Perhaps this is influenced by PGD_2 metabolism, but venous E_2 levels are normal. Are we dealing with "trigger-happy" mast cells in each case?

There is also an association between aspirin-evoked urticaria (or asthma) and sensitivity reactions to one or more foods. It would be interesting to know whether this is seen in mastocytosis. It seems, incidentally, that if you give increasing doses of aspirin to patients with aspirin-evoked urticaria, they may become tolerant not only to aspirin but also to the foods that previously caused reactions.

Turner-Warwick: From this discussion it would appear that none of these subgroups of patients with mastocytosis have obvious asthma. Is this correct?

Oates: Wheezing detectable by auscultation is rare and was found in only two of our patients, both of whom have the aspirin-evoked type of mastocytosis. However, dyspnea is a common concomitant of the attacks of many patients, and we do not yet know whether small airway constriction is responsible.

Morley: You have used high-dose aspirin for therapy, and it is debatable whether effects at this dose can be specifically attributed to cyclooxygenase inhibition. Do you have efficacy with an equivalent dose of sodium salicylate, which lacks significant cycloxygenase inhibition, or with a low dose (25 mg) of indomethacin, which is a selective inhibitor of cyclooxygenase?

Piper: Is PGD_2 metabolized if it is given into the airways or does this only happen in the circulation? In the respiratory tract, does PGD_2 act as PGD_2 or because it has been converted to $PGF_{2\alpha}$?

Oates: Our metabolism studies examined the fate of PGD_2 given intravenously. Whereas the fate of PGD_2 administered by aerosol into the airways has not been examined, I would think it likely that its effects by this route would be principally those of PGD_2 itself.

Holgate: In reply to Dr. Piper's question, we have given nebulized PGD_2 and $PGF_{2\alpha}$ to normal and mild asthmatic subjects and followed the airway response as specific conductance. PGD_2 was about 30 times as potent as $PGF_{2\alpha}$ in both subject groups and was 500 times more potent in the asthmatic compared to the normal subjects.

Kay: Have you had the opportunity to compare dispersed human mastocytoma cells with normal human mast cells in terms of morphology, different triggers for mediator release, and quantative and qualitative difference in mediators? Also, what are the effect of drugs on these variables?

Oates: Dispersed mast cells from these patients have not been studied.

Schwartz: Tryptase has been detected in human cutaneous mastocytosis and mastocytoma tissues.

Austen: The mast cells in skin of patients with mastocytosis contain tryptase and produce PGD_2 with ionophore.

Bach: It may be worth keeping in mind that mast cells may not be the only source of PGD_2. Specifically, Dr. D. E. Tracey has been able to show that several established lines of murine mononuclear cells produce "exclusively" PGD_2 upon stimulation.

Gleich: Can you be confident that the treatment with antihistamines truly is effective? For example, do the doses used block the activity of histamine in skin? Also, have you tried doxepin, which seems to be considerably more effective as an antihistamine than others such as chlorpheniramine.

Nadel: What do you believe to be the sources of bronchorrhea with aspirin?

Oates: The origin is unknown; it may be copious.

Clark: Does aspirin abolition of cyclooxygenase pathways in patients with mastocytoma lead to changes in lipoxygenase metabolism?

Oates: I do not know of effects of inhibiting biosynthesis of PGD_2 on the 5-lipoxygenase pathway specifically. Of course, inhibition of platelet aggregation by PGD_2 will inhibit 12-HETE formation by the platelets.

CHAPTER 5

Mast Cell–Dependent Synthesis of Lipid Mediators of Immediate Hypersensitivity*

ROBERT A. LEWIS, JEAN-MICHEL MENCIA-HUERTA, CHONG W. LEE,
and K. FRANK AUSTEN

Department of Medicine
Harvard Medical School
and Department of Rheumatology and Immunology
Brigham and Women's Hospital
Boston, Massachusetts, U.S.A.

MAST CELL FUNCTION AND HETEROGENEITY

In rats, mast cells of the small bowel are histochemically divisible into two subsets: those that contain a type I neutral protease initially termed chymase in their metachromatic granules, stain pink with azure A/safranin, and reside in the deep connective tissue resemble mast cells of the serosal cavities (1–7); and those that contain a separate neutral chymotryptic protease (type II), stain light blue with the same dyes, and are mucosal or intraepithelial in location (2,4,5,7). In formalin-fixed sections, toluidine blue stains the connective tissue mast cells but does not fix to the mucosal mast cells (5). Furthermore, the mucosal or type II neutral protease-containing rat mast cells are under T-cell regulation *in vivo* and

* This work was supported by Grants AI-07722, AI-10356, AI-20081, HL-13262, HL-17382, GM-10374, and RR-05669 from the National Institutes of Health and in part by grants from the Lillia Babbitt Hyde Foundation and the New England Peabody Home for Crippled Children. R. A. L. is the recipient of an Allergic Diseases Academic Award (AI-00399) from the National Institutes of Health. J.-M. M.-H. is a research Fellow of the Institut National de la Santé et de la Recherche Medicale, France, and partly supported by the Ministère de la Recherche et de l'Industrie. C. W. L. is a research Trainee supported by Training Grant AM-07098 from the National Institutes of Health.

ASTHMA: Physiology,
Immunopharmacology,
and Treatment
THIRD INTERNATIONAL SYMPOSIUM

63

also when generated from bone marrow *in vitro* (5). Human small bowel mast cells similarly are divisible into these two categories according to their staining properties in formalin-fixed sections (8). In the mouse, chemical differences have been described for two mast cell populations, a serosal mast cell population (9) which, like that of the rat (10,11), contains heparin proteoglycan, and a T cell-dependent bone marrow-derived mast cell population, which contains proteoglycan chondroitin sulfate E (9,12,13). The finding that the mast cell subtype that can be differentiated from mouse bone marrow *in vitro* when incubated with a T cell-derived lymphokine (14–16) has granules that contain chondroitin sulfate E proteoglycan (9) rather than heparin appears to account for the relatively decreased affinity of these cells for analine blue dyes.

Mast cell heterogeneity in human lung has been demonstrated on the basis of size. When mast cells from enzymatically dispersed lung tissue (17) are fractionated on an elutriator, the quantities of cell-associated histamine and its releasability by IgE-mediated activation increase with cell size (18). Human mast cells dispersed by the same enzymatic process (17) but isolated by gradient methods may well have lost the pool of cells not staining red violet with toluidine blue dye and retained those with heparin as their major granule-associated proteoglycan (19). The major neutral protease of this cell population is a trypsin-like enzyme, termed *tryptase,* which differs from trypsin in its lack of inhibition by aprotinin and by lima bean, soybean, and ovomucoid trypsin inhibitors and in its tetrameric structure (20,21). Tryptase is a tetramer with an apparent molecular weight of 144,000 that is composed of two subunits of 37,000 daltons and two subunits of 35,000 daltons, each of which may have an active site (21). Although this partially characterized human lung mast cell population appears homogeneous with regard to its granule-associated mediators, technologies that could define nonheparin, highly sulfated proteoglycans (e.g., chondroitin sulfate E) or assess the heterogeneity of tryptase distribution have not yet been utilized.

An additional biochemical difference in mast cell subtypes has been recognized by comparing rat serosal heparin proteoglycan-containing mast cells and mouse bone marrow-derived chondroitin sulfate E proteoglycan-containing mast cells for their major metabolites of arachidonic acid, that are generated subsequent to IgE-dependent activation (Table I). Both cell types possess enzymes of the cyclooxygenase pathway, including prostaglandin (PG) H_2-PGD_2 isomerase, as PGD_2 is a product of each after IgE-dependent activation, but only the heparin-containing rat serosal mast cell produces substantial amounts (12,22). Conversely, only the bone marrow-derived murine mast cells contain substantial amounts of the enzymes of the 5-lipoxygenase pathway; when they are activated with

TABLE I
Heterogeneity of Mast Cells by Defined Mediator Content and Generation

Biochemical mediators	Cell sources			
	Rat serosal	Mouse bone marrow-derived	Rat mucosal	Human pulmonary
Histamine content ($\mu g/10^6$ cells)	8–24	0.1–0.45	0.16	1.7
Proteoglycan content ($\mu g/10^6$ cells)				
Heparin	25–50	—[a]	—	4.0
Chondroitin sulfate E	—	2	ND[b]	ND
Neutral protease content ($\mu g/10^6$ cells)				
RCMP I (chymase)	24	ND	—	—
RCMP II	—	ND	+[c]	—
Carboxypeptidase A	~10	ND	ND	—
Tryptase	—	ND	ND	6–19
Arachidonic acid metabolites, immunologically generated ($ng/10^6$ cells)				
LTB$_4$	—	4.5	ND	<4
LTC$_4$	—	23	ND	25
PGD$_2$	13	<0.7	ND	39

[a] —, Undetectable.
[b] ND, not determined.
[c] +, Detected but not quantitated.

A23187 or by IgE-dependent mechanisms, they release substantial quantities of (5S)-hydroxy-(6R)-S-glutathionyl-7,9-$trans$-11,14-cis-eicosatetraenoic acid, leukotriene C$_4$ (LTC$_4$), as well as (5S,12R)-dihydroxy-6,14-cis-8,10-$trans$-eicosatetraenoic acid, leukotriene B$_4$ (LTB$_4$) (12,23,24). The marked difference in the relative expression of the cyclooxygenase and 5-lipoxygenase pathways in the two mast cell subclasses, as assessed by production of PGD$_2$ [the predominant cyclooxygenase product identified from rat serosal mast cells (22)] and of LTC$_4$ [the dominant leukotriene product of the bone marrow-derived mast cells (12,23,24)], yields ratios of LTC$_4$: PGD$_2$ for the murine bone marrow-derived cells of >25 : 1 and, for the serosal rat mast cells, of <1 : 40.

Human mast cells partially purified by gradient methods, or more highly purified by elutriation and an affinity procedure, biosynthesize large quantities of PGD$_2$ after IgE-dependent activation (22,25), averaging a net of 39 ng/10^6 cells in the earlier study (22). Cells purified by the combined elutriation-affinity method generate a wide range of amounts of sulfidopeptide leukotriene/10^6 cells (26), whereas cells obtained by the gradient method yield reduced quantities of leukotriene, measured as SRS-A, relative to the starting dispersed lung preparation (27,28), when compared in terms of SRS-A units per μg histamine. Bronchoalveolar macrophages are now known to have low affinity IgE receptors (29) and to produce substantial quantities of LTB_4 after A23187 ionophore (30,31) and zymosan-dependent activation (30), but only small quantities of LTC_4 (30). The sources of IgE-dependent biosynthesis of LTC_4 in human lung may include the alveolar macrophage or pulmonary interstitial macrophage responding directly or cooperatively to precursor from activated mast cells, as typified by PGI_2 synthesis by endothelial cells in the presence of activated platelets (32). It is more likely, however, that human lung contains a mast cell subclass comparable to that derived by interleukin regulation of a mouse bone marrow precursor.

An additional mediator of immediate hypersensitivity events, platelet-activating factor (PAF), 1-*O*-alkyl-2-acetyl-*sn*-glyceryl-3-phosphorylcholine (33–35), derives from a specific membrane 1-*O*-alkyl-2-acylphospholipid pool most probably following deacylation of arachidonic acid by a phospholipase A_2 and transfer of an acetyl group to the site previously occupied by arachidonic acid (36). The demonstrated activities of PAF include aggregation of washed rabbit and human platelets and the release of their α-granule contents independently of arachidonic acid and ADP (37,38); aggregation (39) and enhancement of random migration (40) of human neutrophils and enhancement of secretion of their specific and azurophilic granules (40,41); and bronchoconstriction, vasoconstriction, and increased permeability when administered intravenously to guinea pig or baboon (42,43). The generation of PAF by IgE-dependent activation of the mouse bone marrow-derived mast cell subclass reveals this cell to be the initial example of a cell generating structurally unrelated lipid mediators in response to a physiologic stimulus (44).

The antigen-activated bone marrow-derived sensitized mouse mast cell is a useful model cell for studying biochemical modulation in the generation of 5-lipoxygenase products, 5-HETE, 6-*trans*-LTB_4 diastereoisomers, LTC_4, and LTB_4, as well as of PAF and the cyclooxygenase product PGD_2, since it generates each of these in measurable quantities, although PGD_2 is clearly a minor product (12,23,24,44). Each biologically active product derived from the 5-lipoxygenase pathway by the actions of a cascade of enzymes may be separately quantitated: 5-HETE by β-scintillation at its R_f on thin layer chromatography or its retention time on HPLC, after prelabeling the phospholipid pool of the generating cells with [^{3}H]- or [^{14}C]arachidonic acid; LTB_4 and LTC_4, LTD_4 and LTE_4 by class-

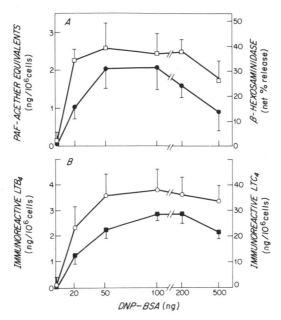

Fig. 1. Antigen-dependent release of β-hexosaminidase ($\square$) and PAF-acether ($\bullet$) in TBSA (A) and of immunoreactive LTC$_4$ ($\blacksquare$) and immunoreactive LTB$_4$ ($\bigcirc$) in TG (B) from sensitized mouse bone marrow-derived mast cells after 10 min at 37°C. Results are expressed as mean ± SD of three experiments.

specific radioimmunoassays (RIAs) after RP-HPLC (45,46); and the non-enzymatic hydrolysis products of LTA$_4$, 5,6-dihydroxy-eicosatetraenoic acids (5,6-diHETEs) and 6-*trans*-LTB$_4$ diastereoisomers by their respective retention times on RP-HPLC and their separate UV absorbances at 280 nm (24). PGD$_2$ is measurable by RIA and PAF by platelet aggregation in the presence of a cyclooxygenase inhibitor and ADP scavengers, with confirmation of its physical properties by retention time on HPLC.

The dose and time dependence of IgE-dependent granule secretion and *de novo* generation of LTB$_4$, LTC$_4$, and PAF from mouse bone marrow-derived mast cells is depicted in Figs. 1 and 2. Bone marrow-derived mast cells, sensitized with IgE-anti-dinitrophenol-BSA (DNP-BSA) and challenged with DNP-BSA over a dose range from 0 to 500 ng, release β-hexosaminidase and generate and release up to 3.8 ± 0.8 ng LTB$_4$, 28.5 ± 2.3 ng LTC$_4$, and 2.1 ± 0.6 ng PAF/10^6 cells (mean ± SD, $n = 3$) with the maximal response for release of each mediator occurring between 50 and 100 ng of antigen (Fig. 1). Antigen challenge activates the cells for maximum release of β-hexosaminidase by 3 min and for maximal generation and release of LTB$_4$, LTC$_4$, and PAF by 4–6 min (Fig. 2).

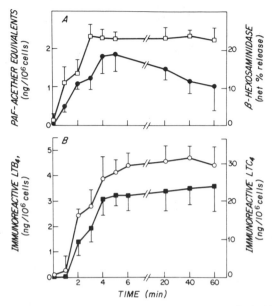

Fig. 2. Release of β-hexosaminidase ($\square$) and PAF-acether ($\bullet$) in TBSA (A) and of immunoreactive LTC$_4$ ($\blacksquare$) and immunoreactive LTB$_4$ ($\bigcirc$) in TG (B) from sensitized mouse bone marrow-derived mast cells after activation with 100 ng DNP-BSA. Results are expressed as mean $\pm$ SD of three experiments.

BIOSYNTHESIS OF PRODUCTS OF THE 5-LIPOXYGENASE PATHWAY

In rat basophilic leukemic cells (RBL-1) (47,48), mouse bone marrow-derived mast cells (12), human and rabbit neutrophils (49,50), and human alveolar macrophages (30,31), there is evidence that the 5-lipoxygenase is the initial enzyme required for the production of noncyclized biologically active compounds from arachidonic acid; thus, the role of the 5-lipoxygenase is analogous to that played by cyclooxygenase in the production of prostaglandins (PG). The 5-lipoxygenase catalyzes the stereospecific addition of molecular oxygen to arachidonic acid to form 5-L-hydroperoxy-6-*trans*-8,11,14-*cis*-eicosatetraenoic acid (5-HPETE), which is converted to 5-L-hydroxy-6-*trans*-8,11,14-*cis*-eicosatetraenoic acid (5-HETE), or alternatively to the unstable intermediate epoxide LTA$_4$ (5,6-*trans*-oxido-7,9-*trans*-11,14-*cis*-eicosatetraenoic acid) by an uncharacterized dehydrase (51). LTA$_4$ is enzymatically metabolized to LTB$_4$ by a soluble epoxide hydrolase (52) or to the sulfidopeptide leukotriene, LTC_4, by a glutathione-S-transferase (53). LTA_4 may be nonenzymatically hydrolyzed to isomers of 6-*trans*-LTB_4 and of 5,6-dihydroxy-eicosatetraenoic acid. LTC_4 is sequentially cleaved by γ-glutamyl transpeptidase to (5S)-hydroxy-(6R)-S-cysteinylglycyl-7,9-*trans*-11,14-*cis*-eicosatetraenoic acid, leukotriene D_4 (LTD_4) (47), and by an additional dipeptidase(s) to (5S)-hydroxy-(6R)-S-cysteinyl-7,9-*trans*-11,14,-*cis*-eicosatetraenoic acid, leukotriene E_4 (LTE_4) (54,55) in plasma and some tissues.

RP-HPLC allows the resolution of all products deriving from LTA_4, as well as quantitation at their separate retention times by ultraviolet absorbance at 280 nm and by RIAs for LTB_4, LTC_4, LTD_4, and LTE_4. One million mouse bone marrow-derived mast cells, when sensitized with monoclonal IgE and subsequently activated under optimal conditions with 100 ng DNP-BSA for 5 min at 37°C, generate 6-*trans*-LTB_4 diastereoisomers in addition to LTB_4 and LTC_4. A product profile that differs quantitatively, but not qualitatively, is obtained after activation of the same cells for 40 min with 0.2 μM A23187, the optimal ionophore concentration and time. As there is neither peptide cleavage of LTC_4 to LTD_4 or LTE_4 (12,24), nor sulfoxidation of LTC_4 to LTC_4 sulfoxides, nor ω-oxidation of LTB_4 to 20-hydroxy or 20-COOH LTB_4 (E. Razin, R. A. Lewis, and K. F. Austen, unpublished observations), the summation of LTC_4, 6-*trans*-LTB_4 diastereoisomers, and LTB_4 is equivalent to the total LTA_4 that was utilized. For the mouse bone marrow-derived mast cell, whether activated by antigen or ionophore, the 6-*trans*-LTB_4 diastereoisomers are generated by nonenzymatic hydrolysis of LTA_4 in quantities greater than that of LTB_4 and approximately 20% that of LTC_4, indicating that although most of substrate LTA_4 derived from the endogenous pool of arachidonic acid is processed enzymatically, a significant proportion is degraded by a noncatalytic process. Human polymorphonuclear (PMN) leukocytes (2 × 10^7) activated by 1 μM A23187 for 5 min, which maximizes both LTB_4 generation and LTB_4 recovery during ongoing ω-oxidation, also incompletely utilizes substrate LTA_4 by enzymatic pathways, so that as much as 15% of the total products represent nonenzymatic hydrolysis of the epoxide; the same amounts of the 6-*trans*-LTB_4 diastereoisomers are also recovered at 30 min, despite virtually complete ω-oxidation of LTB_4. Human alveolar macrophages activated for 30 min by 1 μM A23187 metabolize almost all the LTA_4 that is processed to LTB_4 with little nonenzymatic hydrolysis. Although ω-oxidation of either LTB_4 or its 6-*trans* diastereoisomers has not been ruled out by addition of these moieties as radiolabeled substrates, it is more likely that the alveolar macrophages, which generate four to eight times more leukotriene products/10^6 cells than do mouse bone marrow-derived mast cells or human neutrophils (12,30,46), are more efficient in enzymatically converting LTA_4 to a biologically active product.

It is possible that not all mammalian cellular 5-lipoxygenases are identical *in situ,* since 5,8,11,14-eicosatetraynoic acid (ETYA), a potent inhibitor of the cyclooxygenase and platelet 12-lipoxygenase (56,57), also inhibits the 5-lipoxygenase in rabbit PMNs, human PMNs and eosinophils, and RBL-1 cells (58–61), but not in human lymphocytes or guinea pig PMNs (62,63). In intact human neutrophils (64), 15-HETE inhibits the subsequent formation of [^{14}C]5-HETE from labeled arachidonic acid, possibly by serving as a substrate for formation of 5-hydroperoxy-15-hydroxy-eicosatetraenoic acid with concomitant inhibition of the 5-lipoxygenase. Conversely, in PT-18 cells (65), 15-HETE has been shown to increase 5-lipoxygenase activity. Further, whereas the cellular 5-lipoxygenase pathway of rabbit PMNs is capable of generating 5-HETE and LTB_4 from exogenous arachidonic acid without an added stimulus for cell activation and is inhibited by either 12-HETE or 15-HETE (66), the 5-lipoxygenase of the PT-18 murine mast cell/basophil line does not metabolize exogenous arachidonic acid to pathway products unless the cell is specifically activated (65).

The effects of inhibiting or enhancing the catalytic function of a particular enzyme in the 5-lipoxygenase pathway can be assessed from the product profile. For example, whereas an inhibitor of the 5-lipoxygenase, such as 5,6-dehydroarachidonic acid (5,6-DHA) (67,68), would be expected to decrease all of the products of the 5-lipoxygenase pathway, an apparent inhibitor of the conversion of 5-HPETE to LTA_4, such as ETYA for guinea pig PMNs (63) or diethylcarbamazine for A23187-activated murine mastocytoma cells (69), should decrease the generation of products distal to LTA_4 in the cascade while increasing or failing to alter 5-HETE production. In contrast, 6,9-deepoxy-6,9-(phenylimino)-$\Delta^{6,8}$-PGI_1 (U-60,257), an inhibitor of the glutathione-*S*-transferase responsible for converting LTA_4 to LTC_4 in ionophore-activated rat mononuclear cells (70), should specifically decrease synthesis of LTC_4, LTD_4, and LTE_4 and possibly increase generation of the other products in the cascade (71).

The phospholipase-initiated pathways that lead to liberation of arachidonic acid from a given cell under a given condition may be different or difficult to define, as exemplified by the various pathways cited for thrombin-activated platelets (72–75). Separate pathways of phospholipid turnover have also been indicated for platelets activated by two different stimuli (76). The mouse peritoneal macrophage metabolizes arachidonic acid via the cyclooxygenase pathway alone or together with the 5-lipoxygenase pathway, according to the stimulus (77), and the arachidonic acid metabolized only by the former pathway, but not by the latter, is apparently derived via the sequential actions of phospholipase C and diacylglycerol lipase (78). Since one of the presumed control enzymes which would regulate PAF biosynthesis, phospholipase A_2, is proximal to arachidonic acid release for utilization in either the cyclooxygenase or 5-lipoxygenase pathway, quantitative measurement of PAF should serve as an additional marker in determining the site of modulation by pharmacologic agents.

INTEGRATED BASIS OF TISSUE RESPONSE TO THE SULFIDOPEPTIDE LEUKOTRIENES

The sulfidopeptide leukotrienes, LTC_4, LTD_4, and LTE_4 together constitute the biological activities ascribed to slow-reacting substance of anaphylaxis (SRS-A) (47,79–84). All three of these compounds have been evaluated for their effects after intradermal injection of 1 nmol in the human and shown to elicit augmented vasopermeability responses, as evidenced by a wheal lasting 2–4 hr (85). LTC_4 and LTD_4, when aerosolized and inhaled by normal humans, evoke small airway responses that compromise flow rates at doses averaging 0.3% that of histamine, which effects the same impairment (86,87). Additionally, LTC_4 and LTD_4 are each 100 times as potent as methacholine in provoking mucus secretions from human bronchial mucosal explants *in vitro* (88,89), but their action is not stereospecific (88). *In vitro* studies of the amounts of agonist that are equally potent in eliciting spasmogenic activity have yielded molar ratios of $LTC_4 : LTD_4 : LTE_4$ for guinea pig ileum of 4.2 : 1 : 5, and for guinea pig parenchymal lung strips of 100 : 1 : 30 (80), and molar ratios of $LTC_4 : LTD_4 : LTE_4$ for equal potency in decreasing human and guinea pig myocardial contractility of 25 : 1 : 265 and 10 : 1 : 2000, respectively (90). Possible explanations for these differences in relative potencies for the sulfidopeptide leukotrienes could relate to both receptor-determined primary and receptor or nonreceptor determined secondary muscle responses.

Substantially different rates of bioconversion for each sulfidopeptide leukotriene by the responding tissue(s) have been shown to represent a separate variable in determining the intensity and time course of the contractile response elicited in guinea pig ileal smooth muscle (55). The effect of ongoing bioconversion of $[^3H]LTC_4$ and $[^3H]LTD_4$ on the contractile response of the guinea pig ileum to each was determined by recording the pattern of the contraction and serially quantitating the initial agonist and its metabolic products by their retention times on reverse phase–high performance liquid chromatography (RP-HPLC). After a latent period of 60 sec, LTC_4 initiated a linear response, followed by a slower, progressive response to a maximum level that was maintained without relaxation. The metabolic conversion of LTC_4 was <5% during the linear phase of contraction, and complete inhibition of bioconversion of LTC_4 to LTD_4 by the presence of serine–borate complex did not alter the pattern of the spasmogenic response. As the maximum response in the presence of serine–borate complex was three-fourths of that obtained without the inhibitor of bioconversion, the predominant response was to LTC_4 itself. The spasmogenic response of the ileum to LTD_4 was immediate, linear to a maximum level, and followed immediately by a marked relaxation. That the failure of LTD_4 to sustain a contraction was the result of its immediate, rapid, and quantitative conversion to the less potent LTE_4 was established by pharmacologically inhibiting and anatomically deleting the converting activity. In the presence of L-cysteine, the conversion of LTD_4 to LTE_4 was largely inhibited and the maximum contractile response was well maintained. After anatomic removal of the mucosa that contained the LTD_4 dipeptidase activity, the smooth muscle preparation gave a maximum response to LTD_4 that was fully maintained. Thus, bioconversion is not a prerequisite for the spasmogenic activity of LTC_4 and accounts for the transient response of the ileum to LTD_4 (55).

The structural determinants of LTC_4 and LTD_4 spasmogenic functions on smooth muscle have been shown to exist in the presence of a hydrophobic omega region and in the spacial relationships of the polar region. Although the precise stereochemistry of the omega region is not essential for modest nonvascular smooth muscle contractile activity, as indicated by potencies of the 14,15-dihydro and 9,10,11,12,14,15-hexahydro analogs of both LTC_4 and LTD_4, the region cannot be deleted. C-9, C-12, and C-14 *apo*-LTD_4 lacking 9, 12, and 14 carbons, respectively, are completely inactive as spasmogens, indicating a possible binding function for the hydrophobic omega region (91–93) as a requisite for receptor activation by the stereochemically appropriate region.

Stereochemical requirements for spasmogenic activity on the guinea pig ileum have been ascertained by use of synthetic chiral isomers at the three optically active centers in the natural C-6 sulfidopeptide leukotrienes: carbon 5 (C-5) of the eicosanoid backbone, which bears the hydroxyl; C-6, to which is conjugated the sulfidopeptide; and the asymmetric carbon of cysteine in the sulfidopeptide. Diastereoisomers at C-5 and C-6 of LTD_4 and that at C-6 of LTC_4 each have <5% of the nonvascular spasmogenic activity of the naturally occurring leukotriene (92). Substitution of D-cysteine for L-cysteine in LTD_4 causes only a modest decrement in potency, whereas D- and L-alanine replacements for the glycine of LTD_4 are relatively similar in effect. Thus, the rigorous relationships of function to the stereochemistry of the C-5 and C-6 polar adducts to the eicosanoid backbone are not expressed more distally in the sulfidopeptide chain, indicating that the critical spatial arrangements exist between the eicosanoid carboxyl and the polar adducts, as would be the case for true receptors.

It is not to be assumed that the receptors for LTC_4, LTD_4, and LTE_4 on any responding tissue need be identical (94). The possibility of receptor heterogeneity for this class of oxidative metabolites of arachidonic acid is consistent with radioligand binding studies demonstrating separate sub-class receptors for LTC_4 and LTD_4 (95,96) and with extensive functional studies (80,94,97). The possibility of subclass receptors for the sulfidopeptide leukotrienes was initially raised by the biphasic LTD_4 dose–response isometric contraction of guinea pig peripheral airway strips *in vitro* and by the capacity of FPL55712 to competitively inhibit only the low-dose phase of this LTD_4-mediated contraction of guinea pig parenchymal strips (94); there was no consistent inhibition of the spasmogenic response of this tissue to LTC_4. Since bioconversion of LTC_4 to LTD_4 to LTE_4 occurs during the ongoing contraction of a responding guinea pig ileum smooth muscle strip and modulates the time-dependent profile of the contractile event (55), the concentration of each sulfidopeptide leukotriene at a given time as well as the concentration and heterogeneity of specific receptors may determine the integrated spasmogenic response.

METABOLIC INACTIVATION OF THE C-6 SULFIDOPEPTIDE LEUKOTRIENES

Enzymatic conversions of LTC_4 to LTD_4 and of LTC_3 to LTD_3 by cleavage of glutamic acid from the S-glutathionyl domain have been shown with purified γ-glutamyl transpeptidase (98,99). The conversion of LTD_4 to LTE_4 decreases its potency as a nonvascular smooth muscle spasmogen as well as its potency as an arteriolar vasoconstrictor, while maintaining or even increasing its efficacy as an augmentor of vasopermeability (80). The cleavage of glycine from the dipeptide side chain has been shown to be catalyzed by dipeptidases from several sources, including one from the specific granules of human neutrophils (54).

Neutrophils possess a second mechanism for modifying the structures and functional activities of the C-6 sulfidopeptide leukotrienes, which depends upon triggering of the respiratory burst (100). Ten million PMNs stimulated with 1000 ng of phorbol myristate acetate (PMA) at 37°C, so as to undergo a respiratory burst, rapidly metabolized 2 μg of exogenous LTC_4 to six products that eluted as three doublets on RP-HPLC; these doublets were readily separable both from one another and from the known sulfidopeptide leukotrienes.

These conversion products, designated I, II, and III in order of elution, constituted 13%, 37%, and 50%, respectively, of the metabolites. Doublet I showed the UV absorption spectrum of a sulfidopeptide leukotriene with λ_{max} at 280 nm but had <4% of the immunoreactivity of LTC_4 with class-specific rabbit antibodies and <1% of the contractile activity of LTC_4 on the guinea pig ileum. Doublet II was identified as the diastereoisomeric sulfoxides of LTC_4, because the doublet constituents and synthetic sulfoxides cochromatographed on RP-HPLC, had a 4.5-nm bathochromic shift in their UV spectra relative to that of LTC_4, and showed immunoreactivity comparable to that of LTC_4. Doublet III was identified as the diastereoisomers of 6-*trans*-LTB$_4$ by comparison with synthetic standards. Identity was demonstrated by the specific retention times on RP-HPLC, a UV absorption spectrum with λ_{max} at 269 nm and shoulders at 259 and 279 nm, and mass spectral analysis of methylester, bis(trimethylsilyl) ether derivatives (100). As the diastereoisomeric sulfoxides of LTC_4 and the diastereoisomers of 6-*trans*-LTB$_4$ retain <1% of the spasmogenic activity of LTC_4, they represent products of inactivation of the leukotriene, as contrasted with the modulation of biological activities effected by the peptide cleavage cascade from LTC_4 to LTD_4 to LTE_4 (79,80,94).

Superoxide dismutase and the hydroxyl radical scavengers, benzoate, ethanol, and dimethylsulfoxide, failed to prevent inactivation of LTC_4 and the formation of these oxidative products, indicating that neither superoxide anion nor hydroxyl radical was involved in the inactivation process. Catalase, which destroys hydrogen peroxide, and azide, an inhibitor of myeloperoxidase, completely inhibited catabolism of LTC_4, suggesting that the action of myeloperoxidase on hydrogen peroxide is necessary in the formation of the oxidizing species. That the critical species was hypochlorous acid (HOCl) was supported by the ability of L-serine and glycine, known scavengers of HOCl, to block metabolic inactivation of LTC_4 by PMA-activated human neutrophils and was proven by the capacity of chemically prepared HOCl to convert LTC_4 to diastereoisomeric LTC_4 sulfoxides and the diastereoisomers of 6-*trans*-LTB$_4$. Thus, metabolic inactivation of LTC_4 by activated human PMNs involves myeloperoxidase–H_2O_2–chloride-dependent generation of HOCl; formation of the LTC_4-chlorosulfonium ion as a theoretical intermediate yields diastereoisomers of LTC_4 sulfoxides, the 6-*trans*-LTB_4-C-12-diastereoisomers, and a pair of chemically undefined S-conjugated leukotrienes (100). The same oxidative mechanism also inactivates the other sulfidopeptide leukotrienes, LTD_4 and LTE_4, such that the 6-*trans*-LTB_4 diastereoisomers are generated from each and the specific diastereoisomeric leukotriene sulfoxides are generated from their respective substrates. Minor oxidative products from LTD_4 include one or both 11-*trans*-LTD_4 sulfoxides. Minor products from LTE_4 include two uncharacterized S-conjugated peptide products that have maximal absorbance at 283.6 nm and are moderately (10% and 50%) reactive in the sulfidopeptide leukotriene RIA, relative to LTE_4. One of these products is derived from one or both of the LTE_4 sulfoxides (101).

CONCLUSION

Whether human lung mast cells exist as a single population that shares all aspects of the two described rodent mast cell populations, or whether there is an analogous dichotomy, remains to be delineated. The appreciation of bioconversion of LTC_4 to LTD_4 and LTE_4 in responding tissues, and the implications for different populations of sulfidopeptide leukotriene receptors in tissues, is relevant to understanding integrated tissue responses. The recognition of the oxidative pathway by which activated PMN leukocytes degrade these biologically active lipid mediators, as distinct from their bioconversion, emphasizes the parameters to be considered during quantitation of their biosynthesis.

REFERENCES

1. Enerbäck, L. Mast cells in rat gastrointestinal mucosa. I. Effects of fixation. *Acta Pathol. Microbiol. Scand.* **66:**289–302, 1966.
2. Enerbäck, L. Mast cells in rat gastrointestinal mucosa. II. Dye-binding and metachromatic properties. *Acta Pathol. Microbiol. Scand.* **66:**303–312, 1966.
3. Lagunoff, D., and Pritzl, P. Characterization of rat mast cell granule proteins. *Arch. Biochem. Biophys.* **173:**554–563, 1976.
4. Befus, A. D., Pearce, F. L., Gauldie, J., Horsewood, P., and Bienenstock, J. Mucosal mast cells. I. Isolation and functional characteristics of rat intestinal mast cells. *J. Immunol.* **128:**2475–2480, 1982.
5. Haig, D. M., McKee, T. A., Jarrett, E. E. R., Woodbury, E., and Miller, H. R. P. Generation of mucosal mast cells is stimulated *in vitro* by factors derived from T cells of helminth-infected rats. *Nature (London)* **300:**188–190, 1982.

6. Yurt, R. W., and Austen, K. F. Preparative purification of the rat mast cell chymase: Characterization and interaction with granule components. *J. Exp. Med.* **146:**1405–1419, 1977.

7. Woodbury, R. G., Gruzienski, G. M., and Lagunoff, D. Immunofluorescent localization of a serine protease in rat small intestine. *Proc. Natl. Acad. Sci. U.S.A.* **75:**2785–2789, 1978.

8. Ruitenberg, E. J., Gustowska, L., Elgersma, A., and Ruitenberg, H. M. Effect of fixation on the light microscopical visualization of mast cells in the mucosa and connective tissue of the human duodenum. *Int. Arch. Allergy Appl. Immunol.* **67:**233–238, 1982.

9. Razin, E., Stevens, R. L., Akiyama, F., Schmid, L., and Austen, K. F. Culture from mouse bone marrow of a subclass of mast cells possessing a distinct chondroitin sulfate proteoglycan with glycosaminoglycans rich in *N*-acetylgalactosamine-4,6-disulfate. *J. Biol. Chem.* **257:**7229–7236, 1982.

10. Metcalfe, D. D., Smith, J. A., Austen, K. F., and Silbert, J. E. Polydispersity of rat mast cell heparin. Implications for proteoglycan assembly. *J. Biol. Chem.* **255:**11753–11758, 1980.

11. Yurt, R. W., Leid, R. W., Jr., Austen, K. F., and Silbert, J. E. Native heparin from rat peritoneal mast cells. *J. Biol. Chem.* **252:**518–521, 1977.

12. Razin, E., Mencia-Huerta, J.-M., Stevens, R. L., Lewis, R. A., Liu, F.-T., Corey, E. J., and Austen, K. F. IgE-mediated release of leukotriene C$_4$, chondroitin sulfate E proteoglycan, β-hexosaminidase, and histamine from cultured bone marrow-derived mouse mast cells. *J. Exp. Med.* **157:**189–201, 1983.

13. Stevens, R. L., Razin, E. Austen, K. F., Hein, A., Caulfield, J. P., Seno, N., Schmid, K., and Akiyama, F. Synthesis of chondroitin sulfate E glycosaminoglycan onto *p*-nitrophenol-β-D-xyloside and its localization to the secretory granules of rat serosal mast cells and mouse bone marrow-derived mast cells. *J. Biol. Chem.* **258:**5977–5984, 1983.

14. Razin, E., Cordon-Cardo, C., and Good, R. A. Growth of a pure population of mouse mast cells *in vitro* with conditioned medium derived from concanavalin A–stimulated splenocytes. *Proc. Natl. Acad. Sci. U.S.A.* **78:**2559–2561, 1981.

15. Schrader, J. W., Lewis, S. J., Clark-Lewis, I., and Culvenor, J. G. The persisting (P) cell: Histamine content, regulation by a T cell-derived factor, origin from a bone marrow precursor, and relationship to mast cells. *Proc. Natl. Acad. Sci. U.S.A.* **78:**323–327, 1981.

16. Tertian, G., Yung, Y.-P., Guy-Grand, D., and Moore, M. A. S. Long-term *in vitro* culture of murine mast cells. I. Description of a growth factor-dependent culture technique. *J. Immunol.* **127:**788–794, 1981.

17. Caulfield, J. P., Lewis, R. A., Hein, A., and Austen, K. F. Secretion in dissociated human pulmonary mast cells: Evidence for solubilization of granule contents before discharge. *J. Cell Biol.* **85:**299–312, 1980.

18. Schulman, E. J., MacGlashan, D. W., Peters, S. P., Schleimer, R. P., Newball, H. H., and Lichtenstein, L. M. Human lung mast cells: Purification and characterization. *J. Immunol.* **129:**2662–2667, 1982.

19. Metcalfe, D. D., Lewis, R. A., Silbert, J. E., Rosenberg, R. D., Wasserman, S. I., and Austen, K. F. Isolation and characterization of heparin from human lung. *J. Clin. Invest.* **64:**1537–1543, 1979.

20. Schwartz, L. B., Lewis, R. A., Seldin, D., and Austen, K. F. Acid hydrolases and tryptase from secretory granules of dispersed human lung mast cells. *J. Immunol.* **126:**1290–1294, 1981.

21. Schwartz, L. B., Lewis, R. A., and Austen, K. F. Tryptase from human pulmonary mast cells. Purification and characterization. *J. Biol. Chem.* **256:**11939–11943, 1981.
22. Lewis, R. A., Soter, N. A., Diamond, P. T., Austen, K. F., Oates, J. A., and Roberts, L. J., II. Prostaglandin D_2 generation after activation of rat and human mast cells with anti-IgE. *J. Immunol.* **129:**1627–1631, 1982.
23. Razin, E., Mencia-Huerta, J.-M., Lewis, R. A., Corey, E. J., and Austen, K. F. Generation of leukotriene C_4 from a subclass of mast cells differentiated *in vitro* from mouse bone marrow. *Proc. Natl. Acad. Sci. U.S.A.* **79:**4665–4667, 1982.
24. Mencia-Huerta, J.-M., Razin, E., Ringel, E. W., Corey, E. J., Hoover, D., Austen, K. F., and Lewis, R. A. Immunologic and ionophore-induced generation of leukotriene B_4 from mouse bone marrow-derived mast cells. *J. Immunol.* **130:**1885–1890, 1983.
25. Schleimer, R. P., Schulman, E. J., MacGlashan, D. W., Jr., Peters, S. P., Hayes, E., Adams, G. K., III, Lichtenstein, L. M., and Adkinson, N. F. Effects of dexamethasone on mediator release from human lung fragments and purified human lung mast cells. *J. Clin. Invest.* **71:**1830–1835, 1983.
26. MacGlashan, D. W., Jr., Schleimer, R. P., Peters, S. P., Schulman, E. S., Adams, G. K., III, Newball, H. H., and Lichtenstein, L. M. Generation of leukotrienes by purified human lung mast cells. *J. Clin. Invest.* **70:**747–751, 1982.
27. Lewis, R. A., Drazen, J. M., Corey, E. J., and Austen, K. F. Structural and functional characteristics of the leukotriene components of slow reacting substance of anaphylaxis (SRS-A). *In* "SRS-A and the Leukotrienes" (P. J. Piper, ed.), pp. 101–117. Wiley, London, 1981.
28. Paterson, N. A. M., Wasserman, S. I., Said, J. W., and Austen, K. F. Release of chemical mediators from partially purified human lung mast cells. *J. Immunol.* **117:**1356–1362, 1976.
29. Joseph, M., Tonnel, A.-B., Torpier, G., Capron, A., Arnous, B., and Benveniste, J. Involvement of immunoglobulin E in the secretory process of alveolar macrophages from asthmatic patients. *J. Clin. Invest.* **71:**221–230, 1983.
30. Godard, P., Damon, M., Michel, F. B., Corey, E. J., Austen, K. F., and Lewis, R. A. Leukotriene B_4 production from human alveolar macrophages. *Clin. Res.* **31:**548A (abstr.), 1983.
31. Fels, A. O. S., Pawlowski, N. A., Cramer, E. B., King, T. K. C., Cohn, Z. A., and Scott, W. A. Human alveolar macrophages produce leukotriene B_4. *Proc. Natl. Acad. Sci. U.S.A.* **79:**7866–7870, 1982.
32. Marcus, A. J., Wekser, R. B., Jaffe, E. A., and Broekman, M. J. Synthesis of prostacyclin endoperoxides by cultured human endothelial cells. *J. Clin. Invest.* **66:**979–986, 1980.
33. Demopoulos, C. A., Pinckard, R. N., and Hanahan, D. J. Platelet-activating factor. Evidence for 1-*O*-alkyl-2-acetyl-*sn*-glyceryl-3-phosphorylcholine as the active component (a new class of lipid chemical mediators). *J. Biol. Chem.* **254:**9355–9358, 1979.
34. Benveniste, J., Tencé, M., Varenne, P., Bidault, J., Boullet, C., and Polonsky, J. Semi-synthèse et structure proposée du facteur activant les plaquettes (P.A.F.): PAF-acéther, un alkyl éther analogue de la lysophosphatidylcholine. *C.R. Hebd. Seances Acad. Sci., Ser. D* **289:**1037–1040, 1979.
35. Blank, M. L., Snyder, F., Byers, L. W., Brooks, B., and Muirhead, E. E. Antihypertensive activity of an alkyl ether analog of phosphatidylcholine. *Biochem. Biophys. Res. Commun.* **90:**1194–1200, 1979.
36. Wykle, R. L., Malone, B., and Snyder, F. Enzymatic synthesis of 1-alkyl-2-acetyl-*sn*-glycero-3-phosphorylcholine, a hypotensive and platelet-aggregating lipid. *J. Biol. Chem.* **255:**10256–10260, 1980.

37. Cazenave, J. P., Benveniste, J., and Mustard, J. F. Aggregation of rabbit platelets by platelet-activating factor is independent of the release reaction and the arachidonate pathway and inhibited by membrane-active drugs. *Lab. Invest.* **41**:275–280, 1979.
38. Chignard, M., Le Couédic, J. P., Tencé, M., Vargraftig, B. B., and Benveniste, J. The role of platelet-activating factor in platelet aggregation. *Nature (London)* **279**:799–800, 1979.
39. Camussi, G., Tetta, C., Bussolino, F., Cappio, F. C., Coda, R., Masera, C., and Segolini, G. Mediators of immune-complex-induced aggregation of polymorphonuclear neutrophils. II. Platelet-activating factor as the effector substance of immune-induced aggregation. *Int. Arch. Allergy Appl. Immunol.* **64**:25–41, 1981.
40. Goetzl, E. J., Derian, C. K., Tauber, A. I., and Valone, F. H. Novel effects of 1-*O*-hexadecyl-2-acyl-*sn*-glycero-3-phosphorylcholine mediators on human leukocyte function: Delineation of the specific roles of the acyl substituents. *Biochem. Biophys. Res. Commun.* **94**:881–888, 1980.
41. O'Flaherty, J. T., Wykle, R. L., Miller, C. M., Lewis, J. C., Waite, M., Bass, D. A., McCall, C. E., and DeChatelet, R. L. 1-*O*-alkyl-*sn*-glyceryl-3-phosphorylcholines: A novel class of neutrophil stimulants. *Am. J. Pathol.* **103**:70–78, 1981.
42. Vargaftig, B. B., LeFort, J., Chignard, M., and Benveniste, J. Platelet-activating factor induces a platelet-dependent bronchoconstriction unrelated to the formation of prostaglandin derivatives. *Eur. J. Pharmacol.* **65**:185–192, 1980.
43. Pinckard, R. N., McManus, L. M., O'Rourke, R. A., Crawford, M. H., and Hanahan, D. J. Intravascular and cardiovascular effects of acetyl-glyceryl ether phorylcholine infusion in the baboon. *Clin. Res.* **28**:258A, (abstr.), 1980.
44. Mencia-Huerta, J.-M., Lewis, R. A., Razin, E., and Austen, K. F. Antigen-initiated release of platelet-activating factor (PAF-acether) from mouse bone marrow-derived mast cells sensitized with monoclonal IgE. *J. Immunol.* **131**:2958–2964, 1983.
45. Levine, L., Morgan, R. A., Lewis, R. A., Austen, K. F., Clark, D. A., Marfat, A., and Corey, E. J. Radioimmunoassay of the leukotrienes of slow reacting substance of anaphylaxis. *Proc. Natl. Acad. Sci. U.S.A.* **78**:7692–7696, 1981.
46. Lewis, R. A., Mencia-Huerta, J.-M., Soberman, R. J., Hoover, D., Marfat, A., Corey, E. J., and Austen, K. F. Radioimmunoassay for leukotriene B₄. *Proc. Natl. Acad. Sci. U.S.A.* **79**:7904–7908, 1982.
47. Örning, L., Hammarström, S., and Samuelsson, B. Leukotriene D: A slow reacting substance from rat basophilic leukemia cells. *Proc. Natl. Acad. Sci. U.S.A.* **77**:2014–2017, 1980.
48. Jakschik, B. A., Falkenhein, S., and Parker, C. W. Precursor role of arachidonic acid in release of slow reacting substance from rat basophilic leukemia cells. *Proc. Natl. Acad. Sci. U.S.A.* **74**:4577–4581, 1977.
49. Borgeat, P., and Samuelsson, B. Arachidonic acid metabolism in polymorphonuclear leukocytes: Effects of ionophore A23187. *Proc. Natl. Acad. Sci. U.S.A.* **76**:2148–2152, 1979.
50. Borgeat, P., Hamberg, M., and Samuelsson, B. Transformation of arachidonic acid and homo-gamma-linolenic acid by rabbit polymorphonuclear leukocytes. Monohydroxy acids from novel lipoxygenases. *J. Biol. Chem.* **251**:7816–7820, 1976; correction: **252**:8772, 1977.
51. Borgeat, P., and Samuelsson, B. Arachidonic acid metabolism in polymorphonuclear leukocytes: Unstable intermediate in formation of dihydroxy acids. *Proc. Natl. Acad. Sci. U.S.A.* **76**:3213–3217, 1979.
52. Jakschik, B. A., and Kuo, C. G. Characterization of leukotriene A₄ and B₄ biosynthesis. *Prostaglandins* **25**:767–782, 1983.

53. Jakschik, B. A., Harper, T., and Murphy, R. C. Leukotriene C_4 and D_4 formation by particulate enzymes. *J. Biol. Chem.* **257:**5346–5349, 1982.

54. Lee, C. W., Lewis, R. A., Corey, E. J., and Austen, K. F. Conversion of leukotriene D_4 to leukotriene E_4 by a dipeptidase released from the specific granule of human polymorphonuclear leukocytes. *Immunology* **48:**27–35, 1983.

55. Krilis, S., Lewis, R. A., Corey, E. J., and Austen, K. F. Bioconversion of C-6 sulfido-peptide leukotrienes by the responding guinea pig ileum determines the time course of its contraction. *J. Clin. Invest* **71:**909–915, 1983.

56. Ahern, D. G., and Downing, D. T. Inhibition of prostaglandin biosynthesis by eicosa-5,8,11,14-tetraynoic acid. *Biochim. Biophys. Acta* **210:**456–461, 1970.

57. Hamberg, M., and Samuelsson, B. Prostaglandin endoperoxides. Novel transformations of arachidonic acid in human platelets. *Proc. Natl. Acad. Sci. U.S.A.* **71:**3400–3404, 1974.

58. Stenson, W. F., and Parker, C. W. Monohydroxyeicosatetraenoic acids (HETEs) induce degranulation of human neutrophils. *J. Immunol.* **124:**2100–2104, 1980.

59. Goetzl, E. J. A role for endogenous mono-hydroxy-eicosatetraenoic acids (HETEs) in the regulation of human neutrophil migration. *Immunology* **40:**709–719, 1980.

60. Goetzl, E. J., Weller, P. F., and Sun, F. F. The regulation of human eosinophil function by endogenous mono-hydroxy-eicosatetraenoic acids (HETEs). *J. Immunol.* **124:**926–933, 1980.

61. Falkenhein, S. F., McDonald, H., Huber, M. M., Koch, D., and Parker, C. W. Effect of the 5-hydroperoxide of eicosatetraenoic acid and inhibitors of the lipoxygenase pathway on the formation of slow reacting substance by rat basophilia leukemia cells; direct evidence that slow reacting substance is a product of the lipoxygenase pathway. *J. Immunol.* **125:**163–168, 1980.

62. Parker, C. W., Stenson, W. F., Huber, M. G., and Kelley, J. P. Formation of thromboxane B_2 and hydroxyarachidonic acids in purified human lymphocytes in the presence and absence of PHA. *J. Immunol.* **122:**1572–1577, 1979.

63. Bokoch, G. M., and Reed, P. W. Evidence for inhibition of leukotriene A_4 synthesis by 5,8,11,14-eicosatetraynoic acid in guinea pig polymorphonuclear leukocytes. *J. Biol. Chem.* **256:**4156–4159, 1981.

64. Vanderhoek, J. Y., Bryant, R. W., and Bailey, J. M. Inhibition of leukotriene biosynthesis by the leukocyte product 15-hydroxy-5,8,11,13-eicosatetraenoic acid. *J. Biol. Chem.* **255:**10064–10066, 1980.

65. Vanderhoek, J. Y., Tare, N. S., Bailey, J. M., Goldstein, A. L., and Pluznik, D. M. New role for 15-hydroxyeicosatetraenoic acid: Activator of leukotriene biosynthesis on PT-18 mast/basophil cells. *J. Biol. Chem.* **257:**12191–12195, 1982.

66. Vanderhoek, J. Y., Bryant, R. W., and Bailey, J. M. Regulation of leukocyte and platelet lipoxygenases by hydroxyeicosanoids. *Biochem. Pharmacol.* **31:**3463–3467, 1982.

67. Corey, E. J., and Park, H. Irreversible inhibition of the enzymatic oxidation of arachidonic acid to 15-(hydroperoxy)-5,8,11(Z),13(E)-eicosatetraenoic acid (15-HPETE) by 14,15-dehydroarachidonic acid. *J. Am. Chem. Soc.* **104:**1750–1752, 1982.

68. Sok, D.-E., Han, C.-Q., Pai, J.-K., and Sih, C. J. Inhibition of leukotriene biosynthesis by acetylenic analogs. *Biochem. Biophys. Res. Commun.* **107:**101–108, 1982.

69. Mathews, W. R., and Murphy, R. C. Inhibition of leukotriene biosynthesis in mastocytoma cells by diethylcarbamazine. *Biochem. Pharmacol.* **31:**2129–2132, 1982.

70. Bach, M. K., Brashler, J. R., Smith, H. W., Fitzpatrick, F. A., Sun, F. F., and McGuire, J. C. 6,9-Deepoxy-6,9-(phenylimino)-$\Delta^{6,8}$-prostaglandin I_1, (U-60,257), a new

inhibitor of leukotriene C and D synthesis. *In vitro* studies. *Prostaglandins* **23:**759–771, 1982.

71. Razin, E., Romeo, L. C., Krilis, S., Liu, F-T., Lewis, R. A., Corey, E. J., and Austen, K. F. Analysis of the relationship between 5-lipoxygenase product generation and the secretion of preformed mediators from mouse bone marrow mast cells. *J. Immunol.* (in press).

72. Rittenhouse-Simmons, S., and Deykin, D. The mobilization of arachidonic acid in platelets exposed to thrombin or ionophore A23187. Effects of adenosine triphosphate deprivation. *J. Clin. Invest.* **60:**495–498, 1977.

73. Rittenhouse-Simmons, S. Production of diglyceride from phosphatidylinositol in activated human platelets. *J. Clin. Invest.* **63:**580–587, 1979.

74. Bell, R. L., Kennerly, D. A., Stanford, N., and Majerus, P. W. Diglyceride lipase: A pathway for arachidonate release from human platelets. *Proc. Natl. Acad. Sci. U.S.A.* **76:**3238–3241, 1979.

75. Lapetina, E. G., Schmitges, C. J., Chandrabose, K., and Cuatrecasas, P. Regulation of phospholipase activity in platelets. *Adv. Prostaglandin Thromboxane Res.* **3:**127–135, 1978.

76. Rittenhouse-Simmons, S., Russel, F., and Deykin, D. Mobilization of arachidonic acid in human platelets: Kinetics and Ca^{2+} dependency. *Biochim. Biophys. Acta* **488:**370–380, 1977.

77. Humes, J. L., Sadowski, S., Galavage, M., Goldenberg, M., Bonney, R. J., and Kuehl, F. A. Evidence for two sources of arachidonic acid for oxidative metabolism by mouse peritoneal macrophages. *J. Biol. Chem.* **257:**1591–1594, 1982.

78. Humes, J. L. Regulation of prostaglandin and leukotriene synthesis in mouse peritoneal macrophages. *Winter Prostaglandin Conf., 1983.*

79. Lewis, R. A., Austen, K. F., Drazen, J. M., Clark, D. A., Marfat, A., and Corey, E. J. Slow reacting substance of anaphylaxis: Identification of leukotrienes C-1 and D from human and rat sources. *Proc. Natl. Acad. Sci. U.S.A.* **77:**3710–3714, 1980.

80. Lewis, R. A., Drazen, J. M., Austen, K. F., Clark, D. A., and Corey, E. J. Identification of the C(6)-*S*-conjugate of leukotriene A with cysteine as a naturally occurring slow reacting substance of anaphylaxis (SRS-A). Importance of the 11-*cis* geometry for biological activity. *Biochem. Biophys. Res. Commun.* **96:**271–277, 1980.

81. Murphy, R. C., Hammarström, S., and Samuelsson, B. Leukotriene C: A slow-reacting substance from murine mastocytoma cells. *Proc. Natl. Acad. Sci. U.S.A.* **76:**4275–4279, 1979.

82. Corey, E. J., Clark, D. A., Goto, G., Marfat, A., Mioskowski, C., Samuelsson, B., and Hammarström, S. Stereospecific total synthesis of a ''slow-reacting substance'' of anaphylaxis, leukotriene C-1. *J. Am. Chem. Soc.* **102:**1436–1479 and 3663, 1980.

83. Bach, M. K., Brashler, J. R., Hammarström, S., and Samuelsson, B. Identification of a component of rat mononuclear cell SRS as leukotriene D. *Biochem. Biophys. Res. Commun.* **93:**1121–1126, 1980.

84. Morris, H. R., Taylor, G. W., Piper, P. J., and Tippins, J. R. Structure of slow-reacting substance of anaphylaxis from guinea pig lung. *Nature (London)* **285:**104–105, 1980.

85. Soter, N. A., Lewis, R. A., Corey, E. J., and Austen, K. F. Local effects of synthetic leukotrienes (LTC_4, LTD_4, LTE_4 and LTB_4) in human skin. *J. Invest. Dermatol.* **80:**115–119, 1983.

86. Weiss, J. W., Drazen, J. M., Coles, N., McFadden, E. R., Jr., Weller, P. F., Corey, E. J., Lewis, R. A., and Austen, K. F. Bronchoconstrictor effects of leukotriene C in humans. *Science* **216:**196–197, 1982.

87. Weiss, J. W., Drazen, J. M., McFadden, E. R., Jr., Weller, P., Corey, E. J., Lewis, R. A., and Austen, K. F. Airway constriction in normal humans produced by inhalation of

leukotriene D: Potency, time course, and effect of acetylsalicylic acid. *JAMA, J. Am. Med. Assoc.* **249**:2814–2817, 1983.

88. Coles, S. J., Neill, K. H., Reid, L. M., Austen, K. F., Nii, Y., Corey, E. J., and Lewis, R. A. Effects of leukotrienes C_4 and D_4 on glycoprotein and lysozyme secretion by human bronchial mucosa. *Prostaglandins* **25**:155–170, 1983.

89. Shelhamer, J. H., Marom, Z., Sun, F., Bach, M. K., and Kaliner, M. The effects of arachinoids and leukotrienes on the release of mucus from human airways. *Chest* **81**:36S–37S, 1982.

90. Burke, J. A., Levi, R., Guo, Z. G., and Corey, E. J. Leukotrienes C_4, D_4, and E_4: Effects on human and guinea pig cardiac preparations *in vitro*. *J. Pharmacol. Exp. Ther.* **221**:235–241, 1982.

91. Drazen, J. M., Lewis, R. A., Austen, K. F., Toda, M., Brion, F., Marfat, A., and Corey, E. J. Contractile activities of structural analogs of leukotrienes C and D: Necessity of a hydrophobic region. *Proc. Natl. Acad. Sci. U.S.A.* **78**:3195–3198, 1981.

92. Lewis, R. A., Drazen, J. M., Austen, K. F., Toda, M., Brion, F., Marfat, A., and Corey, E. J. Contractile activities of structural analogs of leukotrienes C and D: Roles of the polar substituents. *Proc. Natl. Acad. Sci. U.S.A.* **78**:4579–4583, 1981.

93. Lewis, R. A., Lee, C. W., Levine, L., Morgan, R. A., Weiss, J. W., Drazen, J. M., Oh, H., Corey, E. J., and Austen, K. F. Biology of the C-6-sulfidopeptide leukotrienes. *Adv. Prostaglandin, Thromboxane, Leukotriene Res.* **11**:15–26, 1983.

94. Drazen, J. M., Austen, K. F., Lewis, R. A., Clark, D. A., Goto, G., Marfat, A., and Corey, E. J. Comparative airway and vascular activities of leukotrienes C-1 and D *in vivo* and *in vitro*. *Proc. Natl. Acad. Sci. U.S.A.* **77**:4354–4358, 1980.

95. Krilis, S., Lewis, R. A., Corey, E. J., and Austen, K. F. Specific receptors for leukotriene C_4 on a smooth muscle cell line. *J. Clin. Invest.* **72**:1516–1519, 1983.

96. Pong, S.-S., and DeHaven, R. N. Characterization of a leukotriene D_4 receptor in guinea pig lung. *Proc. Natl. Acad. Sci. U.S.A.* **80**:7415–7419, 1983.

97. Lee, T. H., Austen, K. F., Corey, E. J., and Drazen, J. M. LTE_4-inducted airway hyperresponsiveness of guinea pig tracheal smooth muscle to histamine. *Proc. Natl. Acad. Sci. U.S.A.* (in press).

98. Örning, L., and Hammarström, S. Inhibition of leukotriene C and leukotriene D biosynthesis. *J. Biol. Chem.* **255**:8023–8026, 1980.

99. Hammarström, S. Metabolism of leukotriene C_3 in the guinea pig: Identification of metabolites formed by lung, liver, and kidney. *J. Biol. Chem.* **256**:9573–9578, 1981.

100. Lee, C. W., Lewis, R. A., Corey, E. J., Barton, A., Oh, H., Tauber, A. I., and Austen, K. F. Oxidative inactivation of leukotriene C_4 by stimulated human polymorphonuclear leukocytes. *Proc. Natl. Acad. Sci. U.S.A.* **79**:4166–4170, 1982.

101. Lee, C. W., Lewis, R. A., Tauber, A. I., Mehrota, M. M., Corey, E. J., and Austen, K. F. The myeloperoxidase-dependent metabolism of leukotrienes C_4, D_4, and E_4 to 6-*trans*-leukotriene B_4 diastereoisomers and the subclass-specific S-diasteroisomeric sulfoxides. *J. Biol. Chem.* **258**:15004–15010, 1983.

DISCUSSION

Lichtenstein: With your cell surface markers have you looked through the tissues to see the distribution of the two types of mast cells?

Austen: No, not yet.

Holgate: Do you have any data on similarities and differences between the pharmacological regulation of E-type and H-type mast cells?

Austen: Based on our studies to date, the pharmacological regulation of the E-type mast cell is not substantially different from that of the H-type mast cell.

Askenase: What are the comparative effects of cromolyn on the E- and H-type mouse mast cells?

Austen: We have not studied the effect of cromolyn in inhibiting the function of the E-type mast cell.

Askenase: The discovery that monoclonal antibodies distinguish these two mast cells is very important. Can you tell us about any other findings with these antibodies?

Austen: We plan to use monoclonal antibodies to isolate and identify these cells from mouse tissue.

Gleich: First, can you speak to the origin of the H-type mast cell. Are they derived from the bone marrow? Second, can you comment on the precursor frequency of the E-type mast cells in various organs, and if so, is this in turn related to the content of bone marrow-derived precursor cells? Precursor cells are distributed outside the marrow, especially to gut and lymphoid tissues.

Austen: I personally believe that both subclasses of mast cells are derived from bone marrow.

Kaliner: One of the most remarkable differences between mouse serosal mast cells and cultured bone marrow-derived cells is that one is grown *in vitro*. Therefore, I have some hesitation in extrapolating the observations seen in these cells to *in vivo*. In this regard, have you cultured mouse serosal mast cells? Have you exposed them to interleukin-3? What are the effects of introducing culture conditions on mouse serosal mast cells on leukotriene generation and glycosaminoglycan synthesis?

Austen: T cell–dependent mast cells have been developed from fetal marrow and from spleen, liver, and lymph node tissue of the mouse in response to interleukin 3 (IL-3). Indeed, several of these cultures have been cloned and maintained with sources of IL-3.

Schwartz: Is the protein core of heparin proteoglycan and chondroitin sulphate E proteoglycan the same or different?

Austen: We are now preparing large amounts of E-type mast cells in order to chemically define the peptide core of the chondroitin sulphate E proteoglycan.

Ishizaka: S. Galli and co-worker reported that the addition of sodium butyrate to the culture of bone marrow-derived mast cells (E mast cells) induced an increase in histamine content and maturation in granules (S. J. Galli, A. M. Dvorak, J. A. Marcum, T. Ishizaka, G. Nabel, H. D. Simonian, K. Pyne, J. M. Galdin, R. D. Rosenberg, H. Cantor, and H. F. Dvorak, *J. Cell Biol.* **95**:435, 1982). Have you had a chance to examine the biochemical changes in the butyrate-treated E mast cells?

Austen: To the best of my knowledge the use of this or other additives has not resulted in a change in the major proteoglycan class of a mast cell. (L. DuBuske, K. F. Austen, and R. L. Stevens, *J. Immunol.*, in press)

Askenase: Would you like to speculate on what this difference between proteoglycans of E- and H-type mast cells might mean with respect to mediator storage or release or other aspects of mast cell function?

Austen: The E-type mast cell contains proteoglycan E and the H-type mast cell contains heparin. I suspect that the E-type mast cell will be synonymous with the mucosal mast cell and that the two cell subclasses have different biological functions through their content of preformed mediators and the manner in which they process membrane phospholipids into lipid mediators. Both proteoglycans can serve as surfaces for contact activation of coagulation (Y. Hojima, C. G. Cochrane, R. C. Wiggins, K. F. Austen, and R. L. Stevens, *Blood*, in press) and both inhibit formation of the alternative pathway C_3 convertase (J. G. Wilson, D. T. Fearon, R. L. Stevens, N. Seno, and K. F. Austen, *J. Immunol.*, in press).

Wasserman: Do connective tissue and mucosal mast cells coexist in the same tissues, and if so are they differentially distributed in organs such as lung or gut?

Austen: Based upon the studies of Woodbury and colleagues with antiserum capable of recognizing type 1 and type 2 rat mast cell neutral protease, there is evidence that both subclasses of mast cells reside in rat lung tissue (R. G. Woodbury, G. M. Gruzenski, and D. Lagunoff, *Proc. Natl. Acad. Sci. U.S.A.* **75:**2785, 1978; R. G. Woodbury and H. Neurath, *Biochemistry* **17:**4298, 1978).

Lichtenstein: Do the bone marrow-derived cells release histamine somewhat more slowly than the peritoneal cells?

Austen: The rate of histamine release from the E-type mast cell is quite similar to the rate of histamine release from the H-type cell.

Turner-Warwick: You have speculated on the role of the mucosal mast cell in relation to IgE protective mechanisms; would you like to speculate on the role of the connective tissue mast cell?

Austen: I suspect that the role of both types of mast cell is to regulate the microenvironment and to facilitate beneficial host responses to noxious substances at the subclinical level.

Holgate: Rat peritoneal mast cells transport and store 5-hydroxytryptamine in their granules. Do the bone marrow-derived cells have a similar transport and storage mechanism?

Austen: I have no information on this subject.

Kaplan: Can we use biochemical markers (or other criteria) to distinguish a mouse basophil from these two types of mast cells, and does IL-3 have anything to do with their development?

Austen: I have no information on this subject.

Ishizaka: Basophils in mice have been identified only morphologically and so far biochemical characteristics of the cells have not been characterized (A. M. Dvorak, G. Nabel, K. Pyne, H. F. Dvorak, and S. J. Galli, *Blood* **59:**1279, 1982).

CHAPTER 6

Pulmonary Mechanical Response to Leukotriene Administration *in Vivo*

A. G. LEITCH

City Hospital
and Department of Respiratory Medicine
University of Edinburgh,
Edinburgh, Scotland, U.K.

JEFFREY M. DRAZEN

Respiratory Disease Division
Brigham and Women's Hospital
Boston, Massachusetts, U.S.A.

INTRODUCTION

Slow-reacting substance of anaphylaxis (SRS-A) (1,2), a potent smooth muscle contractile activity generated during immediate-type hypersensitivity reactions, is now known to contain leukotrienes (LT) C_4, D_4, and E_4 (3–6). However, before this identification was made, it was known that infusion of partially purified SRS-A in the unanaesthetised guinea pig reduced pulmonary dynamic compliance (C_{dyn}) more than pulmonary conductance (G_L) in comparison with other agonists such as histamine and prostaglandin $F_{2\alpha}$ (7). This profile of activity was consistent with a selective peripheral airway action of SRS-A (7); a similar profile of activity was observed in one (8) of two (8,9) studies in which SRS-A was delivered by the airway route to Rhesus monkeys.

In this chapter we review the airway effects of the leukotriene constituents of SRS-A in a number of *in vivo* models. These include intravenous infusion of LTC_4, D_4, and E_4 and aerosol administration of LTC_4 in the anaesthetised, mechanically ventilated guinea pig with or without pretreatment with the cyclooxygenase inhibitor, indomethacin. In addition,

ASTHMA: Physiology,
Immunopharmacology,
and Treatment
THIRD INTERNATIONAL SYMPOSIUM

85

we have studied the effects of aerosol administration of LTC_4 and LTD_4 in normal human subjects and of aerosol administration of LTD_4 to asthmatic subjects.

STUDIES IN GUINEA PIGS

Intravenous Infusion of Leukotrienes C_4, D_4, and E_4

Intravenous infusion of 0.01–10 $\mu g/kg$ of LTC_4, LTD_4, or LTE_4 in the anaesthetised guinea pig results in dose-dependent decrements of both C_{dyn} and G_L (10,11). The interpolated dose required to achieve a 50% fall in C_{dyn} was calculated from dose–response curves and found to be 0.6, 0.3 and 1.4 $\mu g/kg$ for LTC_4, LTD_4, and LTE_4, respectively. However, the effects on G_L and C_{dyn} differed among the various leukotrienes studied. For example, the ratios of the percentage change in conductance to the percentage change in compliance (% ΔG_L/% ΔC_{dyn}) observed after intravenous infusion of LTC_4, LTD_4, or LTE_4 are 0.36, 0.56, and 1.04, respectively (11). Although the apparent sites of pulmonary response varied among leukotrienes, the time courses of the pulmonary mechanical response to intravenous infusion of LTC_4 (1 $\mu g/kg$) and LTD_4 (0.5 $\mu g/kg$) are quite similar. These are shown in Fig. 1 and are characterised by maximal decrements in G_L and C_{dyn} 30 sec after infusion; G_L returned to preinfusion values 15–20 min after infusion while C_{dyn} was still reduced 30 min after infusion.

Our results are similar to those reported by others. For example, Weichman and co-workers (12) found that intravenous infusion of LTD_4 decreased G_L and C_{dyn} in anaesthetised guinea pigs. From their data one can calculate that intravenous infusion of 1.8 μg of LTD_4 resulted in a 50% fall in C_{dyn}. Furthermore, the ratio of the percentage decrease in G_L to that of C_{dyn} was 0.80 for LTD_4. Although other workers have not measured G_L and C_{dyn} separately, the amounts of LTC_4 or LTD_4 required by intravenous infusion to increase total pulmonary impedance are similar to those required in our model (13–15).

Effect of Indomethacin on the Pulmonary Response to Intravenous LTC_4 and LTD_4

Indomethacin pretreatment (30 mg/kg ip) 1 hr before the intravenous infusion of LTC_4 (1 $\mu g/kg$) or LTD_4 (0.5 $\mu g/kg$) resulted in distinctly different patterns of pulmonary mechanical response. After indometha-

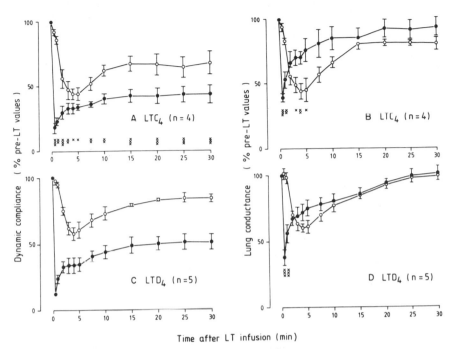

Fig. 1. Pulmonary mechanical response, measured as dynamic compliance and lung conductance and expressed as a percentage of preinfusion values, to intravenous infusion of LTC$_4$ (A and B) or LTD$_4$ (C and D) to control (●) and indomethacin pretreated (○) guinea pigs. Values shown are means ± SEM. The number of animals studied is shown in parentheses. The significance of differences between the group means is shown by *$p < .05$, $p < .01$, and $p < .001$.

cin, leukotriene infusion was accompanied by a significantly smaller decrement in C_{dyn} at all time points, but the abolition of the maximal decrement in C_{dyn} which occurred 30 sec after leukotriene infusion in control animals was more striking (Fig. 1). As a result, after indomethacin pretreatment the maximal fall in C_{dyn} occurred 5 min after the infusion. Similarly, the maximal decrement in G_L observed in control animals 30 sec after leukotriene infusion was abolished by indomethacin pretreatment (Fig. 1). Beginning 2 min after the LT infusion, however, the fall in G_L was greater in indomethacin-pretreated animals, and this difference achieved statistical significance 3–5 min after infusion of LTC$_4$ (Fig. 1) (16).

Other investigators have reported somewhat similar effects of cyclooxygenase inhibition on the pulmonary mechanical response to leukotriene infusion. For example, Weichman *et al.* (12) found that pretreat-

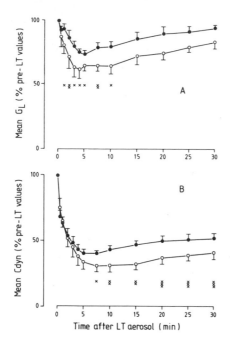

Fig. 2. Mean pulmonary response to 30 tidal breaths of LTC_4 aerosol, 1 μg/ml, before ($\bullet$) and 1 hr after ($\circ$) indomethacin 30 mg/kg ip. Values shown are mean values $\pm$ SEM for four separate experiments expressed as a percentage of preaerosol values for G_L (A) and C_{dyn} (B). Significant differences between responses are indicated by $^*p < .005$, $^{\S}p < .01$, and $^{\S}p < .001$.

ment with meclofenamic acid shifted the dose–response curve of LTD_4 on G_L and C_{dyn} to the right by one-half log. They, however, did not appreciate an enhanced G_L response after meclofenamic acid pretreatment. An inhibitory effect of cyclooxygenase inhibition on the response to intravenous infusion of LTC_4 or LTD_4 was also noted by other workers, who determined total pulmonary impedance rather than G_L or C_{dyn} separately (14,15).

Aerosol Administration of LTC_4

Aerosol administration of LTC_4 to anaesthetised mechanically ventilated guinea pigs resulted in significant dose-dependent decrements in G_L and C_{dyn} when the concentration of LTC_4 in the nebuliser jar (Collison nebuliser driven by oxygen, 20 psi at 2 litres/min) is in the range 0.5–5.0 μg/ml (17). A 50% fall in C_{dyn} resulted from inhalation of an aerosol containing 0.5 μg/ml of LTC_4. The time course of response to aerosol LTC_4 (1 μg/ml), shown in Fig. 2, is characterised by maximal falls in G_L and C_{dyn} 5 min after administration of LTC_4 with G_L returning to baseline in 15 to 20 min, while C_{dyn} remains significantly decreased at 30 min. Five minutes after aerosol exposure, the % ΔG_L/% ΔC_{dyn} ratio was 0.43.

Weichman et al. (12) and Hamel et al. (18) also examined the effects of LTD$_4$ aerosol on pulmonary mechanics in the guinea pig. The former group found that 1000-fold greater concentrations of LTD$_4$ were required to achieve a response similar to that resulting from 0.5 μg/ml of LTC$_4$ in our study. Although Hamel et al. (18) reported a similar qualitative response, their data are not quantitatively comparable.

Effect of Indomethacin on Pulmonary Response to Aerosol LTC$_4$

Indomethacin pretreatment (30 mg/kg ip) 1 hr before aerosol administration of LTC$_4$ (1 μg/ml) significantly increased the resulting decrements in G_L and C_{dyn} (Fig. 2), and at 5 min after aerosol the % ΔG_L/% ΔC_{dyn} ratio was 0.55.

Weichman et al. (12) reported similar potentiation of the pulmonary mechanical response (expressed as G_L and C_{dyn}) to aerosol administration of much higher concentrations (0.03–1 mg/ml) of LTD$_4$.

STUDIES IN HUMAN SUBJECTS

The airway effects of inhalation of leukotrienes C$_4$ and D$_4$ have been studied in normal (19,20) and asthmatic human subjects (21). In these experiments, maximal expiratory flow volume curves initiated from 60% of vital capacity were used to derive indices of airway obstruction as decrements in the flow observed at 30% of vital capacity. This particular combination of tests was used for three reasons: (a) by avoiding a maximal inspiratory manoeuvre the effects of a deep breath on induced airway constriction could be minimised; (b) by using a forced expiratory manoeuvre the effects of subject effort on the result achieved could be minimised; and (c) by measuring flows at 30% of vital capacity we could be fairly certain that the site of flow limitation in the control and bronchoconstriction studies was in the peripheral airways. In control studies, a saline aerosol was inhaled and forced expiratory manoeuvres were performed. Following these studies, 1.0 ml of solution containing a low concentration of bronchoconstrictor was placed in the reservoir of a DeVilbiss nebuliser driven by oxygen at 15–20 psi with the aerosol generator triggered for 0.8 sec by inhalation using a Rosenthal–French dosimeter. The experimental subject breathed in from the nebuliser until the reservoir was emptied and then performed forced expiratory maneuvers from 60% of vital capacity to residual volume for the next 20–60 min. If a decrease in expiratory flow at 30% of vital capacity ($\dot{V}_{30}$) to at least 70% of the control $\dot{V}_{30}$ was not achieved, the concentration of the bronchoconstrictor agent was increased and the inhalation repeated until an effect of the appropriate magnitude was achieved.

Five normal volunteers were studied with this protocol using histamine, LTC_4, or LTD_4 as the bronchoconstrictor agent. All three agents induced bronchoconstriction as evidenced by a decrement in the $\dot{V}_{30}$, but LTC_4 and LTD_4 were substantially more potent in this action than histamine. The concentrations of LTC_4 and LTD_4 in the nebuliser required to achieve a 30% reduction in $\dot{V}_{30}$ ranged from 2 to 32 μM and 1 to 9 μM, respectively. In contrast, to achieve a similar effect concentrations of histamine between 10 and 90 mM were required. Thus LTC_4 and LTD_4 were almost 4000 times more potent on a molar basis than histamine as bronchoconstrictors. Another distinction between the effects of the leukotrienes and histamine was that cough and hoarseness of voice accompanied inhalation of histamine in concentrations high enough to cause a decrease in $\dot{V}_{30}$, but these symptoms were not present after leukotriene inhalation.

Despite the similar potencies of LTC_4 and LTD_4, each of these agents had substantially different time courses of effect from each other and from histamine. After histamine inhalation, maximal effects occurred within 2 min and waned over the ensuing 15 min; the effects of LTC_4 were maximal for 10 to 20 min after inhalation and those of LTD_4 from 4 to 10 min after inhalation. Furthermore, the effects of each of these latter agents were apparent for substantially longer than those of histamine.

Our results in normal subjects are similar to those reported by Holroyde *et al.* (22) in normal subjects. Similar concentrations of leukotriene were required to achieve a response, and the overall time course was also similar. One difference observed is that these investigators reported prominent cough after leukotriene inhalation, which was not observed in our study.

Qualitatively similar effects of LTD_4 inhalation were observed in six otherwise healthy asthmatic subjects; inhalation produced a rapid onset of prolonged bronchoconstriction. An unexpected finding in this group of asthmatic subjects was the absence of the expected hyperreactivity to LTD_4. As shown in Fig. 3, airway constriction in these asthmatic subjects was induced by inhalation of 1/100 to 1/300 of the concentration of histamine required to achieve a similar overall response in normal subjects. In contrast, concentrations of LTD_4 approximately one-third of those re-

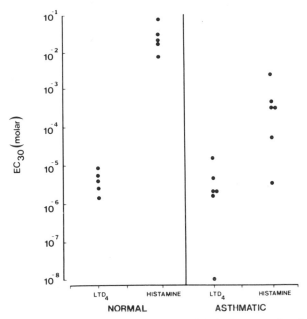

Fig. 3. Comparison of EC_{30} for histamine and LTD_4 in five normal and six asthmatic subjects.

quired in normal subjects were required to achieve a similar bronchoconstrictor response in the asthmatic subjects.

DISCUSSION

Intravenous infusion of LTC_4, LTD_4, or LTE_4, the leukotriene constituents of SRS-A, produce dose-dependent decrements of G_L and C_{dyn} in the anaesthetised mechanically ventilated guinea pig. The time course of effect is prolonged for all three leukotriene constituents, but the $\% \Delta G_L / \% \Delta C_{dyn}$ ratio is substantially lower following LTC_4 and LTD_4 than following LTE_4. A possible interpretation of these results is that, in comparison with LTE_4, LTC_4 and LTD_4 have a selective action on peripheral pulmonary tissues.

This effect may not be entirely direct; some (12,23,24) or perhaps all (14) of these pulmonary effects can be attributed to the elicited synthesis and subsequent action of cyclooxygenase products of arachidonic acid metabolism. The most likely products are PGG_2, PGH_2, TXA_2, or $PGF_{2\alpha}$ which are documented constrictors of guinea pig peripheral lung tissues *in vitro* (25) and *in vivo* (26). The modulation of the pulmonary responses resulting from LTC_4 and LTD_4 infusion by indomethacin indicates that cyclooxygenase products are important in shaping the time course and relative overall site of pulmonary response, but it is necessary to point out that LTC_4 and LTD_4 have substantial pulmonary effects independent of these pathways.

Pretreatment with indomethacin 30 mg/kg ip, a dose known to inhibit cyclooxygenase in the guinea pig (27,28), resulted in the loss of the marked initial decrease in C_{dyn} and G_L which followed infusion of LTC_4 or LTD_4. These findings suggest that synthesis and release of cyclooxygenase products such as thromboxanes and prostaglandins are responsible for the early pulmonary response to intravenous leukotrienes, the short-lived nature of the response perhaps reflecting the brief half-life of the thromboxanes *in vivo* (26,29). Indomethacin pretreatment attenuates the entire C_{dyn} response to LT infusion while augmenting the G_L response from the second minute after infusion (Fig. 1). It is possible that synthesis and release of bronchoconstrictor ($PGF_{2\alpha}$ and PGD_2) prostaglandins may contribute to the predominant and prolonged peripheral pulmonary (C_{dyn}) response following LT infusion. Another possibility is that the prolonged C_{dyn} response reflects the effect of nonuniform peripheral airway narrowing or closure resulting from the initial cyclooxygenase dependent pulmonary insult under the circumstances of mechanical ventilation at a constant tidal volume, the consequences of which could persist even in the absence of an on-going pharmacological effect. The augmented G_L response seen in the indomethacin-treated animals resembles the potentiation by indomethacin of the tracheal contractile response to histamine, acetylcholine, and LTs reported by others (30–32), which has been attributed to inhibition of local formation of PGE_2 (33,34) that could exert a bronchodilator effect in opposition to the contractile agonists (35).

The source of the released cyclooxygenase products that facilitate and attenuate the immediate and subsequent pulmonary mechanical responses is not known. Indomethacin has a small effect on the guinea pig pulmonary parenchymal and airway responses to leukotrienes *in vitro* (32,36), suggesting that the lungs are not a major source. Other possible sources include blood components, particularly platelets (37), and the vascular tree. A further unresolved issue is the exact stimulus for this synthesis of cyclooxygenase products. It is unlikely to be airway constriction *per se* because the mechanical response precedes the underlying direct leukotriene response. The most likely stimulus is an effect of the leukotrienes on arachidonic acid production independent of any contractile effects, although this possibility still remains speculative.

Inhibition of cyclooxygenase by indomethacin pretreatment reveals a residual pulmonary response to intravenous LTs that is slow in onset, peaks at 4 to 5 min, and persists for 15 to 30 min. In the presence of indomethacin, the percentage changes in C_{dyn} and G_L are similar following infusion of both LTC_4 and LTD_4. Thus, cyclooxygenase inhibition reveals a primary pulmonary effect of intravenous leukotrienes that is less suggestive of a predominant peripheral airways response.

Aerosol administration of LTC_4 to guinea pigs also produced dose-dependent decrements in C_{dyn} and G_L which differed significantly from the effects of intravenously administered LTC_4 by the absence of a marked early (<1 min) pulmonary response. The absence of this early response, which is attributable to bronchoconstrictor cyclooxygenase products released in response to LTC_4 infusion, suggested that such products do not contribute to the pulmonary response to LTC_4 aerosol.

The maximal decrements in G_L and C_{dyn} produced by LTC_4 aerosol (1 μg/ml) (26 and 60%, respectively) were significantly potentiated by indomethacin, reaching 40 and 70%, respectively (Fig. 2). This finding is consistent with generation of a bronchodilator cyclooxygenase product, such as PGE_2, as part of the overall leukotriene response. No component of the pulmonary mechanical response to aerosol LTC_4 was inhibited by the indomethacin in contrast to the findings in the first minute following intravenous administration where the decrements in C_{dyn} and G_L were markedly attenuated by indomethacin pretreatment. If only maximal changes in G_L and C_{dyn} are considered, irrespective of time after administration of LTC_4, the predominant effect of indomethacin is to potentiate the responses to aerosol and to inhibit the responses to intravenous treatment. Thus, thromboxane release, believed to be important in the pulmonary response to intravenous leukotrienes (23), is probably not implicated when leukotrienes are administered by the airway route to guinea pigs.

The % ΔG_L/% ΔC_{dyn} ratio following aerosol LTC_4 was 0.43 without and 0.55 with indomethacin pretreatment, a finding consistent with a predominant action in the pulmonary periphery in both situations. This contrasts with the findings following intravenous administration of LTC_4 in which indomethacin pretreatment substantially altered the ratio from 0.35 to 1.0. The differences may reflect involvement of nonpulmonary cells with intravenous administration, different distributions of LTC_4 throughout the lung or differential rates of metabolism throughout the lung.

There are substantial similarities between the guinea pig and human studies. The leukotrienes produce a potent and prolonged bronchoconstriction in both studies. The time course of onset and resolution is comparable to that elicited by inhaled antigen in each species and is compatible with the leukotrienes having a causative role in allergic asthma. Our findings in asthmatic subjects may also be interpreted in this regard. For example, based on our findings in the normal and asthmatic subjects it is possible that leukotrienes act in such a manner as to enhance the response to other inhaled bronchoconstrictors.

ACKNOWLEDGMENTS

This work was supported in part by grants AI-07722, HC-17382, and RR-05669 from the National Institute of Health, and in part by a grant from the National Science Foundation. AGL was in receipt of Medical Research Council and Wellcome Trust Travelling Fellowships. The secretarial assistance of Miss Joyce Holywell is gratefully acknowledged.

REFERENCES

1. Kellaway, C. H., and Trethewie, E. R. The liberation of a slow-reacting smooth muscle stimulating substance in anaphylaxis. *Q. J. Exp. Physiol. Cogn. Med. Sci.* **30:**121–145, 1940.
2. Brocklehurst, W. E. The release of histamine and formation of a slow reacting substance (SRS-A) during anaphylactic shock. *J. Physiol. (London)* **151:**416–435, 1960.
3. Murphy, R. C., Hammarström, S., and Samuelsson, B. Leukotriene C: A slow reacting substance from murine mastocytoma cells. *Proc. Natl. Acad. Sci. U.S.A.* **76:**4275–4279, 1979.
4. Morris, H. R., Taylor, G. W., Piper, P. J., and Tippins, J. R. Structure of slow reacting substance of anaphylaxis from guinea pig lung. *Nature (London)* **285:**104–106, 1980.
5. Lewis, R. A., Austen, K. F., Drazen, J. M., Clark, D. A., Marfat, A., and Corey, E. J. Slow reacting substance of anaphylaxis: Identification of leukotrienes C_1 and D from human and rat sources. *Proc. Natl. Acad. Sci. U.S.A.* **77:**3710–3714, 1980.
6. Lewis, R. A., Drazen, J. M., Austen, K. F., Clark, D. A., and Corey, E. J. Identification of the C-(6)-S-conjugate of leukotriene A with cysteine as a naturally occurring slow reacting substance of anaphylaxis. Importance of the 11-cis geometry for biological activity. *Biochem. Biophys. Res. Commun.* **96:**271–277, 1980.
7. Drazen, J. M., and Austen, K. F. Effect of intravenous administration of slow-reacting substance of anaphylaxis, histamine, bradykinin and prostaglandin $F_{2\alpha}$ on pulmonary mechanics in the guinea pig. *J. Clin. Invest.* **53:**1679–1685, 1974.
8. Michoud, M.-C., Pare, P. D., Orange, R. P., and Hogg, J. D. Airway sensitivity to slow reacting substance of anaphylaxis, histamine and antigen in ascaris sensitive monkeys. *Am. Rev. Respir. Dis.* **119:**419–424, 1979.
9. Patterson, R., Orange, R. P., and Harris, K. E. A study of the effects of slow reacting substance of anaphylaxis on the rhesus monkey airway. *J. Allergy Clin. Immunol.* **62:**371–377, 1978.
10. Drazen, J. M., Austen, K. F., Lewis, R. A., Clark, D. A., Goto, G., Marfat, A., and Corey, E. J. Comparative airway and vascular activities of leukotrienes C_1 and D *in vivo* and *in vitro*. *Proc. Natl. Acad. Sci. U.S.A.* **77:**4354–4358, 1980.
11. Drazen, J. M., Venugopalan, C. S., Austen, K. F., Brion, F., and Corey, E. J. Effects of leukotriene E on pulmonary mechanics in the guinea pig. *Am. Rev. Respir. Dis.* **125:**290–294, 1982.

12. Weichman, B. M., Muccitelli, R. M., Osborn, R. R., Holden, D. A., Gleason, J. G., and Wasserman, M. A. *In vitro* and *in vivo* mechanisms of leukotriene-mediated broncho-constriction in the guinea pig. *J. Pharmacol. Exp. Ther.* **222:**202–208, 1982.

13. Hedqvist, P., Dahlen, S.-E., Gustafsson, L., Hammarström, S., and Samuelsson, B. Biological profile of leukotrienes C_4 and D_4. *Acta Physiol. Scand.* **110:**331–333, 1980.

14. Vargaftig, B. B., Lefort, J., and Murphy, R. C. Inhibition by aspirin of bronchoconstriction due to leukotrienes C_4 and D_4 in the guinea pig. *Eur. J. Pharmacol.* **72:**417–418, 1981.

15. Schiantarelli, P., Bongrani, S., and Folco, G. Bronchospasm and pressor effects induced in the guinea pig by leukotriene C_4 are probably due to release of cyclo-oxygenase products. *Eur. J. Pharmacol.* **73:**363–366, 1981.

16. Leitch, A. G., Austen, K. F., Corey, E. J., and Drazen, J. M. Inhibition of the pulmonary effects of leukotriene D_4 by indomethacin in the anaesthetised guinea pig. *Am. Rev. Respir. Dis.* **125**(2):66, 1982.

17. Leitch, A. G., Corey, E. J., Austen, K. F., and Drazen, J. M. Indomethacin potentiates the pulmonary response to aerosol leukotriene C_4 in the guinea pig. *Clin. Res.* (in press).

18. Hamel, R., Masson, P., Ford-Hutchinson, A. W., Jones, T. R., Brunet, G., and Piechuta, H. Differing mechanisms for leukotriene D_4-induced bronchoconstriction in guinea pigs following intravenous aerosol administration. *Prostaglandins* **24:**419–432, 1982.

19. Weiss, J. W., Drazen, J. M., Coles, N., McFadden, E. R., Weller, P. F., Corey, E. J., Lewis, R. A., and Austen, K. F. Bronchoconstrictor effects of leukotriene C in humans. *Science* **216:**196–198, 1982.

20. Weiss, J. W., Drazen, J. M., McFadden, E. R., Weller, P. F., Corey, E. J., Lewis, R. A., and Austen, K. F. Comparative bronchoconstrictor effects of histamine, leukotriene C and leukotriene D in normal human volunteers. *Trans. Am. Assoc. Physicians* (in press).

21. Griffin, M. D., Weiss, J. W., Leitch, A. G., McFadden, E. R., Corey, E. J., Austen, K. F., and Drazen, J. M. Airway effects of leukotriene D in asthma. *N. Engl. J. Med.* **308:**436–439, 1983.

22. Holroyde, M. C., Altounyan, R. E. C., Cole, M., Dixon, M., and Elliot, E. V. Bronchoconstriction produced in man by leukotrienes C and D. *Lancet* **2:**17–18, 1981.

23. Omini, C., Folco, T., Vigano, T., Rossoni, G., Brunelli, G., and Berti, F. Leukotriene C_4 induces generation of PGI_2 and TXA_2 in guinea pig *in vivo*. *Pharmacol. Res. Commun.* **13:**633–640, 1981.

24. Piper, P. J., and Samhoun, M. N. The mechanism of action of leukotriene C_4 and D_4 in guinea pig isolated perfused lung and parenchymal strips of guinea pigs, rabbit and rat. *Prostaglandins* **21:**793–803, 1981.

25. Schneider, M. W., and Drazen, J. M. Comparative *in vitro* effects of arachidonic acid metabolism on tracheal spirals and parenchymal strips. *Am. Rev. Respir. Dis.* **121:**835–842, 1980.

26. Hamberg, M., Hedqvist, P., Strandberg, K., Svensson, J., and Samuelsson, B. Prostaglandin endoperoxides IV Effects on smooth muscle. *Life Sci.* **16:**451–462, 1975.

27. Brink, C., Ridgway, P., and Douglas, J. S. Regulation of guinea pig airways *in vivo* by endogenous prostaglandins. *Pol. J. Pharmacol. Pharm.* **30:**157, 1978.

28. Orehek, J., Douglas, J. S., Lewis, A. J., and Bouhuys, A. Contractile responses of the guinea pig trachea *in vitro* Modification by prostaglandin synthesis inhibiting drugs. *J. Pharmacol. Exp. Ther.* **194:**554–564, 1975.

29. Hamberg, M., Svensson, J., and Samuelsson, B. Thromboxanes: A new group of biologically active compounds derived from prostaglandin endoperoxides. *Proc. Natl. Acad. Sci. U.S.A.* **72:**2294–2298, 1975.

30. Adcock, J. J., and Garland, L. G. A possible role for lipoxygenase products as regulator of airway smooth muscle reactivity. *Br. J. Pharmacol.* **69:**167–169, 1980.
31. Brink, C., Duncan, P. G., and Douglas, J. S. Histamine, endogenous prostaglandins and cyclic nucleotides in the regulation of airway muscle responses in the guinea pig. *Prostaglandins* **22:**729–738, 1981.
32. Krell, R. D., Osborn, G., Vickery, L., Falcone, K., O'Donnell, M., Gleason, J., Kinzig, C., and Bryan, D. Contraction of isolated airway smooth muscle by synthetic leukotrienes C_4 and D_4. *Prostaglandins* **22:**387–407, 1981.
33. Burka, J. F., Ali, M., McDonald, J. W. D., and Paterson, N. A. M. Immunological and non-immunological synthesis and release of prostaglandins from isolated guinea pig trachea. *Prostaglandins* **22:**683–691, 1981.
34. Grodzinsak, L., Panczenko, B., and Bryglewski, R. J. Generation of prostaglandin E like material by the guinea pig trachea contracted by histamine. *J. Pharm. Pharmacol.* **27:**88–91, 1975.
35. Orehek, J., Douglas, J. S., Lewis, A. J., and Bouhuys, A. Prostaglandin regulation of airway smooth muscle tone. *Nature (London)* **245:**84–85, 1973.
36. Leitch, A. G., Austen, K. F., Corey, E. J., and Drazen, J. M. Effect of indomethacin on the contractile response of guinea pig lung parenchymal strips to leukotrienes B_4, C_4, D_4 and E_4. *Fed. Proc., Fed. Am. Soc. Exp. Biol.* **41:**1047, 1982.
37. Hammarström, S., and Falardeau, P. Resolution of prostaglandin endoperoxide synthase and thromboxane synthase of human platelets. *Proc. Natl. Acad. Sci. U.S.A.* **74:**3691–3695, 1977.

DISCUSSION

Adams: Does indomethacin potentiate the response of guinea pigs to inhaled histamine?

Leitch: I have not studied that. Indomethacin does not, however, potentiate intravenous histamine dose–response curves in the *in vivo* guinea pig preparation.

Piper: Do you have any positive evidence for the release of a bronchodilator cyclooxygenase product by leukotrienes in guinea pig? An alternative explanation for the potentiating effects of indomethacin when leukotrienes are inhaled is the release of a bronchoconstrictor lipoxygenase product.

Leitch: No measurements of PGE_2 have been made *in vivo* but PGE_2 is known to be released from guinea pig trachea *in vitro* in response to a number of agonists including leukotrienes. We are confident that the bronchoconstrictor cyclooxygenase component of the response is due to TxA_2. Others, including Omini *et al.,* have measured TxA_2 and found increases following LTC_4 infusion to the guinea pig (C. Omini, T. Folco, T. Vigano, G. Rossoni, G. Brunelli, and F. Berti, *Pharmacol. Res. Commun.* **13:**633, 1980).

Lichtenstein: Does the fact that there is not an immediate fall in FEV_1 in man following leukotriene inhalation imply that the putative cyclooxygenase product exists in the guinea pig and not humans?

Leitch: The immediate (<1 min) deterioration following leukotriene administration is seen only following iv infusion to the guinea pig. Aerosol administration to both guinea pigs and man results in slowly developing and prolonged deterioration in pulmonary function. Obviously we have no data on iv infusion in man.

Kay: You showed that the effects of LTD_4, administered by aerosols to humans, was still demonstrable at 30 min. How long did this take to revert to prechallenge values?

McFadden: As I recollect Dr. Drazen's data, the effect lasted 30–40 min. A few patients had to be given a bronchodilator.

Lessof: Can you speculate on the reason why you did not find a hyperreactive bronchial response to leukotrienes in asthmatics?

Leitch: We have no definite explanation for this and I would like to see some further studies before committing myself. However, if the observation is substantiated, then LTD_4 is the only mediator so far described to which asthmatics are not hyperreactive and so it is tempting to speculate, perhaps somewhat illogically, that LTD_4 may have a primary role in causing bronchial hyperreactivity.

Hogg: The changes in conductance which you describe for the guinea pig could be influenced by lung volume. Did you control for lung volume in these studies?

Leitch: Lung volume was not controlled for in the guinea pigs, which were ventilated at a fixed tidal volume and inflation pressure. Changes in lung volume were not studied in detail in the present investigation but Jeff Drazen has previously published data on lung volume changes following antigen challenge (J. M. Drazen and K. F. Austen, *J. Appl. Physiol.* **39:**916, 1975).

Tattersfield: Some of the differences between the asthmatic and normal subjects with respect to inhaled histamine and LTD_4 could be due to differences in the distribution of the stimulus. It is known that with increasing airway obstruction more of the inhaled stimulus is deposited centrally, rather than peripherally. Thus in the asthmatic subjects you would expect a relatively smaller effect with LTD_4 if it is acting peripherally than with histamine which is thought to act centrally. Less of the LTD_4 will actually reach the appropriate receptors in these patients.

Leitch: One possible explanation for the absence of hyperreactivity to LTD_4 is that LTD_4 is delivered preferentially to one part of the lung and that bronchial hyperreactivity resides in another part of the lung. This seems unlikely, however, since the nebulizer we used should have delivered LTD_4 to all parts of the lung.

McFadden: I think Dr. Tattersfield has raised an important point. The effect of the leukotrienes could possibly be related to their site of action or there could be an interaction with some other constrictors.

Hogg: The data on intravenous infusion in the guinea pig is consistent with alveolar duct constriction with resulting fall in compliance. This should produce a decrease in lung volume and the changes in conductance could be secondary to that. If you say there is no change in volume, it suggests constriction of membranous bronchioles and this surprises me, because I would expect that these airways could be perfused by the bronchial rather than the pulmonary circulation.

Nadel: You speculate that leukotrienes may actually be responsible for the increased responsiveness that occurs in asthma. Do you imply that leukotrienes do not act by ''pharmacomechanical coupling'' in the muscle (as other agonists are purported to act)? If leukotrienes cause increased responsiveness they should increase the responsiveness to histamine. Do they?

Leitch: I have no doubt that the bronchoconstrictor activity of the sulfidopeptide leukotrienes is receptor-mediated, possibly by discrete receptors for each leukotriene. The sulfidopeptide leukotrienes have other activities, some identified, such as their effects on permeability and the microcirculation and probably others as yet unidentified. The latter activities could conceivably result in bronchial hyperreactivity.

Bach: In collaboration with Dr. H. G. Johnson at our laboratories, we have been studying the effect of aerosolized leukotrienes on pulmonary mechanics in the rhesus monkey. Three points need to be made. First, the duration of action is as long as 2 to 3 hr; second, depending on mode of administration, changes in compliance are by far greater than changes in resistance; and third, both diphenhydramine and mepyramine, at relatively low doses given iv, markedly inhibit the response to the leukotrienes. Indomethacin has a slight but statistically nonsignificant stimulatory effect.

Clark: What were the clinical effects of inhaled leukotrienes? In particular, did you observe cough?

Leitch: In our studies with both normal and asthmatic subjects histamine produced cough and irritation but the leukotrienes did not. This finding conflicts with the original report by Holroyde *et al.* that leukotriene-induced bronchoconstriction in normal man was associated with significant cough (M. A. Holroyde, R. E. C. Altounyan, M. Cole, M. Dixon, and E. V. Elliot, *Lancet* **2:**17, 1981). We are unable to explain these differences.

Schiffmann: It is possible that the phenomenon of hypo- and/or hypersensitivity to leukotrienes may be related to the "up" or "down" regulation of receptors for these compounds. This could be determined by measuring the number and affinity of receptors for leukotrienes.

Pride: Is there any evidence of a differential effect of leukotrienes on the different sizes of airways in man? Would measuring specific conductance alter the apparent relative potency of histamine and leukotrienes as bronchoconstrictors in humans? The $\dot{V}_{30}$ predominantly measures effects on the small airways.

McFadden: We have not yet systematically evaluated this area.

Morley: Guinea pig tissues are relatively sensitive to inhibition of the cyclooxygenase enzyme by indomethacin (M. A. Bray and D. Gordon, *Br. J. Pharmacol.* **63:**635, 1978). I wonder, therefore, why such a large dose of indomethacin was used in your study. Does this dose of indomethacin affect responses to any other stimulus that is putatively independent of cyclooxygenase involvement?

Leitch: We used 30 mg/kg because Douglas and his co-workers have shown that this was the concentration necessary to inhibit cyclooxygenase in the guinea pig *in vivo* (C. Brink, P. Ridgway, and J. S. Douglas, *Pol. J. Pharmacol. Pharm.* **30:**157, 1978). Small doses (3 mg/kg) had qualitatively similar effects which did not achieve statistical significance. There is no published evidence that any noncyclooxygenase system would be affected by the doses we used.

Austen: The administration of aspirin did not change the response of normal humans to inhalation of leukotrienes C or D, indicating that the role of cyclooxygenase products was not significant as compared with the studies in the guinea pig.

Piper: I think leukotrienes are stimulating release of cyclooxygenase products in guinea pig lung by activating a phospholipase, probably PLA_2, because in isolated lung preparations from guinea pig, which closely resemble the situation when LTs are given intravenously, the LT-induced release of TxA_2 was blocked by mepacrine as well as by indomethacin.

Leitch: I think that this is a very reasonable suggestion. Have you looked at the effect of mepacrine *in vivo*?

Piper: No.

Kay: How reproducible, in terms of magnitude and duration of effect, is leukotriene inhalation in a single individual? There seemed to be a wide scatter of responsiveness in the small number of subjects that you studied.

Leitch: Although there was some variation in the duration of bronchoconstrictor response to inhaled leukotrienes in both normal and asthmatic subjects, the responses were reproducible within subjects. The concentration of leukotriene selected for the duration studies was the concentration which produced a 30% fall in FEV_1 in the dose response studies in the same subject, and the magnitude of this effect was also remarkably reproducible.

Austen: The response in an individual subject was reproducible based upon inhalation of the maximum dose on separate days. This contrasted with the marked subject to subject variation to inhaled leukotrienes.

Kaliner: I am concerned about the interpretation of your human leukotriene effects. Is it possible that your lack of hyperreactivity to leukotrienes reflects the test employed? Flow at 30% avoids a volume history which Orehek has shown to be a major reason normals do not hyperreact (J. Orehek, M. M. Nicoli, S. Delpierre, and A. Beaupre, *Am. Rev. Respir. Dis.* **123:**269, 1981). Thus, is your lack of hyperreactivity real, can you see hyperreactivity to methacholine with this test, and is the hyperreactivity to histamine you displayed in the same range as seen with other measures of reactivity?

Leitch: The volume history was the same for LTD_4 and histamine in both the normals and asthmatics.

McFadden: We do not yet know if there are differences in the volume history effects among the various leukotrienes or between them and histamine.

CHAPTER 7

Arachidonic Acid Metabolism and Airway Smooth Muscle*

G. KENNETH ADAMS III, STEPHEN P. PETERS, and
LAWRENCE M. LICHTENSTEIN

Clinical Immunology Division
The Johns Hopkins University School of Medicine
at the Good Samaritan Hospital
Baltimore, Maryland, U.S.A.

INTRODUCTION

Asthma is a multifactoral disease for which there is no specific treatment. The functionally significant changes in the mechanical properties of the lungs that characterize an acute asthmatic episode most likely result from the direct and reflex effects of endogenous chemicals on tracheobronchial smooth muscle. These chemicals are, at least in part, released from airway mast cells. Identifying the principal chemical mediators involved and defining the mechanisms regulating their synthesis and release within airway tissue is essential in order to develop effectively targeted procedures for the management of asthma.

Isolated sensitized airways studied under carefully regulated *in vitro* conditions have proven to be particularly useful model systems for the investigation of the immunopharmacological fundamentals of anaphylactic bronchospasm. The classic experiments of Schultz (1) and Dale (2) established that exposure of sensitized smooth muscle preparations to specific antigen results in a forceful and persistent contraction. Subsequent investigations by Rosa and McDowall (3) and Schild *et al.* (4)

* Supported in part by grant No. HL-30132 from the National Heart, Lung and Blood Institute, National Institutes of Health, U.S. Public Health Service.

ASTHMA: Physiology,
Immunopharmacology,
and Treatment
THIRD INTERNATIONAL SYMPOSIUM

101

showed that airways from human asthmatic subjects studied postmortem contract when exposed to antigens which produced bronchospasm *in vivo*. Since the release of histamine from the airway tissue was found to accompany the contraction, it was suggested that histamine might mediate the response. This hypothesis, however, was not supported by experiments with antihistamines, since very high concentrations of antagonists failed to block the response of sensitized human (4) and guinea pig (5) airways to antigen while ablating the response to exogenous histamine.

More recent studies have demonstrated that histamine mediates only the initial, rapid increase in smooth muscle tone that follows exposure of sensitized airways to antigen. The later, prolonged phase of the response is not affected by antihistamines but is blocked or reversed by the slow-reacting substance (SRS-A) or leukotriene antagonist FPL 55712 (6–8). The combination of an antihistamine and FPL 55712 administered prior to antigen reduces the amplitude and duration of antigen-induced contraction, affecting both the early and late phases in a dose-related manner. Although complete blockade has been observed, the inhibition is usually incomplete and characterized by a low-amplitude, short-duration "intermediate" phase. This chapter will deal with additional studies on the control of antigen-induced bronchospasm, focusing on the role of arachidonic acid metabolism.

EFFECT OF CYCLOOXYGENASE INHIBITORS

Antigen challenge of human bronchial tissue (9,10) or guinea pig trachea (11) *in vitro* results in the generation of a number of cyclooxygenase (CO) metabolites of arachidonic acid, including PGE_2 and PGI_2, which may act as bronchodilators, and $PGF_{2\alpha}$, PGD_2, and TxA_2, which are bronchoconstrictors (12). In order to explore the possibility that the "intermediate" phase may reflect the involvement of bronchoconstrictor prostaglandins, we have studied the effect of inhibitors of the CO pathway on anaphylactic bronchospasm *in vitro* (13,14).

Treatment of passively sensitized human segmental and subsegmental bronchial strips with indomethacin (3 μM, 30-min incubation) reduced the anaphylactic production of CO metabolites to less than 10% of control, but significantly increased the amplitude of antigen-induced bronchoconstriction, as shown in Fig. 1. Both early (histamine dependent) and late (leukotriene dependent) phases of the contraction were potentiated. Other CO inhibitors, including aspirin and RO 20-5720, produced comparable augmentation of human airway anaphylactic bronchospasm.

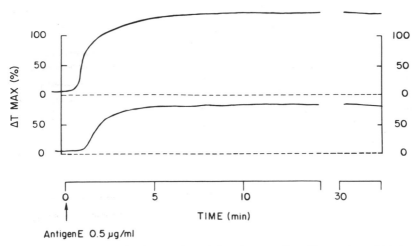

Fig. 1. Effect of indomethacin on antigen-induced contraction of human bronchial strips. Lower tracing is control response to antigen, and tissue depicted in upper tracing was treated with 3 μM indomethacin for 30 min before antigen administration. Note that indomethacin potentiated both early and late phases of anaphylactic bronchospasm, as indicated by the increased contraction amplitude at 3 and 30 min, respectively. T_{max} defined as response to 1 mM methacholine.

Burka and Paterson (15,16) and Hitchcock (17) have demonstrated that CO inhibitors potentiate antigen-induced contraction of tracheal spirals obtained from actively sensitized guinea pigs. Using tracheal rings from passively sensitized guinea pigs, we found that indomethacin (3 μM, 30-min incubation) significantly increased the amplitude of anaphylactic bronchospasm over a wide range of antigen concentrations (Fig. 2). As in the human airway model, both phases of contraction were significantly enhanced. Furthermore, indomethacin (in combination with diphenhydramine and FPL 55712) potentiated the "intermediate" phase of antigen-induced contraction of human bronchial strips and guinea pig tracheal rings (data not shown), suggesting that CO products do not mediate that phase of bronchospasm.

CO inhibitors have been shown to affect several components of the isolated airway system. Orehek *et al.* (18) have reported that indomethacin and aspirin potentiate the response of guinea pig tracheal spirals to high concentrations of histamine, serotonin, acetylcholine, barium, and potassium. They concluded that released prostaglandins may modulate the intensity of the contraction. More recent studies by Adcock and Garland (19) and Mitchell (20,21) have suggested that the potentiation may reflect the diversion of arachidonic acid to the lipoxygenase (LO) path-

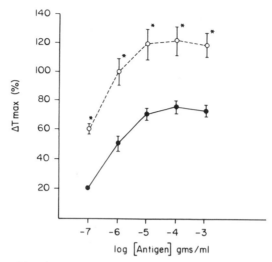

Fig. 2. Effect of indomethacin on antigen-induced contraction of guinea pig tracheal rings. Tension change was measured at 3 min following antigen administration. Indomethacin, 3 μM (O---O); control (●——●). Each data point (mean ± SEM) represents the results from six experiments. Asterisk (*), significantly different from control ($p < .01$, Wilcoxon–Mann–Whitney rank-sum test).

way, favoring the formation of an LO product which facilitates airway smooth muscle contraction.

Similar studies have been carried out with human airways *in vitro.* Brink *et al.* (22) found no evidence of enhanced responsiveness to contractile agonists following CO inhibition in large human bronchi, whereas Adcock and Garland (23) demonstrated potentiation to histamine following indomethacin treatment in small (internal diameter, <3 mm) but not large (internal diameter, 5–8 mm) human bronchi. They also reported that BW 755C and CLI, inhibitors of both the CO and LO pathways, did not enhance histamine responsiveness and did reverse the indomethacin-induced potentiation in small airways. We have found that indomethacin, aspirin, and RO 20-5720 do not increase the response of segmental and subsegmental (internal diameter, >3 mm) human bronchi to histamine, although they dramatically enhance antigen-induced contraction (13,14).

The effect of CO inhibitors on anaphylactic mediator release has been evaluated in many experimental systems, and most studies have demonstrated that these agents augment the release of SRS-A (17,24–28). A concomitant increase in histamine release has been reported in some (17,24–26) but not all (28) cases. In order to further explore the mechanisms underlying the potentiation of anaphylactic bronchospasm by CO

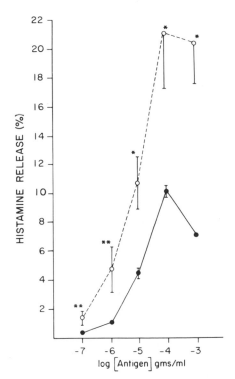

Fig. 3. Effect of indomethacin (3 μM) on antigen-induced histamine release from guinea pig tracheal rings. Percentage of histamine released during a 20-min incubation period following antigen is plotted as a function of antigen concentration. Indomethacin (O---O); control (●——●). Each data point (mean ± SEM) represents the results from at least five experiments. Asterisk (*), significantly different from control ($p < .01$, Wilcoxon–Mann–Whitney rank-sum test); **, significantly different from control ($p < .05$).

inhibitors, we studied the effect of indomethacin on antigen-induced histamine release from airway tissue.

Inhibition of the CO pathway resulted in significant potentiation of histamine release from sensitized human bronchus and guinea pig trachea. In studies with human bronchial strips, indomethacin (3 μM, 30 min incubation) increased histamine release from 8.3 ± 1.3% to 15.6 ± 4.8% (mean ± SEM, $n = 5$). In similar studies with guinea pig trachea, indomethacin significantly potentiated histamine release at every antigen concentration studied (Fig. 3). Although we did not directly measure SRS-A (or leukotriene) release from the airway tissue, potentiation of the FPL 55712-sensitive component of the contraction by CO inhibitors is consistent with an increase in SRS-A generation, particularly with regard to the human bronchial studies, in which smooth muscle responsiveness *per se* was not modified.

The mechanism(s) by which CO inhibitors potentiate anaphylactic mediator release from airway tissue is not clear. Adcock *et al.* (26,29) have studied the effect of inhibitors of arachidonic acid metabolism on mediator release from guinea pig lung. They found that indomethacin augmented release, but CLI did not. They concluded that enhancement of release involves diversion of arachidonic acid to the LO pathway, possibly resulting in the increased production of a hydroperoxy eicosatetraenoic acid which promotes mediator release. Numerous subsequent reports have provided evidence implicating the LO pathways in the release process (30–32).

In regard to the airway, however, the hypothesis that airway mast cell function is regulated by endogenous prostaglandins must be considered. This possibility is supported by the observations that PGE_2 inhibits anaphylactic histamine release from human lung fragments (33) and partially purified human lung mast cells (32). Since PGE_2 is a major metabolite of arachidonic acid generated by human bronchus (9,10) and guinea pig trachea (11), inhibition of the CO pathway would abolish this inhibitory input and might thereby facilitate mediator release.

EFFECT OF LIPOXYGENASE INHIBITORS

We have found that 5,8,11,14-eicosatetraynoic acid (ETYA, 30–100 μM), which blocks both the CO and LO pathways (34), inhibits both the early and late phases of antigen-induced contraction of human and guinea pig airways (Fig. 4). The drug did not interfere with the response of airway smooth muscle to histamine or methacholine, but produced a dose-dependent inhibition of anaphylactic histamine release from the airway tissue (13,35). Because agents that block the CO pathway alone enhance mediator release, the inhibition by ETYA probably results from altered metabolism of arachidonic acid metabolism through the LO pathway. ETYA has been shown to inhibit histamine release from several other tissues, including human basophils (30), and Paterson *et al.* have shown that ETYA inhibits both histamine and SRS-A release from antigen-challenged dispersed pig lung cells (28).

Somewhat in contrast to the effect of ETYA, 1-phenyl-3-pyrazolidone (phenidone, 50 μM), another inhibitor of both the CO and LO pathways (36), preferentially inhibited the late phase of antigen-induced bronchoconstriction (Fig. 5). In addition to phenidone, several other LO inhibitors, including BW 755C and nordihydroguaiaretic acid have shown late-phase selectivity. Each of these compounds demonstrates at least 10-fold greater potency for the late phase of anaphylactic bronchospasm than for the early phase.

Phenidone has been shown to inhibit SRS-A production in dispersed pig lung cells without significantly reducing histamine release (28). Nordihy-

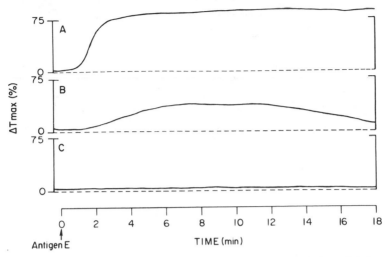

Fig. 4. Effect of ETYA on response of human bronchial strips to antigen E (0.5 μg/ml). Passively sensitized human bronchial tissue was incubated with ETYA for 5 min before antigen administration. (A) Control, duration = 120 min; (B) ETYA, 30 μM; (C) ETYA, 100 μM.

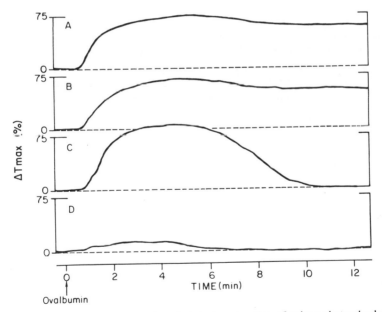

Fig. 5. Effect of phenidone on antigen-induced contraction of guinea pig tracheal rings. Actively sensitized guinea pig tracheal tissue was incubated with phenidone for 5 min before antigen administration (ovalbumin, 0.1 μg/ml). Note that 50 μM phenidone blocked the late (leukotriene-dependent) phase of the contraction without inhibiting the early (histamine-dependent) phase. (A) Control, duration = 83 mm; (B) phenidone, 5 μM; (C) phenidone, 50 μM; (D) phenidone, 500 μM.

droguaiaretic acid and BW 755C inhibit SRS-A release in guinea pig lung (37), and Saad *et al.* have reported that nordihydroguaiaretic acid inhibits the release of LTC_4-like material from guinea pig trachea (38). Furthermore, all of these compounds are potent inhibitors of 5-HETE formation in guinea pig polymorphonuclear leukocytes (W. Pickett, personal communication). The late phase selectivity of these LO inhibitors may, therefore, be the result of physiologically significant inhibition of leukotriene synthesis without comparable inhibition of histamine release from airway mast cells.

SUMMARY

The response of sensitized airways to antigen *in vitro* is a complex process involving multiple mast cell-derived mediators acting upon airway smooth muscle cells to produce a characteristically persistent contraction. Both bronchoconstrictor as well as bronchodilator prostaglandins are released from the airway tissue during anaphylaxis, but functional roles for specific prostaglandins have not been determined. Nevertheless, the results from a wide range of studies with inhibitors suggest that CO pathway products restrain the anaphylactic reaction in some manner, perhaps by modulating both airway smooth muscle responsiveness and mast cell mediator release. Arachidonic acid metabolism through the LO pathway, however, appears to be central to antigen-induced bronchospasm, as it is essential for the biosynthesis of the sulfidopeptide leukotrienes, and LO products may be required for mast cell activation. The LO pathway, therefore, may prove to be a particularly vulnerable link in the pathogenic process and provide a basis for the development of novel and effective drugs for the treatment of asthma.

REFERENCES

1. Schultz, W. H. Physiological studies in anaphylaxis. I. The reaction of smooth muscle of the guinea pig sensitized with horse serum. *J. Pharmacol. Exp. Ther.* **1**:549–567, 1910.
2. Dale, H. H. The anaphylactic reaction of plain muscle in the guinea pig. *J. Pharmacol. Exp. Ther.* **4**:167–223, 1913.
3. Rosa, L. M., and McDowall, R. J. S. The action of local hormones on the isolated human bronchus. *Acta Allergol.* **4**:293–304, 1951.
4. Schild, H. O., Hawkins, D. F., Mongar, J. L., and Herxheimer, H. Reactions of isolated human asthmatic lung and bronchial tissue to a specific antigen. Histamine release and muscular contraction. *Lancet* **2**:376–382, 1951.
5. Castillo, J. D. The tracheal chain. II. The anaphylactic guinea pig trachea and its response to antihistamine and drugs. *J. Pharmacol. Exp. Ther.* **94**:412–415, 1948.

6. Adams, G. K., Lichtenstein, L. M. Antagonism of antigen-induced contraction of guinea pig and human airways. *Nature (London)* **270:**255–257, 1977.
7. Adams, G. K., III, and Lichtenstein, L. M. *In vitro* studies of antigen-induced broncho-spasm: Effect of antihistamine and SRS-A antagonist on response of sensitized guinea pig and human airways to antigen. *J. Immunol.* **122:**555–562, 1979.
8. Adams, G. K., III *In vitro* studies of antigen-induced bronchospasm. *Monogr. Allergy* **14:**95–105, 1979.
9. Adkinson, N. F., Jr., Newball, H. H., Findlay, S. Adams, K., and Lichtenstein, L. M. Anaphylactic release of prostaglandins from human lung *in vitro*. *Am. Rev. Respir. Dis.* **121:**911–920, 1980.
10. Schulman, E. S., Adkinson, N. F., Jr., and Newball, H. H. Cyclo-oxygenase metabo-lites in human lung anaphylaxis: Airway vs. parenchyma. *J. Appl. Physiol.* **53:**589–595, 1982.
11. Burka, J. F., Ali, M., McDonald, J. W. D., and Paterson, N. A. M. Immunological and non-immunological synthesis and release of prostaglandins and thromboxanes from isolated guinea pig trachea. *Prostaglandins* **22:**683–691, 1981.
12. Horton, E. W. Prostaglandins and smooth muscle. *Br. Med. Bull.* **35:**295–390, 1979.
13. Adams, G. K., Adkinson, N. F., Jr., and Lichtenstein, L. M. Arachidonic acid metabo-lism and antigen-induced bronchospasm. *Fed. Proc., Fed. Am. Soc. Exp. Biol.* **40:**1024, 1981.
14. Adams, G. K., III, and Lichtenstein, L. M. Indomethacin enhances response of human bronchus to antigen. *Am. Rev. Respir. Dis.* in press.
15. Burka, J. F., and Paterson, N. A. M. Evidence for lipoxygenase pathway involvement in allergic tracheal contraction. *Prostaglandins* **19:**499–515, 1980.
16. Burka, J. F., and Paterson, N. A. M. Enhancement of antigen-induced tracheal contrac-tion by cyclo-oxygenase inhibition. *Adv. Prostaglandin Thromboxane Res.* **8:**1755–1758, 1980.
17. Hitchcock, M. Effect of inhibitors of prostaglandin synthesis and prostaglandins E_2 and $E_{2\alpha}$ on the immunologic release of mediators of inflammation from actively sensitized guinea-pig lung. *J. Pharmacol. Exp. Ther.* **207:**630–640, 1978.
18. Orehek, J., Douglas, J. S., and Bouhuys, A. Contractile responses of the guinea pig trachea *in vitro:* Modification by prostaglandin synthesis-inhibiting drugs. *J. Pharmacol. Exp. Ther.* **194:**554–564, 1975.
19. Adcock, J. J., and Garland, L. G. A possible role for lipoxygenase products as regula-tors of airway smooth muscle reactivity. *Br. J. Pharmacol.* **69:**167–169, 1980.
20. Mitchell, H. W. Effect of ETYA and BW 755c on arachidonate-induced contractions in the guinea-pig isolated trachea. *Br. J. Pharmacol.* **76:**527–529, 1982.
21. Mitchell, H. W. The effect of mixed inhibitors of cyclo-oxygenase and lipoxygenase on the indomethacin-induced hyper-reactivity in the isolated trachea of the pig. *Br. J. Pharmacol.* **77:**701–705, 1982.
22. Brink, C., Grimaud, C., Guillot, C., and Orehek, J. The interaction between indometha-cin and contractile agents on human isolated airway muscle. *Br. J. Pharmacol.* **69:**383–388, 1980.
23. Adcock, J. J., and Garland, L. G. Modification of human airway smooth muscle reactiv-ity by drugs that interfere with arachidonic acid metabolism. *Br. J. Pharmacol.* **77:**570–572, 1982.
24. Engineer, D. M., Niederhauser, U., Piper, P. J., and Sirois, P. Release of mediators of anaphylaxis: Inhibition of prostaglandin synthesis and the modification of release of slow-reacting substance of anaphylaxis and histamine. *Br. J. Pharmacol.* **62:**61–66, 1978.

25. Hitchcock, M. Stimulation of the antigen-induced contraction of guinea-pig trachea and immunological release of histamine and SRS-A from sensitized guinea-pig lung by (2-isopropyl-3-indolyl)-3 pyridyl ketone (L8027) and indomethacin. *Br. J. Pharmacol.* **71:**65–73, 1980.

26. Adcock, J. J., Garland, L. G., Moncada, S., and Salmon, J. A. The mechanism of enhancement by fatty acid hydroperoxides of anaphylactic mediator release. *Prostaglandins* **16:**179–187, 1978.

27. Burka, J. F., and Flower, R. J. Effects of modulators of arachidonic acid metabolism on the synthesis and release of slow-reacting substance of anaphylaxis. *Br. J. Pharmacol.* **65:**35–41, 1979.

28. Paterson, N. A. M., Burka, J. F., and Craig, I. D. Release of slow-reacting substance of anaphylaxis from dispersed pig lung cells: Effect of cyclo-oxygenase and lipoxygenase inhibitors. *J. Allergy Clin. Immunol.* **67:**426–434, 1981.

29. Adcock, J. J., Garland, L. G., Moncada, S., and Salmon, J. A. Enhancement of anaphylactic hydroperoxides. *Prostaglandins* **16:**163–177, 1978.

30. Marone, G., Kagey-Sobotka, A., and Lichtenstein, L. M. Effects of arachidonic acid and its metabolites on antigen-induced histamine release from human basophils *in vitro.* *J. Immunol.* **123:**1669–1677, 1979.

31. Stenson, W. F., Parker, C. W., and Sullivan, T. J. Augmentation of IgE-mediated release of histamine by 5-hydroxyeicosatetraenoic acid and 12-hydroxyeicosatetraenoic acid. *Biochem. Biophys. Res. Commun.* **96:**1045–1052, 1980.

32. MacGlashan, D. W., Jr., Schleimer, R. P., Peters, S. P., Schulman, E. S., Adams, G. K., Sobotka, A. K., Newball, H. H., and Lichtenstein, L. M. Comparative studies of human basophils and mast cells. *Fed. Proc., Fed. Am. Soc. Exp. Biol.* **42:**2504–2509, 1983.

33. Peters, S. P., Schulman, E. S., Schleimer, R. P., MacGlashan, D. W., Jr., Newball, H. H., and Lichtenstein, L. M. Dispersed human lung mast cells. Pharmacologic aspects and comparisons with human lung tissue fragments. *Am. Rev. Respir. Dis.* **126:**1034–1039, 1982.

34. Tobias, L. D., and Hamilton, J. G. The effect of 5,8,11,14-eicosatetraynoic acid on lipid metabolism. *Lipids* **14:**181–193, 1978.

35. Schulman, E. S., Adams, G. K., and Lichtenstein, L. M. Inhibition of antigen-induced bronchospasm *in vitro* by 5,8,11,14-eicosatetraynoic acid. *Am. Rev. Respir. Dis.* **121:**92, 1980.

36. Blackwell, G. J., and Flower, R. J. 1-phenyl-3-pyrazolidone: An inhibitor of cyclo-oxygenase and lipoxygenase pathways in lung and platelets. *Prostaglandins* **16:**417–425, 1978.

37. Morris, H. R., Piper, P. J., Taylor, G. W., and Tippins, J. R. The effect of arachidonate lipoxygenase substrates and inhibitors on SRS-A release in the guinea-pig lung. *Br. J. Pharmacol.* **66:**452P, 1979.

38. Saad, M. H., Wilson, M. A., and Burka, J. F. Release of leukotriene C_4 from guinea pig trachea. *Prostaglandins* **25:**741–752, 1983.

DISCUSSION

Kay: The concentration of FPL 55712 ($5 \times 10^{-5} M$) you used was about 10,000 times more than in the original studies with SRS-A–induced contraction of the guinea pig ileum. Would you comment on this?

Adams: The high concentration of FPL 55712 required to produce inhibition of the late phase may reflect a high local concentration of SRS-A (leukotrienes) generated within the tissue following mast cell activation.

Austen: Can you quantitate your comments, that is, the concentration of antihistamine used relative to the concentration of histamine released? I suspect the concentration of FPL 55712 is many logs higher than the amount of sulfidopeptide leukotriene produced and may not be specific in its action.

Adams: The concentration of antihistamine required to inhibit the early phase of anaphylactic bronchospasm suggests that following antigen challenge (resulting in 1% histamine release and a tension change of 50% of maximum), the peak tissue histamine concentration in the region of the airway smooth muscle may approach 10^{-4} M. Our interpretation of the FPL 55712 data as being consistent with the possibility that the leukotrienes contribute to antigen-induced airway contraction *in vitro,* and our explanation for the high antagonist requirement, are not based on the measurement of tissue leukotriene concentration. We agree that the specificity of FPL 55712 limits its usefulness as a pharmacological probe and additional experimental approaches must be used to define the role of leukotrienes in the response of sensitized airways to antigen.

Piper: When you showed the HPLC data from human bronchus challenged with antigen, did you have any idea of the quantity of leukotriene D_4 represented by the peak of the trace, perhaps by comparison with standard LTD$_4$?

Adams: We have not yet quantified the leukotriene activity in the peaks from HPLC. Nevertheless, in preliminary studies in collaboration with Dr. Ed Hayes we have found that antigen challenged guinea pig trachea generates approximately 20 pg of immunoreactive leukotriene per mg tissue (wet weight) per 20 min, greater than 50% of which is associated with the tissue pellet.

Nadel: Perhaps you could consider delivery of the agonist/antagonist via the bloodstream in the isolated bronchus (rather than by superfusion).

Kaplan: Did you add cyclooxygenase inhibitors to tracheal (bronchial) preparations already inhibited with a combination of antihistamine and FPL 55712 to determine whether the intermediate residual contraction is affected?

Adams: Cyclooxygenase inhibitors potentiate antigen-induced contraction of airways treated with a combination of diphenhydramine and FPL 55712, suggesting that the "intermediate phase" of the response is not mediated by a cyclooxygenase product.

Bach: As you know, FPL 55712 inhibits mediator release as well as antagonizing leukotriene responses. Have you tested the effects of disodium cromoglycate to control for this? Also, in terms of the effects of lipoxygenase inhibitors in your system, I wonder if you have tested their effect on leukotriene responses in your tissue. In the guinea pig ileum they selectively inhibit leukotriene responses.

Adams: We and others have found that cromolyn has no effect on the response of guinea pig trachea to antigen. In one of seven experiments with human bronchus, cromolyn produced approximately 50% inhibition of the response to antigen E.

Holgate: The tritium of [³H]arachidonic acid of high specific activity may undergo exchange reactions with hydrogen. How do you know that the peaks of radioactivity eluting from the HPLC are oxidative products of arachidonate?

Adams: Antigen challenge of human bronchus that has been incubated with [³H]arachidonic acid, followed by chloroform–ethanol extraction of the tissue and fluid phase, yields radioactive HPLC fractions which coelute with the PGs and thromboxane, with 5-, 11-, 12-, and 15-HETE, and with leukotrienes C_4 and D_4. We have not yet further characterized the material in any of the fractions.

Askenase: Have you added exogenous LTC$_4$ or LTD$_4$ standards to your bronchial or tracheal muscle preparations and then performed extraction and HPLC to see what your recoveries are like?

Adams: Using [³H]LTC₄, we have obtained nearly 100% recovery from the fluid phase and approximately 70% recovery from the tissue pellet through the extraction procedure. Recovery of tritiated LTC₄ from HPLC has averaged approximately 75%.

Oates: Were the human airways from which the arachidonate metabolite migrating with 15-HETE was derived obtained from patients who had asthma?

Adams: The airway tissue was a surgical specimen obtained from a lung cancer patient without asthma.

Clark: Have you studied bronchial muscle taken from asthmatic patients, and have you studied the effects of glucocorticoids on your preparation?

Adams: We have not yet had the opportunity to study airway smooth muscle from asthmatic patients. In experiments with Dr. Schleimer we have found that incubation for 24 hr with dexamethasone (1 μM) produced significant inhibition of the late phase without significantly inhibiting the early phase of the guinea pig tracheal response to antigen.

CHAPTER 8

Bronchial Secretory and Cardiac Smooth Muscle Responses to Leukotrienes

PRISCILLA J. PIPER

Department of Pharmacology
Institute of Basic Medical Sciences
Royal College of Surgeons of England
London, U.K.

P. S. RICHARDSON

Department of Physiology
St. George's Hospital Medical School
London, U.K.

L. G. LETTS

Merck Frosst Laboratories
Pointe Claire-Dorval, Quebec, Canada

Discovery and study of the 5-lipoxygenase metabolites of arachidonic acid, the leukotrienes (1), has led to important advances in the field of allergic mediators. During the past 3 years, the structure of the slow-reacting substance of anaphylaxis (SRS-A) has been elucidated (2), and SRS-A from various species has been shown to contain various leukotrienes (LTs). Leukotriene D_4 accounts for the major biological activity of guinea pig SRS-A (assayed on guinea pig ileum) (2); human SRS-A contains LTC_4 and LTD_4 (3), and LTC_4, LTD_4, and LTE_4 are present in rat SRS-A (4). Guinea pig SRS-A also contains substantial amounts of LTB_4 (5).

Generation of mediators by the lung and other tissues is thought to play an important role in the manifestation of allergic airway disease such as asthma. In addition to direct action on bronchial smooth muscle to cause narrowing of the airways (described in Chapter 6, this volume), leukotrienes may act in other ways to cause respiratory embarrassment.

ASTHMA: Physiology,
Immunopharmacology,
and Treatment
THIRD INTERNATIONAL SYMPOSIUM

113

STIMULATION OF MUCUS SECRETION

Blocking of the airways with thick, viscid mucus often occurs in the lungs of patients dying from asthma (6). There is also evidence that patients with mild asthma have a patchy narrowing of the lumen of the airways due to the presence of the same material (7). Clearance of airway mucus by cilia is unusually slow, even at times not associated with asthmatic bronchospasm, and antigen challenge causes further slowing of mucociliary clearance (8). Indirect evidence showing that the LT antagonist FPL-55712 caused reversal of the slowing of mucociliary transport produced by antigen challenge suggested that LTs might impair airway clearance (9). This might result from the stimulation of the secretion of mucins, the impairment of ciliary beating, the change in the physical properties of airway mucus that cause it to be less readily transported by the cilia, or from a combination of these effects.

In order to investigate one of the above effects, the actions of LTs on secretion of mucous glycoproteins was studied in tracheae from specific pathogen-free cats *in vivo* and *in vitro* (10–12).

In Vivo Experiments

Cats (either sex) were anaesthetised with pentobarbitone sodium (42 mg · kg^{-1}, given intraperitoneally) and maintained with further intravenous injections as required. A segment of cervical trachea was isolated with its blood and nerve supply intact and cannulated at both ends so that mucus could be flushed from the lumen and drugs could be administered. At the beginning of each experiment, sodium [^{35}S]sulfate (2.0 mCi) and [^{3}H]glucose (0.5 mCi) were placed in the tracheal segment to be taken up by the secretory cells and incorporated into mucins. Subsequent tracheal washings contained radiolabelled mucins, which were separated from unbound radiolabel by exhaustive dialysis.

When LTC$_4$ (6×10^{-8} to 6×10^{-5} M) or LTD$_4$ (6×10^{-8} to 1.2×10^{-4} M) was placed in the tracheal segment for 15 min at hourly intervals, significant dose-related increases in mucus secretion occurred. Doses of LTC$_4$ above 6×10^{-7} M increased the output of ^{3}H-labelled mucins, and doses from 6×10^{-6} M increased the output of ^{35}S-labelled mucins (Fig. 1). LTD$_4$ in doses from 6×10^{-7} M stimulated mucus output.

The LT antagonist FPL-55712 (incubated in the trachea with LTC$_4$) only significantly reduced the output of ^{3}H-labelled mucins stimulated by the highest dose of LTC$_4$. It did not alter release of ^{35}S-labelled mucins or cause a parallel shift in the dose–response curve (Fig. 2) (10).

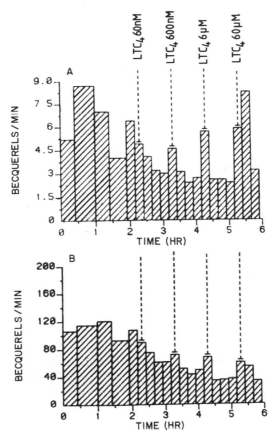

Fig. 1. Graphs showing the rate of output of ^{35}S-labelled mucins (A) and ^{3}H-labelled mucins (B) against time. Four doses of LTC_4 were given as indicated. Reproduced from Richardson *et al.* (11), with permission.

In Vitro Experiments

Sections of cat trachea were pinned flat between two halves of an Ussing chamber (13) and LTC_4 (6×10^{-8} to 6×10^{-6} M) or LTD_4 (1×10^6 to 1×10^{-7} M) added to both sides. In these experiments LTs failed to stimulate output of mucins although other agonists such as methacholine or phenylephrine increased release of ^{35}S-sulfated mucins.

The above observations show that high doses of both LTC_4 and LTD_4 caused secretion of mucins into the cat trachea. The doses required were higher than those necessary to cause bronchoconstriction (14), vasoconstriction (15), or exudation of plasma (16), and even at high doses were

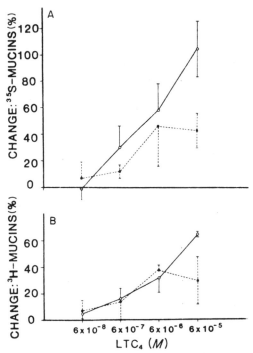

Fig. 2. Graphs showing the percentage changes in ^{35}S-labelled mucins (A) and ^{3}H-labelled mucins (B) in response to four concentrations of LTC$_4$: effect of LTC$_4$ in the absence of antagonist (O——O, $n = 5$); effect of LTC$_4$ in the presence of FPL 55712 at 9.5×10^{-6} M (●----●, $n = 3$). The bars show standard errors. Reproduced from Richardson *et al.* (11), with permission.

smaller than those produced by adrenoceptor agonists (12), cholinergic agonists (17), or prostaglandins (18). The fact that LTs were inactive in cat trachea *in vitro* suggested their action *in vivo* might be indirect, perhaps via action on the nervous system or local circulation, but the failure of LTs to alter respiration while incubated in the trachea did not provide evidence of a reflex mechanism. The report (19) that doses of LTC$_4$ or LTD$_4$ (as low as 4×10^{-10} M) stimulated the output of mucins from human bronchial strips cultured *in vitro* is of considerable interest. The difference in threshold doses may be caused by species difference or due to the fact that the bronchial tissue was removed from patients undergoing surgery for bronchial carcinoma. These airways were probably bronchitic and thus the bronchial mucous glands could have an increased number of receptors for agonists stimulating mucin output (20), an altered sensitivity to such agonists (21), or may have produced other mediators such as prostaglandins that could have acted synergistically with LTs (16). Such human isolated bronchial strips may easily generate mucins *in vitro,* because output of mucus from strips of human bronchus has been observed following stimulation with LTs (K. Barnett and P. J. Piper, unpublished observations). Although LTC$_4$ and LTD$_4$ are only weak stimulators of mucin output in the normal cat, they are probably one of several mediators that influence secretion of mucus into the inflamed airway. In inflamed airways, they may have a more important role, especially if they cause secretion of mucus with physical properties unsuitable for ciliary transport (22).

EFFECT OF LEUKOTRIENES ON CORONARY AND PULMONARY CIRCULATION

Antigen challenge of human or guinea pig lung tissue leads to the generation of LTs (2,3) and the heart has been described as a target organ for mediators released in the lung (23). In addition, substantial quantities of SRS-A or LTs are generated from the heart during cardiac anaphylaxis (23,24). In cardiac anaphylaxis, there is an abrupt change in rate and rhythm of the heart, a transient increase followed by prolonged decrease in contractility and a rapid and sustained reduction in coronary flow. Systemic anaphylaxis in guinea pig includes severe prolonged bronchospasm and primary cardiac participation including a decrease in cardiac output (23). Besides bronchospasm, changes in heart rate and systemic blood pressure occur during human anaphylaxis and include systemic hypotension, increased heart rate, arrhythmias, and changes in the S–T segment of the ECG, which might be indicative of coronary constriction (25). Chest pain, possibly resulting from angina, has been reported during allergic response to bee sting (26,27).

An important primary mechanism and site of action of peptidolipid leukotrienes is a potent constriction of small-diameter blood vessels of the skin (16,28) and hamster cheek pouch (29). Leukotrienes also exhibit powerful vasoconstrictor actions in the coronary circulation of various species both *in vitro* (30,31) and *in vivo* (30–35) and are more active than other vasoconstrictors such as angiotensin.

In Vitro Experiments

The actions of leukotrienes were investigated in isolated perfused hearts from various species. The hearts were perfused either under constant pressure or under constant flow (30,32), and LTs administered as single 5-min infusions or as bolus injections.

LTC$_4$, LTD$_4$ (4×10^{-10} to $2 \times 10^{-8} M$), or LTE$_4$ ($9 \times 10^{-8} M$) infused into guinea pig, rat, rabbit, or cat hearts caused a dose-dependent decrease in coronary flow (30,32). Leukotrienes administered to hearts perfused under constant flow caused a dose-related increase in perfusion pressure. LTC$_4$ was the most active LT in both guinea pig and rat, the order of potency being LTC$_4$ > LTD$_4$ > LTE$_4$. In guinea pig hearts, LTC$_4$ caused a maximum reduction in coronary flow of 70%. LTB$_4$ in doses of up to $5.9 \times 10^{-8} M$ was inactive in the isolated perfused hearts of either species. Although LTC$_4$ and LTD$_4$ reduced coronary flow in the two species, their actions on spontaneous rate and contractility varied., LTD$_4$ ($2.8 \times 10^{-8} M$) produced a greater reduction in coronary flow in rat hearts than in guinea pig hearts (Fig. 3A,B). In guinea pig LTs caused a significant reduction in contractility but little change in heart rate while in rat hearts, reduced coronary flow was associated with a marked reduction in spontaneous rate with little change in contractility. Leukotrienes had no action on spontaneously beating paired atria or driven ventricular strips and did not cause arrhythmias in isolated hearts.

A cyclooxygenase product(s) appeared to be involved in LT-induced reduction in coronary flow and contractility in guinea pig hearts, because indomethacin ($1.4 \times 10^{-5} M$) partially inhibited these effects. No such inhibition occurred in rat hearts. The cyclooxygenase product(s) remains unidentified, because there was no biological evidence of thromboxane A$_2$ release and a thromboxane synthetase inhibitor UK 37248 did not inhibit the cardiac actions of LTs. The coronary constrictor actions of LTs were partially antagonised by the leukotriene antagonist FPL-55712 ($3.8 \times 10^{-6} M$) in higher doses than those required to antagonise LT action on guinea pig ileum.

The doses of LTs causing potent coronary constrictor actions in guinea pig hearts were higher than those required to constrict the airways, whereas in the rat LTs produced marked vasoconstriction in coronary arteries in doses which had no action in the lung.

In Vivo Experiments

Coronary vasoconstriction induced by LTC$_4$ and LTD$_4$ was investigated in two series of experiments in anaesthetised greyhounds and pigs (33,35). After thoracotomy, the left anterior descending coronary artery was cannulated and perfused with the animal's carotid arterial blood, the perfusion pressure being adjusted to equal systemic arterial pressure.

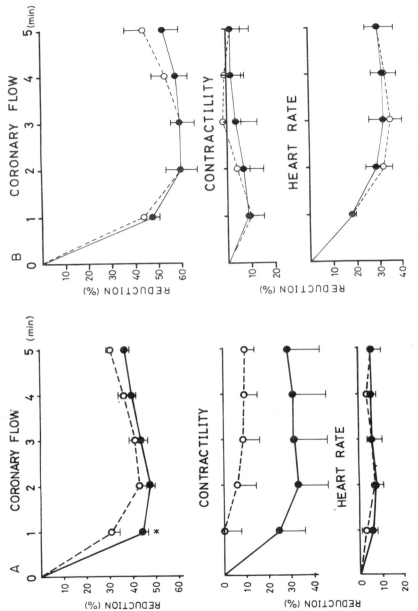

Fig. 3. Percentage in coronary flow, contractility, and heart rate in guinea pig and rat isolated hearts following administration of LTD$_4$ (2×10^{-8} M) (●——●). Values from hearts pretreated with indomethacin (1.4×10^{-5} M) (○----○). (A) Guinea pig hearts; (B) rat hearts.

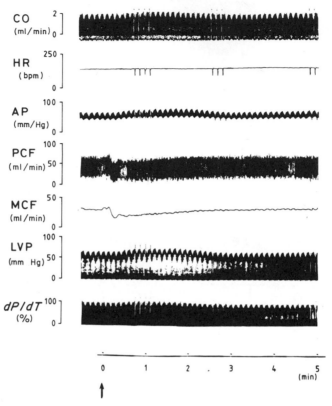

Fig. 4.   Effects of intracoronary bolus injections at time zero (note arrow) of LTD$_4$, 2 × 10^{-8} *M*, in greyhounds. CO, cardiac output; HR, heart rate; AP, arterial pressure; PCF, phasic coronary flow; MCF, mean coronary flow; LVP, left ventricular pressure; *dP/dt*, first differential of LVP, and time expressed as percentage of predose level. Reproduced from Greenwald *et al.* (35).

Blood flow in the coronary artery, systemic arterial pressure, cardiac output, *dP/dt*, and heart rate were monitored. Leukotrienes were administered into the perfusion line supplying the coronary artery as bolus injections.

In both the pig and the dog, LTC$_4$ and LTD$_4$ caused long-lasting reduction in coronary flow (Fig. 4). A species difference in responses to LTs clearly exists, because the pig is more sensitive to LT-induced coronary constriction than the greyhound. Similar results have been reported in the dog by Woodman and Dusting (36). Pig coronary arteries were more sensitive to the constrictor actions of LTs than were dog coronaries (Fig. 5A,B), and (in the pig) high doses sometimes caused irreversible spasm. Michelassi *et al.* (34) have also described potent coronary constrictor

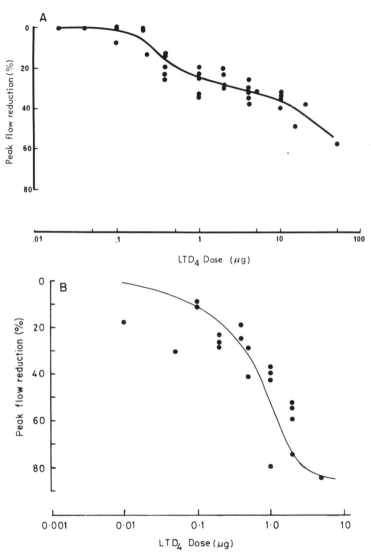

Fig. 5. Percentage reduction in flow in left anterior descending coronary artery of (A) dog, and (B) pig, following intracoronary administration of LTD_4.

effects of LTs in the sheep. The reduction in coronary flow lasted 10–15 min, but there were few other changes in the cardiac parameters measured and no development of arrhythmias. In the dog, small discrete haemorrhages occurred on the surface of the heart over the vascular bed perfused. These haemorrhages were visible within 5 to 10 min of adminis-

TABLE I
Release of LT-Like Material from Porcine Tissues Incubated
with A23187

Tissue	LT-like material (ng equivalent, g^{-1})[a]	n
Pulmonary artery (+ adventitia)	29.00 ± 11.9	8
Pulmonary artery (+ adventitia)[b]	16.00 ± 5.60	3
Adventitia	27.00 ± 10.00	6
Pulmonary artery (− adventitia)	19.00 ± 13.90	6
Coronary artery	19.61 ± 6.48	16
Mesenteric artery	9.71 ± 4.01	5
Renal artery	9.45 ± 2.55	6
Femoral artery	8.46 ± 1.81	3
Carotid artery	4.36 ± 2.56	5
Abdominal aorta	2.33 ± 1.23	3
Aortic arch	7.55 ± 1.88	5
Thoracic aorta	None detected	4
Bronchus	6.00 ± 3.46	3
Parenchyma	9.30 ± 2.10	3
Ventricle	None detected	3
Atrium	1.15	3

[a] Activity is expressed as ng equivalents of LTD_4.
[b] Incubated without indomethacin or sodium aspirin.

tration of LTs and were not accompanied by plasma leakage, as was demonstrated by extravasation of Evan's blue dye. The small areas of bleeding did not occur in those dogs in which the chest remained closed, or in pigs. It is of interest that surface haemorrhages have been recorded in the heart and lungs of animals that have suffered lethal anaphylactic shock (37–39). Indomethacin (5 mg · kg^{-1}) given intravenously did not affect the coronary constrictor actions of LTs in either pig or dog.

The finding that LTs cause potent coronary constriction in all species investigated, *in vitro* and *in vivo,* and that they are more active than vasoconstrictors such as angiotensin, suggests they may have a role in myocardial ischaemia and angina whether of allergic or other origin. As LTs do not appear to be circulating hormones (40), these results would support the hypothesis that a localised release of leukotriene-like substances in the close proximity of the vessel wall would decrease coronary flow.

Brocklehurst (24) demonstrated the release of SRS-A from blood vessels from sensitised guinea pigs during antigen challenge. Recently, we showed the generation of a leukotriene-like substance(s) from vascular tissue from pig, dog, rabbit, and rat incubated with the calcium ionophore A23187 and confirmed its release during antigen challenge of guinea pig aorta and pulmonary artery (41,42). There was considerable variation in the amounts of leukotriene-like material released from the coronary and pulmonary arteries and their surrounding adventitia (Table I). The material generated by the vascular tissue had biological characteristics that were similar to those of LTD_4, and its release was inhibited by BW 755c (42).

The fact that a 5-lipoxygenase system is present in coronary vascular tissue and that a leukotriene-like substance(s) may be released from the tissue supports the hypothesis that a local release of leukotrienes may have a role in myocardial ischaemia or angina. Since the pulmonary arteries of pig and guinea pig also generate 5-lipoxygenase products, and increased pulmonary arterial pressure has been demonstrated in following administration of LTC_4 (43), LTs released in the lung may act locally to cause vasoconstriction. Therefore, in addition to their constrictor action in the airways, LTs might cause constriction of peripheral vessels and thus influence respiratory parameters such as compliance.

CONCLUSION

The LTs have potent biological actions which suggest that, in addition to their action on airway smooth muscle, they may have a role in the stimulation of bronchial secretion and in the cardiac responses which occur during allergic responses. Leukotrienes may only be weak agonists in the stimulation of mucin output in the airways, but they are more active than other vasoconstrictors in causing constriction of coronary arteries.

REFERENCES

1. Samuelsson, B. The leukotrienes: An introduction. *Adv. Prostaglandin, Thromboxane, Leukotriene Res.* **9:**1–17, 1982.
2. Morris, H. R., Taylor, G. W., Piper, P. J., and Tippins, J. R. Structure of slow reacting substance of anaphylaxis from guinea-pig lung. *Nature (London)* **285:**105–106, 1980.
3. Lewis, R. A., Austen, K. F., Drazen, J. M., Clark, D. A., Marfat, A., and Corey, E. J. Slow reacting substances of anaphylaxis: Identification of leukotrienes C-1 and D from human and rat sources. *Proc. Natl. Acad. Sci. U.S.A.* **77:**3710–3714, 1980.
4. Bach, M. K., Brashler, J. R., Hammarström, S., and Samuelsson, B. Identification of a component of rat mononuclear cell SRS as leukotriene D. *Biochem. Biophys. Res. Commun.* **93:**1121–1126, 1980.

5. Morris, H. R., Taylor, G. W., Piper, P. J., and Tippins, J. R. Slow-reacting substances of anaphylaxis: Studies on purification and characterisation. *Agents Actions Suppl.* **ASS6:**27–36, 1979.
6. Dunnill, M. S. The pathology of asthma, with special reference to changes in the bronchial mucosa. *J. Clin. Pathol.* **13:**27–33, 1960.
7. Dunnill, M. S. The morphology of the airways in bronchial asthma. *In* (M. Stein, ed.), "Asthma" pp. 214–221. Park Ridge, Illinois, 1973.
8. Mezey, R. J., Cohn, M. A., Fernandez, R. J., Januszkiewicz, A. J., and Wanner, A. Mucociliary transport in allergic patients with antigen-induced bronchospasm. *Am. Rev. Respir. Dis.* **118:**677–684, 1978.
9. Ahmed, T., Greenblatt, D. W., Birth, S., Marchette, B., and Wanner, A. Abnormal mucociliary transport in allergic patients with antigen-induced bronchospasm: Role of slow reacting substance of anaphylaxis. *Am. Rev. Respir. Dis.* **124:**110–114, 1981.
10. Peatfield, A. C., Piper, P. J., and Richardson, P. S. The effect of leukotriene C_4 on mucin release into the cat trachea *in vivo* and *in vitro*. *Br. J. Pharmacol.* **77:**391–393, 1982.
11. Richardson, P. S., Peatfield, A. C., Jackson, D. M., and Piper, P. J. The effect of leukotrienes on the output of mucins from the cat trachea. *In* "Leukotrienes and Other Lipoxygenase Products" (P. J. Piper, ed.), pp. 178–187. Wiley, New York, 1983.
12. Peatfield, A. C., and Richardson, P. S. The control of mucin secretion into the lumen of the cat trachea by α- and β-adrenoceptors and their relative involvement during sympathetic nerve stimulation. *Eur. J. Pharmacol.* **81:**617–626, 1982.
13. Phipps, R. J., Nadel, J. A., and Davis, B. Effect of α-adrenergic stimulation on mucus secretion and on ion transport in cat trachea *in vitro*. *Am. Rev. Respir. Dis.* **121:**359–365, 1980.
14. Piper, P. J., Samhoun, M. N., Tippins, J. R., Williams, T. J., Palmer, M. A., and Peck, M. J. Pharmacological studies of pure SRS-A, and synthetic leukotrienes C_4 and D_4. *In* "SRS-A and Leukotrienes" (P. J. Piper, ed.), pp. 81–99. Wiley, New York, 1981.
15. Letts, L. G., and Piper, P. J. The actions of leukotrienes C_4 and D_4 on guinea-pig isolated hearts. *Br. J. Pharmacol.* **76:**169–176, 1982.
16. Peck, M. J., Piper, P. J., and Williams, T. J. The effects of leukotrienes C_4 and D_4 on the microvasculature of guinea-pig skin. *Prostaglandins* **21:**315–321, 1981.
17. Gallagher, J. T., Kent, P. W., Passatore, M., Phipps, R. J., and Richardson, P. S. The composition of tracheal mucus and the nervous control of its secretion in the cat. *Proc. R. Soc. London, Ser. B* **192:**49–76, 1975.
18. Richardson, P. S., Phipps, R. J., Balfre, K., and Hall, R. L. The roles of mediators, irritants and allergens in causing mucin secretion from the trachea. *Ciba Found. Symp.* **54:**111–131, 1978.
19. Marom, Z., Shelhamer, J. H., Bach, M. K., Morton, D. R., and Kaliner, M. Slow reacting substances, leukotrienes C_4 and D_4 increase the release of mucus from human airways *in vitro*. *Am. Rev. Respir. Dis.* **126:**449–451, 1982.
20. Sturgess, J., and Reid, L. An organ culture study of the effects of drugs on the secretory activity of the human bronchial submucosal gland. *Clin. Sci.* **43:**535–543, 1972.
21. Cole, S. J., Said, S. I., and Reid, L. M. Inhibition by vasoactive intestinal polypeptide of glycoconjugates and lysozyme secretion by human airways *in vitro*. *Am. Rev. Respir. Dis.* **124:**531–536, 1981.
22. King, M. Interrelation between mechanical properties of mucus and mucociliary transport: Effect of pharmacologic interventions. *Biorheology* **16:**57–68, 1979.
23. Capurro, N., and Levi, R. The heart as a target organ in systemic allergic reactions: Comparison of cardiac anaphylaxis *in vivo* and *in vitro*. *Circ. Res.* **36:**520–528, 1975.

24. Brocklehurst, W. E. The release of histamine and formation of a slow-reacting substance (SRS-A) during anaphylactic shock. *J. Physiol. (London)* 151:416–435, 1960.
25. Smith, P. L., Kagey-Sobotka, A., Bleecker, E. R., Traystman, R., Kaplan, A. P., Gralnick, H., Valentine, M. D., Permutt, S., and Lichtenstein, L. M. Physiologic manifestations of human anaphylaxis. *J. Clin. Invest.* 66:1072–1080, 1980.
26. Patterson, R., and Valentine, M. Anaphylaxis and related allergic emergencies including reactions due to insect stings. *JAMA, J. Am. Med. Assoc.* 248:2632–2636, 1982.
27. Hirsch, S. A. Acute allergic reaction with coronary vasospasm. *Am. Heart J.* 103:928, 1982.
28. Drazen, J. M., Austen, K. F., Lewis, R. A., Clark, D. A., Goto, G., Marfat, A., and Corey, E. J. Comparative airway and vascular activities of leukotrienes C-1 and D *in vivo* and *in vitro*. *Proc. Natl. Acad. Sci. U.S.A.* 77:4354–4358, 1980.
29. Dahlén, S.-E., Bjork, J., Hedqvist, P., Arfors, K.-E., Hammarström, S., Lindgren, N.-A., and Samuelsson, B. Leukotrienes promote plasma leakage and leukocyte adhesion in postcapillary venules: *In vivo* effects with relevence to the acute inflammatory response. *Proc. Natl. Acad. Sci. U.S.A.* 78:3887–3891, 1981.
30. Letts, L. G., and Piper, P. J. Cardiac actions of leukotrienes B_4, C_4, D_4 and E_4 in guinea pig and rat *in vitro*. *Adv. Prostaglandin, Thromboxane, Leukotriene Res.* 11:391–396, 1983.
31. Terashita, Z., Fukui, H., Hirata, M., Terao, S., Ohkawa, S., Nishikawa, K., and Shintaro, K. Coronary vasoconstriction and PGI_2 release by leukotrienes in isolated guinea-pig hearts. *Eur. J. Pharmacol.* 73:357–361, 1981.
32. Letts, L. G., and Piper, P. J. Actions of LTC_4, LTD_4 in guinea-pig isolated hearts and the effect of indomethacin and FPL-55712. *Br. J. Pharmacol.* 76:169–176, 1981.
33. Letts, L. G., Piper, P. J., and Newman, D. L. Leukotrienes and their action in the coronary circulation. *In* "Leukotrienes and Other Lipoxygenase Products" (P. J. Piper, ed.), pp. 94–107. Wiley, New York, 1983.
34. Michelassi, F., Landa, L., Hill, R. D., Lowenstein, E., Watkins, W. D., Petkau, A. J., and Zapol, W. M. Leukotriene D_4: A potent coronary artery vasoconstrictor associated with impaired ventricular contraction. *Science* 217:841–843, 1982.
35. Greenwald, S. E., Letts, L. G., Newman, D. L., and Piper, P. J. Effects of intracoronary administration of leukotriene D_4 in the anaesthetised dog. *Prostaglandins* 26:563–572, 1983.
36. Woodman, O. L., and Dusting, G. J. Coronary vasoconstriction induced by leukotrienes in the anaesthetized dog. *Eur. J. Pharmacol.* 86:125–128, 1983.
37. Auer, J., and Lewis, P. A. The physiology of the immediate reaction of anaphylaxis in the guinea pig. *J. Exp. Med.* 12:151–175, 1910.
38. Auer, J. Lethal cardiac anaphylaxis in the rabbit. *J. Exp. Med.* 14:476–495, 1911.
39. Suzuki, T. Ultrastructural changes in heart muscle associated with anaphylaxis in the guinea pig. *Tohoku J. Exp. Med.* 106:109–123, 1972.
40. Hammarström, S. Metabolism of leukotriene C_3 in the guinea pig. *J. Biol. Chem.* 256:9673–9578, 1981.
41. Piper, P. J., Letts, L. G., Tippins, J. R., and Barnett, K. Generation of a substance with the biological properties of a leukotriene from porcine vascular tissue. *In* "Leukotrienes and Other Lipoxygenase Products" (P. J. Piper, ed.), pp. 299–306. Wiley, New York, 1983.
42. Piper, P. J., Letts, L. G., and Galton, S. A. Generation of a leukotriene-like substance from porcine vascular and other tissues. *Prostaglandins* 25:591–599, 1983.
43. Smedegård, G., Hedqvist, P., Dahlén, S.-E., Revenas, B., Hammarström, S., and Samuelsson, B. Leukotriene C_4 affects pulmonary and cardiovascular dynamics in monkey. *Nature (London)* 295:327–329, 1982.

DISCUSSION

Flenley: In my experience neither angina nor bradycardia are common features of clinical asthma in man. This leads me to ask if leukotrienes are released into the pulmonary venous circulation, as I presume would occur if they were released from mast cells in alveoli, or in respiratory, or even terminal bronchioles. If so, and if indeed the blood does move "as it were in a circle" as Harvey said, then the left heart and the coronary circulation would get the mediators at about the same time as the muscle of trachea and bronchi that are perfused by the bronchial circulation and which we know *are* constricted in the asthmatic attack. How do leukotrienes get to the tracheal and major airway muscle?

Piper: Leukotrienes probably act locally in or near the tissues in which they are generated; they do not appear to be circulating hormones.

Hogg: Guerzon *et al.* showed that the mast cell numbers increased markedly from the trachea to the parenchyma, and that the majority of these cells were in the submucosa and around the cartilage (G. M. Guerzon, P. D. Pare, M. C. Michaud, and J. C. Hogg, *Am. Rev. Respir. Dis.* **119**:59, 1979). Although there are many mast cells in the airways perfused by the bronchial circulation, most of them appear to be in tissue that is probably perfused by the pulmonary circulation.

Gleich: I believe it appropriate to point out that there is a cell type, namely the eosinophil, which is richly represented in the airways of patients with asthma and which produces leukotrienes. As I shall discuss (Chapter 12), the eosinophil seems to be in the correct anatomic locations and possesses the requisite capabilities to be an important contributor to the pathogenesis of asthma.

Hogg: Mucus in asthma is viscous and this is in part related to high protein concentration in the plugs. It seems to me that the leukotrienes could play a role in this if they produce exudation as a result of their effect on the bronchial microvasculature.

Nadel: In relation to gland secretion and mast cells, it is of some interest that the glands are concentrated in major airways, whereas mast cells increase in concentration with decreasing size of airways. Also, few stimuli release goblet cell contents. In our hands, no autonomic agonists or arachidonate metabolites that we have tested release goblet cell contents.

Hogg: An inflammatory reaction induced by cigarette smoke causes goblet cells in the lung mucosa to discharge (W. C. Hulbert, D. C. Walker, A. Jackson, and J. C. Hogg, *Am. Rev. Respir. Dis.* **123**:320, 1981). I believe that Florey found similar results in inflammatory reactions induced in the colon (M. A. Jennings and H. W. Florey, *Q. J. Exp. Physiol. Cogn. Med. Sci.* **41**:131, 1956; H. W. Florey, *ibid.* **45**:329, 1960).

Kaliner: Victor Ferrans (O. Kawanami, V. Ferrans, J. D. Fulmer, and R. G. Crystal, *Lab. Invest.* **40**:717, 1979) has carefully analysed the topographical content and distribution of human lung mast cells and reported these data several years ago. Mast cells are found in rich concentration just beneath the basement membrane of bronchi and bronchioles, although the largest number is in the intraalveolar spaces. It is possible that peripheral mast cells may be involved in SRS production, and that its release into the alveolar space may make it available to more proximal airways.

Clark: Mast cells are unlikely to remain localised to any site and I would like further information on the mobility of mast cells. For example, do mast cells move to the epithelium or lumen following the initial challenge where they can then augment their alleged protective role?

Lichtenstein: I think that the importance of the mast cell in the asthmatic episode was well illustrated by Roy Patterson's experiments with monkeys (R. Patterson, I. M. Susko, and K. E. Harris, *J. Clin. Invest.* **62:**519, 1978). You will recall that he had a colony of ascaris-sensitive monkeys. Some responded to bronchial challenge (with ascaris) and others did not. He could make the unreactive animals respond by taking mast cells obtained at bronchial lavage from a responsive monkey and placing them in the airways of the previously unresponsive animal.

Morley: The potency of LTC_4 and LTD_4 as stimulants of mucus secretion is unimpressive. Is $PGF_{2\alpha}$ more potent? It is reported to be an effective stimulus to secretion in man.

Piper: In the specific pathogen-free cat, LTC_4 and LTD_4 are much weaker than prostaglandins in stimulating mucus secretion.

Askenase: Have you studied non-SPF cats with background infection and inflammation to test your hypothesis that this leads to increased sensitivity to leukotrienes? This could be clinically important, as it might be another reason to treat asthma with antibiotics and antiinflammatory drugs.

Piper: We did not test the effect of LTD_4 or LTD_4 on mucus secretion in cats that might have had inflammation or infection of the airways.

Platts-Mills: Have you looked at the relationship between coronary artery spasm induced by leukotrienes and changes in the ST segment on the ECG of your animals?

Piper: We did not look at changes in S–T segment of ECG in dogs or pigs. It was in a series of experiments on anaesthetised guinea pigs that we observed S–T changes after administration of luekotrienes.

Grant: What is the evidence that FPL 55712 is a specific antagonist?

Austen: We do not feel that FPL 55712 is a specific receptor antagonist. In inhibiting mucous secretions from human bronchial explants, we found no stereochemical requirements, that is, no evidence for a specific receptor.

Piper: FPL 55712 is not a specific antagonist of leukotrienes. If left in contact with tissues for, say, 45 min or so, it will antagonise prostaglandins as well as leukotrienes.

Turner-Warwick: Is it true that the major duration of leukotrienes on human bronchial smooth muscle is between ~5 and 30 min? Is this as immediately reversible by β-agonists, as is seen in the clinical situation when these drugs will rapidly and usually completely reverse the immediate reaction (when given at the point of maximum response)?

Leitch: There have been studies with human bronchial strips (Davis *et al.*) in which leukotriene-induced contractions were rapidly reversed by isoprenaline (C. Davis, T. R. Jones, and E. E. Daniel, *Am. Rev. Respir. Dis.* **125:**65, 1982).

Lee: Adam Wanner's group [W. M. Abraham, J. C. Delehurst, E. Russi, A. Wanner, L. Yerger, and G. A. Chapman, *Am. Rev. Respir. Dis.* **127**(Suppl.):65, 1983] has shown that the administration of aerosolized LTD_4 to sheep produced an early and a late asthmatic reaction. Since the late asthmatic response is associated with increased bronchial reactivity, it was interesting that the administration of LTD_4 by itself could produce a nonimmediate reaction.

CHAPTER 9

Regulation of Airway Responsiveness and Secretion: Role of Inflammation*

JAY A. NADEL and MICHAEL J. HOLTZMAN

Cardiovascular Research Institute
and Departments of Medicine and Physiology
University of California
San Francisco, California, U.S.A.

INTRODUCTION

An abnormal responsiveness of the airways (evidenced by increased contractile responsiveness of the airway smooth muscle) and an abnormal generation and clearance of airway secretions (evidenced by increased amounts, increased viscosity, and decreased clearance of airway secretions) are fundamental features of asthma (1-4). Therefore, it is likely that improved treatment of asthma will be based on determination of the possible cause(s) of these abnormalities. An important possibility is that the abnormal airway responsiveness and the abnormal generation and clearance of airway secretions are caused by airway inflammation. This possibility is suggested by the observation that the airways of patients with asthma not only show abnormal amounts of smooth muscle and secretory cells (5), but also show that the airway lumen is plugged with a heterogeneous exudate and that the airway wall is intensely inflamed (6). Similarly, the sputum of asthmatic patients contains clusters of desquamated epithelial cells (7,8), and bronchoalveolar lavage fluid from asthmatic airways may contain increased numbers of epithelial cells and neutrophils (9). Thus, there is evidence of an inflammatory reaction characterized by

* This work was supported in part by National Institutes of Health Program Project Grant HL-24136.

ASTHMA: Physiology,
Immunopharmacology,
and Treatment
THIRD INTERNATIONAL SYMPOSIUM

129

injury to epithelial cells and influx of neutrophils into the airways in asthmatic patients, but there is not yet direct evidence that these events lead to hyperresponsiveness and to abnormal generation and clearance of secretions in these patients.

The lack of evidence is due, at least in part, to the difficulty in obtaining airway tissue from asthmatic patients for histologic studies, and the consequent difficulty in relating inflammatory changes to the changes in airway function in these patients. For this reason, experimental models of airway inflammation that might also lead to abnormal airway function are essential. The fact that certain inflammatory stimuli can cause both the abnormal responsiveness of airways (e.g., ref. 10) and the abnormal clearance of airway secretions (e.g., ref. 11) in experimental models makes it possible to investigate which features of airway inflammation may be responsible for causing these abnormalities in asthma.

This chapter will describe some of the studies in our laboratory and in other laboratories carried out in humans and in animals that support the hypothesis that airway inflammation is linked to the abnormalities of airway responsiveness and secretion that are characteristic of asthma. Although substantial information is accumulating on the regulation of airway secretion, only limited studies are related to the effect of inflammation. On the other hand, although many of our own studies focus on the effect of inflammation on airways, these studies were carried out on airway smooth muscle. Therefore, we have divided the chapter into two parts. First, we will review the studies on the role of inflammation in airway responsiveness. With that as a background, we will review the studies on airway secretions and relevant studies on inflammation and inflammatory mediators.

INFLAMMATION AND AIRWAY RESPONSIVENESS

The hypothesis that increased airway responsiveness can be caused by airway inflammation was first suggested by the observation that each stimulus that has been used to cause hyperresponsiveness experimentally in humans may also cause airway inflammation or the release of inflammatory mediators. Thus, viral respiratory infection causes hyperresponsiveness (12–14) and also causes airway inflammation (15); exposure to allergen causes hyperresponsiveness (16–19) and also may cause airway inflammation (20) and release inflammatory mediators (21,22); and exposure to ozone causes hyperresponsiveness (11,23–25) and also may cause airway inflammation (26–29). Therefore, it is possible that these stimuli caused hyperresponsiveness, not by acting directly on airway smooth muscle or on its innervation, but by acting indirectly via airway inflammation.

Several investigators have found that viral respiratory infection causes hyperresponsiveness in humans (12–14). The evidence that viral respiratory infection may cause inflammation is available from other studies of humans with influenza, in which there is inflammation of the airways characterized by epithelial cell injury and by early neutrophil influx (15). The latter finding is supported by the observation that viruses may generate chemotactic factors for neutrophils (30). Because infection with influenza virus (14) and inoculation with live, attenuated influenza viruses (31) causes transient airway hyperresponsiveness in otherwise healthy humans, a link between viral-induced inflammation and hyperresponsiveness, at least due to influenza virus, is likely. The exact features of the inflammatory response and the mechanism by which inflammation could lead to hyperresponsiveness is uncertain.

Other investigators have studied the airway inflammation and hyperresponsiveness associated with inhalation of antigen. Although it was known that patients with more severe asthma more often develop a "delayed" response to antigen inhalation (32–34), it has been reported that the delayed response following antigen inhalation is accompanied by increased airway responsiveness whereas the immediate response is not (18). As yet, evidence of airway inflammation has not been obtained in these patients, but it has been suggested that the inflammatory response of the airways to antigen is similar to the delayed response in the skin, in which a large percentage of the cells are neutrophils (35,36). Of interest is the finding that neutrophil chemotactic activity (presumed to be generated by mast cells) appears in the blood of asthmatic subjects during delayed responses (37). Thus, there is some evidence that the delayed response to antigen is accompanied by increased airway responsiveness and possibly airway inflammation involving neutrophils. An animal model of the delayed response to antigen has been developed (38), but the characteristics of the inflammatory response and their link to an increase in responsiveness have not yet been reported.

Over the past 6 years, our group has concentrated on the mechanism of airway inflammation and hyperresponsiveness induced by exposure to ozone. The possibility that ozone exposure could lead to hyperresponsiveness came from the observation that it caused airway inflammation in a variety of animal species (see ref. 29 for review). Thus, an acute exposure to ozone caused airway inflammation characterized by damage and loss of airway epithelial cells and influx of neutrophils into the airways in rats (26,28), cats (39), and rabbits (27). Exposure to ozone also caused reversible hyperresponsiveness both in dogs (10) and in otherwise healthy humans (23–25). It was evident from these studies in our laboratories that the increase in responsiveness was associated with an increase in the response of airway smooth muscle to stimulation of its muscarinic receptors. It was likely that the responses both to direct stimulation of the muscle (24,40,41) and to indirect stimulation via nervous activity (10,42,43) were increased and combined to produce the increased smooth muscle response during the hyperresponsive state. Because we did not obtain evidence of airway inflammation in these studies, the mechanism by which inflammation might have enhanced the response of the smooth muscle to stimulation was uncertain.

Our subsequent studies have focused on ozone exposure as an experimental model to determine the link between hyperresponsiveness and airway inflammation. The studies were carried out first to establish that ozone-induced inflammation occurred during hyperresponsiveness and then to determine what types of cells were involved in the inflammatory response. The studies were carried out in dogs, because the techniques for studying airway inflammation are difficult to carry out in humans.

The studies in dogs suggested a close link between ozone-induced hyperresponsiveness and an airway inflammatory response involving airway epithelial cells and neutrophils. Thus, increases in airway responsiveness after ozone are accompanied by an inflammatory response characterized by increases in the numbers of epithelial cells and of neutrophils recovered in bronchoalveolar lavage (Fig. 1), without significant changes in the numbers of macrophages, lymphocytes, or eosinophils (44). Furthermore, increases in airway responsiveness develop only in dogs that also exhibit increases in the number of neutrophils in the airway epithelium, whereas increases in responsiveness do not develop in dogs that do not develop increases in neutrophils in the epithelium (45) (Fig. 2). In fact, the time course of the increase in responsiveness is similar to the time course of epithelial cell desquamation and of neutrophil influx into the airways (44–46). Because the desquamation of epithelial cells and the influx of neutrophils signaled the development of acute inflammation, the results suggested that ozone-induced hyperresponsiveness may depend on the development of acute airway inflammation.

The studies in dogs also suggested the source of the inflammatory mediators that caused neutrophils to enter the airway. Thus, we found that the increase in neutrophil number during hyperresponsiveness was greatest in the epithelium, less in the subepithelium, and least in the circulation (Fig. 2). This finding implied that the greatest concentration of mediators chemotactic for neutrophils was generated in the epithelium and suggested that cell type(s) present in the inflamed epithelium were the major

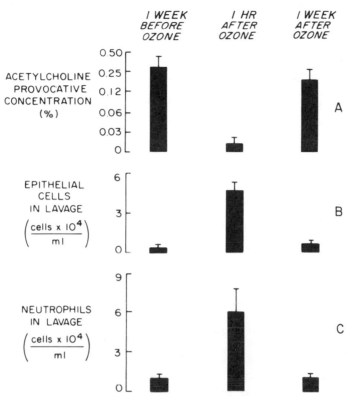

Fig. 1. Effect of ozone exposure on the airway responsiveness to acetylcholine (A) and on the numbers of epithelial cells (B) and neutrophils (C) in bronchoalveolar lavage fluid in dogs. Airway responsiveness is expressed as acetylcholine provocative concentration (the concentration of acetylcholine aerosol needed to increase pulmonary resistance by 5.0 cm H_2O liter^{-1} s^{-1}). Provocative concentration and numbers of cells in lavage were determined 1 week before exposure and 1 hr and 1 week after exposure. Each bar represents the values for mean and SEM. Ozone exposure decreased the provocative concentration (signifying increased responsiveness) and increased the numbers of epithelial cells and neutrophils. Modified from Fabbri *et al.* (44).

source of the mediators. For example, either the epithelial cells or the neutrophils themselves may release chemotactic mediators in response to ozone or other inflammatory stimuli. Whether chemotactic mediators or other types of mediators released by activation of these cells then enhanced the responsiveness of smooth muscle was uncertain.

To follow up the possibility that epithelial cells may generate potent chemotactic factors for neutrophils, and possibly other inflammatory mediators, we studied the generation of inflammatory mediators by airway epithelial cells isolated from dogs (47). That the introduction of ozone into

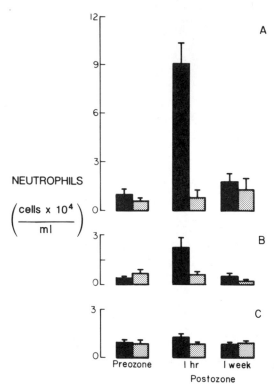

Fig. 2. Effect of ozone exposure on the number of neutrophils in the airway epithelium (A), or subepithelium (B), and in the venous circulation (C) for dogs that became hyperresponsive after ozone (solid bars) and for dogs that did not (stippled bars). The numbers of epithelial and subepithelial neutrophils were determined in biopsies of the airway mucosa before ozone and 1 hr and 1 week after ozone. Ozone exposure caused a marked and reversible increase in the number of epithelial and subepithelial neutrophils only in the dogs that became hyperresponsive. Reprinted from Holtzman *et al.* (45).

the airways releases arachidonic acid (48) suggested that oxygenation products of arachidonic acid might be important mediators of the inflammatory response. In fact, we found that epithelial cells convert arachidonic acid to the potent chemotactic factor leukotriene B_4 with only small quantities of leukotrienes C_4, D_4, and E_4, and generated several monohydroxyeicosatetraenoic acids (HETEs) of which 15-HETE was the predominant product (Table I). The results suggested that the airway epithelial cells may be an important source of inflammatory mediators derived from the lipoxygenase pathway of arachidonic acid. Some of the lipoxygenase products, such as leukotriene B_4, may amplify the inflammatory response in airways by causing chemotaxis of leukocytes (49). Other

TABLE I
Conversion of Arachidonic Acid to Lipoxygenase Products by Canine Tracheal Epithelial Cells[a]

Concentration of arachidonic acid added (μg/ml)	Quantities of lipoxygenase products (pmol/10^6 cells)[b]			
	LTB$_4$	15-HETE	12-HETE	5-HETE
0	0.2 ± 0.1[c]	<1	<1	<1
25	1.8 ± 1.2	12 ± 7	5 ± 3	18 ± 11
50	4.8 ± 0.7	46 ± 7	41 ± 5	83 ± 29
100	18.0 ± 5.3	218 ± 51	121 ± 55	162 ± 59
200	36.2 ± 9.1	1030 ± 463	767 ± 500	324 ± 100

[a] From Holtzman et al. (in press).

[b] Quantities were determined by high performance liquid chromatography after incubating the cells for 90 min with or without arachidonic acid.

[c] Each value is the mean ± SEM (n = 4–8). Abbreviations used: LTB$_4$, leukotriene B$_4$; HETE, monohydroxyeicosatetraenoic acid.

lipoxygenase products, such as 15-HETE, may also amplify inflammatory and allergic responses in airways by selectively activating other airway cells, such as mast cells, which in turn generate and release lipoxygenase products (50).

Since the two types of cells that are prominently involved in the inflammatory response to ozone are epithelial cells and neutrophils, we speculated that either type might release mediators that cause hyperresponsiveness (45). To better determine whether the increased responsiveness after ozone was due to mediators released from epithelial cells or from neutrophils, we studied the effect of neutrophil depletion by hydroxyurea treatment on ozone-induced hyperresponsiveness in dogs (51). We found that although the desquamation of epithelial cells persisted during hydroxyurea treatment, the absence of neutrophils was associated with the loss of hyperresponsiveness after ozone. This finding has two important implications. First, it implies that epithelial cell desquamation and injury may be an initial event after ozone exposure and may not depend on neutrophil influx. Second, it implies that epithelial cell desquamation does not by itself result in the release of mediators that cause hyperresponsiveness. Since the introduction of ozone into the airways releases arachidonic acid (48), it is possible that the desquamation of epithelial cells after exposure to ozone in vivo is similar to the toxicity of epithelial cells after exposure to arachidonic acid in vitro (47). The latter exposure results in the generation and release of leukotriene B$_4$ from these cells. Together the studies

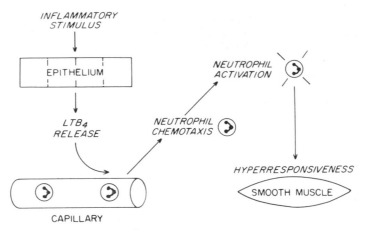

Fig. 3. Possible steps by which inflammatory stimuli lead to the hyperresponsiveness of airway smooth muscle. Inflammatory stimuli (e.g., ozone) interact initially with airway epithelial cells, causing these cells to generate and release lipid chemotactic factors (e.g., LTB_4). These factors mediate the infiltration of neutrophils from the microcirculation and into the airway epithelium, where neutrophils in turn can also interact with stimuli and become activated. The next step may involve the generation and release from neutrophils of other lipid factors (cyclooxygenase and lipoxygenase products). These factors may then act on smooth muscle (and on the nerves that regulate the muscle) to cause increased contractile responsiveness.

suggest that, although epithelial cells may produce chemotactic mediators that cause neutrophils to enter the airway, neutrophils may in turn produce mediators that cause hyperresponsiveness of the airways.

Even though the exact mechanism by which airway inflammation induced by ozone (and by other inflammatory stimuli) leads to hyperresponsiveness is still not certain, our results and those of others suggest some possible steps involved (Fig. 3). Ozone's properties as a potent oxidant and free radical generator allow it to initiate cell damage rapidly and locally (52,53). In the process, ozone may generate arachidonic acid (48), a substance that is readily converted by airway epithelial cells to lipoxygenase products with potent chemotactic activity for neutrophils (47,49). These reactions would fit with our own observations and the observations of others that ozone causes damage and loss of airway epithelial cells (26,39) and causes chemotaxis of neutrophils into the airways (26–29).

Although the mobilization of neutrophils appears necessary for hyperresponsiveness to develop, the next step is uncertain. It is likely, however, that it involves activation of neutrophils (by epithelial cell products or by ozone itself) so that additional cyclooxygenase or lipoxygenase products are released, increasing airway responsiveness. The potential for these events is based on the observations that neutrophils may be activated by a variety of stimuli to release cyclooxygenase and lipoxygenase products (54), that these products can increase airway smooth muscle responsiveness (55,56), and that inhibitors of these products also inhibit the increased responsiveness induced by ozone (57). The precise nature of such events in airways can only be determined from further studies of the mediators generated and released by epithelial cells and neutrophils. These studies may also provide a basis for understanding the importance of epithelial cell–neutrophil interaction for hyperresponsiveness due to other inflammatory stimuli or for hyperresponsiveness in asthma.

INFLAMMATION AND AIRWAY SECRETION

The fluid that lines the airways consists of a liquid sol phase in contact with the cell surface and a superficial mucous gel phase in contact with the air. The cilia move easily through the sol phase. Their tips make contact with the viscous mucus and propel it up the airways along with entrapped foreign materials. Two major functions exist in the secretory system: mucus secretion and ion transport. These will be discussed separately.

Mucus Secretion

Approximately 95% of airway secretions is water. The remaining 5% is carbohydrates, proteins, lipids, and inorganic materials, much of which is incorporated into mucins by cells in the superficial epithelium (e.g., goblet cells) and in the submucosal glands. Because the glands normally occupy ~40 times more volume than surface goblet cells in human conducting airways, the glands are likely to be the major contributors to the total secretion of mucus.

Submucosal Glands

Autonomic Regulation. Submucosal glands are under parasympathetic, sympathetic, and nonadrenergic noncholinergic nervous control.

The parasympathetic nerve supply to the glands is via the vagus nerves. Blocking conduction in the vagus nerves in cats decreased the rate of gland fluid secretion into micropipets slightly (58) and decreased fluid collection rate in dogs (59), indicating that vagal nervous activity plays a small role in the production of gland secretions in the resting state. However, the reduction in resting secretory rate by nerve blockade or by the muscarinic antagonist atropine is small, indicating that most of the basal secretion is independent of parasympathetic nervous control. Electrical stimulation of these nerves increased the rate of fluid secretion into micropipets (58), produced "hillocks" or small elevations in the airway lumen produced by fluid and mucin secretion (60), and caused radiolabelled mucin release from glands (61). Most reflexes that affect mucus secretion travel via the vagus nerves. The most potent secretomotor responses occur on mechanical or chemical stimulation of the airways. Thus, touching the laryngeal mucosa in cats increased the rate of fluid secretion from glands (62) and increased the rate of radiolabelled mucin secretion (61). Chemical stimulation of the airway mucosa with ammonia (63) or with sulfur dioxide (64) also increased mucus secretion via a vagal reflex. Secretion into the airway thus appears to be a part of the normal cough reflex. Presumably, the secreted fluid dilutes the irritant and assists in its removal during cough.

Chronic inflammation present in asthma (65) and in bronchitis may, by chronically stimulating gland secretion reflexly, contribute to the abnormal secretions in these diseases. Stimulation of bronchial C fibers with capsaicin or bradykinin also increases mucus production in dogs via a vagal reflex (66). Because these nerve-fiber endings are located in the airway epithelium, inflammatory changes in the epithelium could cause a chronic reflex secretomotor response and excessive or abnormal secretions. Steroids could produce a salutory effect on secretions in status asthmaticus by their antiinflammatory effects on the airway epithelium, thus decreasing the stimulation of airway submucosal gland secretion. Hypoxia stimulates submucosal gland secretion via a vagal reflex originating in the carotid bodies in dogs (67). If this reflex exists in humans, then the hypoxia present in diseases such as asthma and bronchitis could intensify the airway obstruction by adding reflexly stimulated secretions to the original airway obstruction. Chronic reflex gland stimulation caused by the stimulation of cough receptors, C-fiber endings, or carotid bodies could also play a role in producing the gland hypertrophy that is so characteristic of asthma and bronchitis (65).

The sympathetic nervous system can influence gland secretion by the release of circulating catecholamines from chromaffin cells and by direct nervous innervation of the airways. The sympathetic nerves, like the parasympathetic nerves, mostly exist in interstitial bundles between gland acini; few motor nerve varicosities make close contact with gland cells. Electrical stimulation of the thoracic sympathetic nerves *in vivo* (61) or field stimulation *in vitro* (68) increased gland secretion. Reflexes mediated via sympathetic nerves are rarely studied. Nevertheless, it appears that sympathetic motor pathways play a role in reflex secretomotor responses to irritation of the nose, pharynx, and larynx (63). Stimulation of the vagus nerves or administration of muscarinic agonists stimulated the release of secretions from both mucous and serous cells and thus does not appear to be selective (69). On the other hand, there is much information that indicates that although both α- and β-adrenergic agonists stimulate gland secretion, their effects are more selective and differ from one another. A summary of their effects is shown in Table II. Both α- and β-adrenergic agonists stimulate the release of radiolabelled mucins (70), indicating that mucus secretion is regulated by both types of agonists. α-Adrenergic agonists are potent in causing fluid secretions from glands (58,71,72) but β-adrenergic agonists are not (71). Micropipet studies showed biochemical selectivity: Ueki and Nadel showed that α-adrenergic stimulation decreased the protein concentration in gland secretions, while β-adrenergic stimulation increased fluid protein concentration (73). Quinton (72) showed that α-adrenergic agonists produce fluid with lower concentrations of sulfur than do β-adrenergic agonists.

Morphometric methods have been used to determine the cells of origin of the secretions. Lysozyme is localized within the serous granules of serous, but not mucous, cells (74). The fact that α-adrenergic agonists cause the release of large amounts of lysozyme compared to β-adrenergic agonists suggests that alpha receptors selectively regulate the release of secretions from serous cells (74). Morphometric studies indicated that α-adrenergic agonists preferentially deplete serous cells, sparing mucous cells (69). The morphologic and biochemical differences are also reflected in differences in the viscoelastic properties of the mucus produced. Thus, Leikauf found that α-adrenergic stimulation produced secretions of low apparent viscosity, whereas β-adrenergic stimulation produced secretions of higher apparent viscosity and lower elasticity than controls (75).

Several clinical implications of sympathetic regulation emerged. Since nerves release mainly norepinephrine, it would be expected that sympathetic nervous stimulation would produce profuse fluid of low apparent viscosity. Therapeutic intervention with adrenergic agonists could change the viscoelastic properties of mucus and thus modify mucociliary clearance. Chronic stimulation with β-adrenergic agonists leads to hypertrophy of the submucosal gland cells, especially mucous cells (76). The physiologic implications of this hypertrophy are unknown. Some evidence suggests that chronic β-adrenergic stimulation leads to an acceleration of uptake of mucin precursors by the gland cells and a down-regulation of mucus secretion by the cells (M. Tom-Moy, personal communication). Because β-adrenergic agonists are the mainstay of therapy in asthma, it will be important to determine the clinical implications of this gland hypertrophy on mucociliary clearance.

TABLE II

Relative Activities of Autonomic Agonists on Gland Secretion

Agonist	Actions					
	Radiolabelled mucin secretion	Lysozyme release	Fluid output	Protein concentration	Sulfur concentration	Morphologic evidence of cell depletion
Muscarinic	High	Higher	Higher	Lower	Lower	Serous and mucous
α-Adrenergic	High	Higher	Higher	Intermediate	Higher	Primarily serous
β-Adrenergic	High	Lower	Lower	Highest	Lower	Primarily serous

There is anatomic and physiologic evidence that a third nervous system innervates the airways. Thus, electron microscopic evidence showing varicosities in nerves in the airway submucosa containing large dense-cored vesicles suggests the presence of noncholinergic nonadrenergic nerves (77). Transmural electrical stimulation of the nerves to the submucosal glands increased radiolabelled mucin release, even after atropine, phentolamine, and propranolol. The effect was abolished by tetrodotoxin, indicating that a nonmuscarinic, non-α-adrenergic, and non-β-adrenergic nervous effect was responsible for the secretion (68).

The mediator of this response is unknown. Vasoactive intestinal peptide (VIP) has been suggested as the mediator of this system and is a likely candidate because (a) immunocytochemical studies have demonstrated the presence of VIP-containing nerves in airway ganglia and in the submucosa of cats (78) and ferrets (79); (b) anatomic studies revealed the presence of VIP-containing nerve vesicles in the airways; and (c) VIP caused the secretion of radiolabelled mucins into the airway (80). The role of this system in modulating secretions in health and disease is unknown.

Effects of Drugs and Mediators. In addition to autonomic mediators, many substances affect mucus secretion, but little is known about the mechanism or even the source of the secretions (e.g., glands versus surface epithelial cells). There are many reasons for this confusion: species vary widely in anatomic features in responses to drugs (81). The structures involved are small and relatively inaccessible, and only more recently have techniques been developed to harvest secretions from specific structures and isolate specific cell types (82). Because the amounts of secreted materials are small and the constituents (e.g., mucins) biochemically complicated, methods for measuring secretory responses are presently limited.

Most reported studies of possible secretagogue effects have examined mediators known to be released from only some "fixed" airway cells (i.e., the mast cell) and circulating cells (e.g., macrophages, neutrophils). Cells such as the airway epithelial cells, glands, Clara cells, sensory nerve endings, gland secretions, smooth muscle, and vascular cells may also play important roles in modulating secretory (and other target cell) responses, but few investigators have investigated this possibility. The substances studied include preformed mediators (e.g., histamine), whose sources and metabolism are well known, and mediators generated by stimulation. The sources and pathways of these mediators in various cells (e.g., arachidonate metabolites) are still poorly understood.

Studies have usually involved the measurement of the response of secretory tissue to an agonist *in vitro,* and this design suffers from many deficiencies. The administered material could be converted by airway cells to another more or less potent material. Important interactions among cells might not occur *in vitro*. Studies of administered mediators are frequently limited by the small amounts available (e.g., lipoxygenase products). Physiologic studies of release of mediators from tissue have been handicapped in the past by the lack of specific assays and specific antagonists. The structures of many of the mediators derived from arachidonic acid have been described, and specific immunoassays have been developed. As specific assays for various mediators become available, as specific antagonists to these are developed, and as more knowledge about the action of each cell and cell-to-cell interactions becomes known, a better understanding of the regulation of secretion will be possible.

Histamine is a preformed mediator released from mast cells; its effects on secretion are variable (83). Histamine was reported to have no effect on secretion in dogs or humans *in vitro,* but it stimulated mucus production in geese and cats. One study reported that histamine released mucins from human airways, an effect that was less potent than leukotrienes or prostaglandins (84).

Mediators have also been described that act indirectly to produce mucus secretion by activating nervous pathways. Thus, bradykinin reflexly stimulated fluid production from airway submucosal glands via a reflex (66), but had no significant effect on mucin release from explants (85). Bradykinin is released endogenously and produces inflammatory changes (86). In the gut, kinins activate cyclooxygenase pathways and produce prostaglandins (87); a similar effect in airways could modify secretion. Basic polypeptides (e.g., kallidin and substance P) stimulated mucus secretion in dogs, and hexadrimethrine, a kallidin antagonist, decreased secretion (88).

The two metabolic pathways of arachidonic acid metabolism have been implicated in the regulation of airway secretions, but these systems are not well understood. The cyclooxygenase pathway is most studied. Prostaglandins PGA_2, PGD_2, and $PGF_{2\alpha}$ increased mucin secretion by human airway tissue, and PGE_2 reduced release (89). Indomethacin is reported to decrease baseline mucin release, suggesting that lipoxygenase products generated by the airways modulate resting mucin production (90). It is not known whether this release is normal or whether it is due to the handling of tissue, nor are the cells of origin of the cyclooxygenase products known. No study has examined the release of arachidonic acid metabolites from the secretory cells alone.

Lipoxygenase products have been shown to affect mucin secretion. Thus, mono-HETEs stimulated mucin secretion in human bronchi, and several mono-HETEs increased mucin release (84). The leukotrienes C_4 and D_4 increased mucin production even more potently than the mono-HETEs.

The role of these mediators in mucociliary clearance in disease is unclear. The fact that nonselective antagonists of the lipoxygenase pathway prevent changes in mucociliary clearance produced experimentally in dogs with anaphylaxis suggests that these products might have serious deleterious effects on either ciliary or secretory function (91).

Inflammation and Hypertrophy of Secretory Tissues. Mucus gland hypertrophy has been observed in asthma (65). While the cause is unknown, there are compelling reasons to consider the possibility that inflammation plays an important role. First, inflammation plays a conspicuous role in the pathology of the various diseases associated with gland hypertrophy (i.e., chronic bronchitis, bronchiectasis, cystic fibrosis), and asthma is no exception (9). Second, most successful animal models of experimental hypertrophy of mucus-secreting cells involve the administration of an irritating material to the airways. These materials include formalin (92), sulfur dioxide (93), tobacco smoke (94), chlorine gas (95), and nitrogen dioxide (96). Because hypertrophy occurs with chronic stimulation, even in pathogen-free animals (97), bacterial infection cannot be the sole cause. Perhaps, activation of the epithelium by irritants releases mediators that stimulate growth of secretory cells. Studies with antiinflammatory drugs suggest that inflammatory mediators play a role in the overgrowth of secretory cells; phenylmethyloxadiozole inhibited the goblet cell proliferation that usually occurs after exposure to tobacco smoke (98). Indomethacin inhibited the increase in numbers of epithelial mucous cells caused by chronic inhalation of tobacco smoke in rats, suggesting that cyclooxygenase products might be involved in the hypertrophic response (99).

In each case of experimental hypertrophy, the irritant was delivered into the airway lumen, exposing the surface epithelial cells to the highest concentrations of the irritant. Perhaps stimulation of these surface epithelial cells results in the production of arachidonate metabolites, which in turn stimulate growth of the mucus-secreting cells.

Inflammation could cause increased growth by the release of mediators that act on cell growth and/or on secretory cell division. Alternatively, chronic irritation could cause hypertrophy in a manner similar to the work hypertrophy of skeletal muscle. Similar neural mechanisms have been implicated in experimental salivary gland hypertrophy (100). Acute irritation of the respiratory tract causes reflex secretion of mucus. Chronic release of autonomic mediators from nerve endings could, by chronic activation of mucous cell secretions, cause cell growth. Compatible with this hypothesis is the fact that chronic administration of both β-adrenergic and muscarinic agonists caused secretion cell hypertrophy (101).

Surface Mucin Secretion

Of the various cells lining the airways, the goblet cells, serous cells, Clara cells, and ciliated cells contribute to secretion. As with submucosal glands, the concentration and distribution of these cells vary widely among species (81). Goblet cells are normally limited to the major airways, but chronic inflammation results in an increase in their number (97). Little is known about airway goblet cell secretion. Epithelial serous cells are most common in the fetus and in specific pathogen-free rats (102); their function in healthy and diseased individuals is uncertain. There is evidence that suggests that irritation with tobacco smoke causes these cells to transform into goblet cells (97). Clara cells are generally found in bronchioles and have anatomic features suggesting a secretory function (103), but their function is unknown. Some authors believe they secrete a lipoprotein (104), perhaps a surfactant (105). Tobacco smoke appears to convert them into goblet cells (97), or they may be precursors of ciliated and brush cells (95). Ciliated cells are the most common surface cells. Although they do not contain secretory granules, they contain a layer of alcianophilic material close to the surface of the cell (106). This surface mucosubstance is believed to be an integral component of the cell.

There is no motor nerve supply to the surface cells, and autonomic agonists do not stimulate their activity (107). A variety of irritants cause mucus secretion (81). In many cases, these irritants cause reflex secretion from glands.

In many cases in which goblet cell secretion is claimed, the studies are inconclusive because there was no satisfactory method of demonstrating goblet cell secretion. However, some studies do suggest that irritants affect goblet cells. Jeffery found that treatment with ammonia resulted in fewer goblet cells in tracheal segments (106), and Adler reported similar results after application of cholera toxin to airway explants (108). Serum caused secretion from surface cells (109). It appears that ammonia and serum remove surface mucosubstance from ciliated cells (110), so surface secretions previously believed to be derived from goblet cells may in fact come from ciliated cells. Thus, regulation of surface-cell secretions is almost entirely unknown. Separation and culture of the various cell types and development of monoclonal antibodies to specific secretory materials should assist in understanding the contribution of various substances from different cells to the airway secretions.

Active Ion Transport

The coupling of cilia and surface mucus requires a delicate adjustment of the thickness of the sol layer. In 1975, we demonstrated a mechanism for regulating secretion or reabsorption of fluid locally (111). As in other epithelia, water crosses passively as the result of osmotic gradients created by active ion transport. In dog tracheal epithelium, we showed that there was a net movement of Cl^- toward the airway lumen and a smaller net movement of Na^+ toward the submucosa. The reader is referred to reviews of mechanisms of airway ion transport (81,112). In dogs in the resting condition, the net flux toward the lumen exceeds the net flux of Na^+ toward the submucosa. In resting tissue of rabbits (113) and perhaps humans (114), only reabsorption is demonstrable. Results of fluid sampling suggest that regional differences exist in airway of different sizes (115); net Cl^- movement toward the lumen predominates in the trachea, and net Na^+ movement toward the submucosa predominates in the bronchi (114).

We measured fluid flow directly and showed that net volume flow was usually not demonstrable in the resting state. However, upon stimulation of Cl^- transport, flow toward the airway lumen was markedly stimulated (116). The tissue can be transformed into an absorbing surface by adding a drug that inhibits Cl^- transport (117). Thus, the degree and the direction of fluid movement can be modified by drugs, and perhaps by disease.

Although there are no motor nerves in the airway epithelium (81), autonomic agonists affect active ion transport in airways. Acetylcholine increased net transport toward the airway lumen in dogs (118). Similarly, β-adrenergic agonists terbutaline (119), epinephrine, (120) and theophylline (121) increased net flux toward the lumen, presumably via cAMP (122). Vasoactive intestinal peptide, a putative mediator of the nonadrenergic, noncholinergic nervous system, also increased net flux toward the lumen by increasing intracellular levels of cAMP (123).

Mediators also have potent effects on the ion transport system, but there have been few studies. Histamine was observed to increase net fluxes toward the lumen, an effect prevented by an H_1-antagonist (124). Prostaglandin $F_{2\alpha}$ also stimulated tracheal ion transport (125). The resting net flux toward the epithelial lumen was decreased by indomethacin in dogs, suggesting that cyclooxygenase products were actively secreted at rest, at least *in vitro* (122).

Inflammatory processes could have potent effects on active ion transport. Alteration of prostaglandin release by the epithelium could have potent effects. Epithelial irritation, by increasing prostaglandin release, could stimulate fluid movement toward the lumen and thus dilute the irritant. Bradykinin has also been incriminated in inflammatory processes (126). Bradykinin stimulates increased net ion movement toward the airway lumen (G. Leikauf, personal communication), probably by the release of prostaglandins (127). Circulating plasma kinins are reported to be increased in severe asthma (128), and nasal secretions of asthmatic subjects are also reported to contain bradykinin (129). Kinins are released from the lungs of guinea pigs during anaphylaxis (130); IgE-mediated reactions in asthma could result in a similar generation of kinins.

Mucociliary Abnormalities in Asthma and in Experimental Anaphylaxis

Postmortem findings of mucous gland hypertrophy, increased numbers of goblet cells, and excessive airway secretions all point to serious abnormalities of mucociliary clearance in asthma (5). In patients who die in status asthmaticus, the ciliated epithelium is often denuded (131), and mucous plugs are seen (132,133). Abnormal mucociliary clearance occurs in some asymptomatic asthmatic subjects (3,4), while normal clearance is found in other studies (134). Asthmatic sputum has been reported to be more viscous than sputum from other patients (2).

Pharmacologic studies suggest mechanisms that might be involved in asthma. In sensitive dogs, inhalation of *Ascaris suum* aerosols decreased tracheal mucus velocity (91), and in asthmatic subjects inhalation of specific antigen had similar effects (135). The fact that the decreased clearance in sensitive asthmatics after inhaled ragweed antigen was prevented by cromolyn (136) suggests that the release of mast cell mediators was involved in the impaired clearance. The fact that FPL 55712 also prevented the impaired clearance (91,135) suggests that lipoxygenase products of arachidonic acid metabolism were involved in the abnormal clearance.

REFERENCES

1. Boushey, H. A., Holtzman, M. J., Sheller, J. R., and Nadal, J. A. State of the art. Bronchial hyperreactivity. *Am. Rev. Respir. Dis.* **121**:389–413, 180.
2. Charman, J., and Reid, L. Sputum viscosity in chronic bronchitis, bronchiectasis, asthma and cystic fibrosis. *Biorheology* **9**:185–199, 1972.
3. Santa-Cruz, R., Landa, J., Hirsch, J., and Sackner, M. A. Tracheal mucous velocity in normal man and patients with obstructive lung disease; effects of terbutaline. *Am. Rev. Respir. Dis.* **109**:458–463, 1974.
4. Mezey, R. J., Cohn, M. A., Fernandez, R. J., Januszkiewicz, A. J., and Wanner, A. Mucociliary transport in allergic patients with antigen-induced bronchospasm. *Am. Rev. Respir. Dis.* **118**:677–684, 1978.

5. Huber, H. L., and Koessler, K. K. Pathology of bronchial asthma. *Arch. Intern. Med.* **30:**689–760, 1922.

6. Dunnill, M. S., Mossarella, G. R., and Anderson, J. A. A comparison of the quantitative anatomy of the bronchi in normal subjects, in status asthmaticus, in chronic bronchitis, and in emphysema. *Thorax* **24:**176, 1969.

7. Sanerkin, N. G., and Evans, D. M. D. The sputum in bronchial asthma: Pathognomonic patterns. *J. Pathol. Bacteriol.* **89:**535–541, 1965.

8. Dunnill, M. S. The pathology of asthma. *In The identification of Asthma.* (R. Porter and J. Birch, eds.), pp. 35–46. Churchill, London, 1971.

9. Rottoli, P. Cellule mediatrici e epitelio bronchiale. *In* "Medicina Respiratoria Oggi" (S. C. Lees, P. Sestini, and L. Zignego, eds.), pp. 87–90. Siena, Grafica Pistolesi, 1983.

10. Lee, L.-Y., Bleecker, E. R., and Nadel, J. A. Effect of ozone on bronchomotor response to inhaled histamine aerosol in dogs. *J. Appl. Physiol.* **43:**626–631, 1977.

11. Abraham, W. M., Januszkiewicz, A. J., Mingle, M., Welker, M., Wanner, A., and Sackner, M. A. Sensitivity of bronchoprovocation and tracheal mucous velocity in detecting airway responses to O_3. *J. Appl. Physiol.* **48:**789–793, 1980.

12. Parker, C. D., Bilbo, R. E., and Reed, C. E. Methacholine aerosol as test for bronchial asthma. *Arch. Intern. Med.* **115:**452–458, 1965.

13. Empey, D. W., Laitinen, L. A., Jacobs, L., Gold, W. M., and Nadel, J. A. Mechanisms of bronchial hyperreactivity in normal subjects after upper respiratory tract infection. *Am. Rev. Respir. Dis.* **113:**131–139, 1976.

14. Little, J. W., Hall, W. J., Douglas, R. G., Jr., Mudholkar, G. S., Speers, D. M., and Patel, K. Airway hyperreactivity and peripheral airway dysfunction in influenza A infection. *Am. Rev. Respir. Dis.* **118:**295–303, 1978.

15. Walsh, J. J., Dietlein, L. F., Low, F. N., Bunch, G. E., and Mogabgab, W. J. Tracheobronchial response in human influenza. *Arch. Intern. Med.* **108:**376–382, 1961.

16. Popa, V., Douglas, J. S., and Bouhuys, A. Airway response to histamine, acetylcholine, and propranolol in anaphylactic hypersensitivity in guinea pigs. *J. Allergy Clin. Immunol.* **51:**344–356, 1973.

17. Patterson, R. W., and Harris, K. E. The effect of cholinergic and anticholinergic agents on the primate model of allergic asthma. *J. Lab. Clin. Med.* **87:**65–72, 1976.

18. Cockcroft, D. W., Ruffin, R. E., Dolovich, J., and Hargreave, F. E. Allergen-induced increase in non-allergic bronchial reactivity. *Clin. Allergy* **7:**503–513, 1977.

19. Boucher, R. C., Pare, P. D., and Hogg, J. C. Relationship between airway hyperreactivity and hyperpermeability in Ascaris-sensitive monkeys. *J. Allergy Clin. Immunol.* **64:**197–201, 1979.

20. Schlueter, D. P. Response of the lung to inhaled antigens. *Am. J. Med.* **57:**476–492, 1974.

21. Atkins, P. C., Norman, M., Weiner, H., and Zweiman, B. Release of neutrophil chemotactic activity during immediate hypersensitivity reactions in humans. *Ann. Intern. Med.* **86:**415–418, 1977.

22. Atkins, P. C., Norman, M. E., and Zweiman, B. Antigen-induced neutrophil chemotactic activity in man. Correlation with bronchospasm and inhibition of disodium cromoglycate. *J. Allergy Clin. Immunol* **62:**149–155, 1978.

23. Golden, J. A., Nadel, J. A., and Boushey, H. A. Bronchial hyperirritability in healthy subjects after exposure to ozone. *Am. Rev. Respir. Dis.* **118:**287–294, 1978.

24. Holtzman, M. J., Cunningham, J. H., Sheller, J. R., Irsigler, G. B., Nadel, J. A., and Bushey, H. A. Effect of ozone on bronchial reactivity in atopic and nonatopic subjects. *Am. Rev. Respir. Dis.* **120:**1059–1067, 1979.

25. DiMeo, J. J., Glenn, M. G., Holtzman, M. J., Sheller, J. R., Nadel, J. A., and

Boushey, H. A. Threshold concentration of ozone causing an increase in bronchial reactivity in humans and adaptation with repeated exposures. *Am. Rev. Respir. Dis.* **124**:245–248,1981.

26. Scheel, L. D., Dobrogorski, O. J., Mountain, J. T., Svirbely, J. L., and Stokinger, H. E. Physiologic, biochemical, immunologic, and pathologic changes following ozone exposure. *J. Appl. Physiol.* **14**:67–80, 1959.

27. Coffin, D. L., Gardner, D. E., Holzman, R. S., and Woolcock, F. J. Influence of ozone on pulmonary cells. *Arch. Environ. Health* **16**:633–636, 1968.

28. Plopper, C. G., Dungworth, W. S., and Tyler, W. S. Pulmonary lesions in rats exposed to ozone. A correlated light and electron microscopic study. *Am. J. Pathol.* **71**:375–394, 1973.

29. Bils, R. F., and Christie, B. R. The experimental pathology of oxidant and air pollutant inhalation. *Int. Rev. Exp. Pathol.* **21**:195–293, 1980.

30. Ward, P. A., Cohen, S., and Flanagan, T. D. Leukotactic factors elaborated by virus-infected tissues. *J. Exp. Med.* **135**:1095–1103, 1972.

31. Laitinen, L. A., Elkin, R. B., Empey, D. W., Jacobs, L., Mills, J., Gold, W. M., and Nadel, J. A. Changes in bronchial reactivity after administration of live attenuated influenza virus. *Am. Rev. Respir. Dis.* **113**:194, 1976.

32. Herxheimer, H. The late bronchial reaction in asthma. *Int. Arch. Allergy Appl. Immunol.* **3**:323–328, 1952.

33. Booij-Noord, H., Ovie, N. G. M., and de Vries, K. Immediate and late bronchial obstructive reactions to inhalation of house dust and protective effects of disodium cromoglycate and prednisolone. *J. Allergy Clin. Immunol.* **48**:344–354, 1971.

34. Hargreave, F. E., Dolovich, J., Robertson, D. G., and Kerigan, A. T. The late asthmatic responses. *Can. Med. Assoc. J.* **110**:415–421, 1974.

35. Dolovich, J., Hargreave, F. E., Chalmers, R., Shies, K. J., Gauldie, J., and Bienenstock, J. Late cutaneous allergic responses in isolated IgE-dependent reactions. *J. Allergy Clin. Immunol.* **52**:38–46, 1973.

36. Solley, G. O., Gleich, G. J., Jordan, R. E., and Schroeter, A. L. The late phase of the immediate wheal and flare skin reaction. *J. Clin. Invest.* **58**:408–420, 1976.

37. Nagy, L., Lee, T. H., and Kay, A. B. Neutrophil chemotactic activity in antigen-induced late asthmatic reactions. *N. Engl. J. Med.* **306**:497–501, 1982.

38. Shampain, M. P., Behrens, B. L., Larsen, G. L., and Henson, P. M. An animal model of late pulmonary responses to alternaria challenge. *Am. Rev. Respir. Dis.* **126**:493–498, 1982.

39. Boatman, E. S., Sato, S., and Frank, R. Acute effects of ozone on cat lungs. II. Structural. *Am. Rev. Respir. Dis.* **110**:157–169, 1974.

40. Holtzman, M. J., Sheller, J. A., DiMeo, M. D., Nadel, J. A., and Boushey, H. A. Effect of ganglionic blockade on bronchial reactivity in atopic subjects. *Am. Rev. Respir. Dis.* **122**:17–25, 1980.

41. Dumont, C. G., Kirkpatrick, M. B., and Nadel, J. A. Airway hyperreactivity to acetylcholine aerosol after ozone in anesthetized dogs. *Clin. Res.* **29**:67A, 1980.

42. Lee, L.-Y., Dumont, C., Djokic, T. D., Menzel, T. E., and Nadel, J. A. Mechanism of rapid, shallow breathing after ozone exposure in conscious dogs. *J. Appl. Physiol.* **46**:1108–1114, 1979.

43. Lee, L.-Y., Djokic, T. D., Dumont, C., Graf, P. D., and Nadel, J. A. Mechanism of ozone-induced tachypneic response to hypoxia and hypercapnia in conscious dogs. *J. Appl. Physiol.* **48**:163–168, 1980.

44. Fabbri, L. M., Aizawa, H., Alpert, S. E., Walters, E. H., O'Byrne, P. M., Gold, B.

D., Nadel, J. A., and Holtzman, M. J. Hyperreactivity and changes in cell counts in bronchoalveolar lavage after ozone in dogs. *Am. Rev. Respir. Dis.* **127:**244, 1983.

45. Holtzman, M. J., Fabbri, L. M., O'Byrne, P. M., Gold, B. D., Aizawa, H., Walters, E. H., Alpert, S. E., and Nadel, J. A. Importance of airway inflammation for hyperresponsiveness induced by ozone. *Am. Rev. Respir. Dis.* **127:**686–690, 1983.

46. Holtzman, M. J., Fabbri, L. M., Skoogh, B.-E., O'Byrne, P. M., Walters, E. H., Aizawa, H., and Nadel, J. A. Time course of ozone-induced hyperresponsiveness in dogs. *J. Appl. Physiol.* **55:**1232–1236, 1983.

47. Holtzman, M. J., Aizawa, H., Nadel, J. A., and Goetzl, E. J. Selective generation of leukotriene B$_4$ by tracheal epithelial cells from dogs. *Biochem. Biophys. Res. Commun.* **114:**1071–1076, 1983.

48. Shimasaki, H., Takatori, T., Anderson, W. R., Horten, H. L., and Privett, O. S. Alteration of lung lipids in ozone exposed rats. *Biochem. Biophys. Res. Commun.* **68:**1256–1262, 1976.

49. Goetzl, E. J., and Pickett, W. C. The human PMN leukocyte chemotactic activity of complex hydroxyeicosatetraenoic acids (HETES). *J. Immunol.* **125:**1789–1791, 1980.

50. Goetzl, E. J., Phillips, M. J., and Gold, W. M. Stimulus specificity of the generation of leukotrienes by dog mastocytoma cells. *J. Exp. Med.* **158:**731–737, 1983.

51. O'Byrne, P., Walters, E., Gold, B., Aizawa, H., Fabbri, L., Alpert, S., Nadel, J., and Holtzman, M. Neutrophil depletion inhibits airway hyperresponsiveness induced by ozone. *Physiologist* **26:**A35, 1983.

52. Cross, C. E., DeLucia, A. J., Reddy, A. K., Hussain, M. Z., Chow, C.-K., and Mustafa, M. G. Ozone interactions with lung tissue. Biochemical approaches. *Am. J. Med.* **60:**929–935, 1976.

53. Mustafa, M. G., Tierney, D. F. State of the Art. Biochemical and metabolic changes in the lung with oxygen, ozone, and nitrogen dioxide toxicity. *Am. Rev. Respir. Dis.* **118:**1061–1090, 1978.

54. Goetzl, E. J. Oxygenation products of arachidonic acid as mediators of hypersensitivity and inflammation. *Med. Clin. North Am.* **65:**809–828, 1981.

55. Walters, E. H., Parrish, R. W., Bevan, C., and Smith, A. P. Induction of bronchial hypersensitivity: Evidence for a role for prostaglandins. *Thorax* **36:**571–574, 1981.

56. Copas, J. L., Borgeat, P., and Gardiner, P. J. The actions of 5-, 12-, and 15-HETE on tracheobronchial smooth muscle. *Prostaglandins, Leukotrienes Med.* **8:**105–114, 1982.

57. Fabbri, L. M., Aizawa, H., O'Byrne, P. M., Walters, E. H., Holtzman, M. J., and Nadel, J. A. BW755c inhibits airway hyperresponsiveness induced by ozone in dogs. *Physiologist* **26:**A35, 1983.

58. Ueki, I., German, V. F., and Nadel, J. A. Micropipette measurement of airway submucosal gland secretion. Autonomic effects. *Am. Rev. Respir. Dis.* **121:**351–357, 1980.

59. King, M., Cohen, C., and Viires, N. Influence of vagal tone on rheology and transportability of canine tracheal mucus. *Am. Rev. Respir. Dis.* **120:**1215–1219, 1979.

60. Nadel, J. A. Autonomic control of airway smooth muscle and airway secretions. *Am. Rev. Respir. Dis.* **115**(Suppl. 6):117–126, 1977.

61. Gallagher, J. T., Kent, P. W., Passatore, M., Phipps, R. J., and Richardson, P. S. The composition of tracheal mucus and the nervous control of its secretion in the cat. *Proc. R. Soc. London, Ser. B* **192:**49–76, 1975.

62. German, V. F., Ueki, I. F., and Nadel, J. A. Micropipette measurement of airway submucosal gland secretion: Laryngeal reflex. *Am. Rev. Respir. Dis.* **122:**413–416, 1980.

63. Phipps, R. J., and Richardson, P. S. The effects of irritation at various levels of the

airway upon tracheal mucus secretion in the cat. *J. Physiol. (London)* **261:**563–581, 1976.

64. Hahn, H. L., Johnson, H. G., Chow, A. W., Graf, P. D., and Nadel, J. A. Reflex effects of sulfur dioxide on submucosal gland secretion in canine trachea. *Clin. Res.* **30:**71A, 1982.

65. Takizawa, T., and Thurlbeck, W. M. Muscle and mucous gland size in the major bronchi of patients with chronic bronchitis, asthma, and asthmatic bronchitis. *Am. Rev. Respir. Dis.* **104:**331–336, 1971.

66. Davis, B., Roberts, A. M., Coleridge, H. M., and Coleridge, J. C. G. Reflex tracheal gland secretion evoked by stimulation of bronchial C-fibers in dogs. *J. Appl. Physiol.* **53:**985–991, 1982.

67. Davis, B., Chinn, R., Popovac, D., Widdicombe, J. G., and Nadel, J. Hypoxia stimulates mucus gland secretion via a carotid body reflex in dogs. *Am. Rev. Respir. Dis.* **121:**332, 1980.

68. Borson, D. B., Charlin, M., Gold, B. D., and Nadel, J. A. Nonadrenergic noncholinergic nerves mediate secretion of macromolecules by tracheal glands of ferrets. *Fed. Proc., Fed. Am. Soc. Exp. Biol.* **41:**1754, 1982.

69. Basbaum, C. B., Ueki, I., Brezina, L., and Nadel, J. A. Tracheal submucosal gland serous cells stimulated in vitro with adrenergic and cholinergic agonists: A morphometric study. *Cell Tissue Res.* **220:**481–498, 1981.

70. Phipps, R. J., Nadel, J. A., and Davis, B. Effect of alpha-adrenergic stimulation on mucus secretion and on ion transport in cat trachea in vitro. *Am. Rev. Respir. Dis.* **121:**359–365, 1980.

71. Borson, D. B., Chinn, R. A., Davis, B., and Nadel, J. A. Adrenergic and cholinergic nerves mediate fluid secretion from tracheal glands of ferrets. *J. Appl. Physiol.* **49:**1027–1031, 1980.

72. Quinton, P. M. Composition and control of secretions from tracheal bronchial submucosal glands. *Nature (London)* **279:**551–552, 1979.

73. Ueki, I., and Nadel, J. A. Differences in total protein concentration in submucosal gland fluid: Alpha-adrenergic vs cholinergic. *Fed. Proc., Fed. Am. Soc. Exp. Biol.* **40:**622, 1981.

74. Tom-Moy, M., Basbaum, C. B., and Nadel, J. A. Immunocytochemical localization of lysozyme in the ferret trachea. *Physiologist* **178:**99, 1980.

75. Leikauf, G. D., Ueki, I. F., and Nadel, J. A. Selective autonomic regulation of the viscoelastic properties of submucosal gland secretions from cat trachea. *J. Appl. Physiol.* **56:**426–430, 1984.

76. Tom-Moy, M., Basbaum, C. B., and Nadel, J. A. Isoproterenol produces hypertrophic submucosal glands in the ferret trachea. *Fed. Proc., Fed. Am. Soc. Exp. Biol.* **41:**1510, 1982.

77. Uddman, R., and Sundler, F. Vasoactive intestinal polypeptide nerves in human upper respiratory tract. *Oto-, Rhino-, Laryngol. (Amsterdam)* **41:**221–226, 1979.

78. Uddman, R., Alumets, J., Densert, O., Hakanson, R., and Sundler, F. Occurrence and distribution of VIP nerves in the nasal mucosa and tracheobronchial wall. *Acta Otol-Laryngol.* **86:**443–448, 1978.

79. Basbaum, C. B., Barnes, P. J., Grillo, M. A., Widdicombe, J. H., and Nadel, J. A. Adrenergic and cholinergic receptors in submucosal glands of the ferret trachea: Autoradiographic localization. *Eur. J. Respir. Dis.* (in press).

80. Peatfield, A. C., Barnes, P. J., Bratcher, C., Nadel, J. A., and Davis, B. Vasoactive intestinal peptide stimulates tracheal submucosal gland secretion in ferret. *Am. Rev. Respir. Dis.* **128:**89–93, 1983.

81. Nadel, J. A., Widdicombe, J. H., and Peatfield, A. C. Regulation of airway secretions. *In* "Handbook of Physiology" (A. P. Fishman and A. B. Fisher, eds.). *Am. Physiol. Soc.* Bethesda, Maryland (in press).

82. Davis, B., and Nadel, J. A. New methods used to investigate the control of mucus secretion and ion transport in airways. *Environ. Health Perspect.* **35:**121–130, 1980.

83. Nadel, J. A. Regulation of bronchial secretions. *In* "Immunopharmacology of the Lung" (H. H. Newball, ed.), pp. 109–139. Dekker, New York, 1983.

84. Shelhamer, J. H., Marom, Z., Sun, F., Bach, M. K., and Kaliner, M. The effects of arachinoids and leukotrienes on the release of mucus from human airways. *Chest* **81S:**36S–37S, 1982.

85. Sturgess, J., and Reid, L. An organ culture study of the effect of drugs on the secretory activity of the human bronchial submucosal gland. *Clin. Sci.* **43:**533–543, 1972.

86. Regoli, D., and Barabe, J. Pharmacology of bradykinin and related kinins. *Pharmacol. Rev.* **32:**1–46, 1980.

87. Field, M., Musch, W., and Stoff, J. S. Role of prostaglandins in the regulation of intestinal electrolyte transport. *Prostaglandins* **21**(Suppl.):73–79, 1981.

88. Boyd, E. M., and Lapp, M. S. On the expectorant action of parasympathomimetic drugs. *J. Pharmacol. Exp. Ther.* **87:**24–32, 1946.

89. Marom, Z., Shelhamer, J. H., and Kaliner, M. Effects of arachidonic acid, monohydroxyeicosatetraenoic acid and prostaglandins on the release of mucous glycoproteins from human airways in vitro. *J. Clin. Invest.* **67:**1695–1702, 1981.

90. Boat, T. F., and Cheng, P. W. Biochemistry of airway mucus secretions. *Fed. Proc., Fed. Am. Soc. Exp. Biol.* **39:**3067–3074, 1980.

91. Wanner, A., Zarzecki, S., Hirsch, J., and Epstein, S. Tracheal mucous transport in experimental canine asthma. *J. Appl. Physiol.* **39:**950–957, 1975.

92. Florey, H., Carleton, H. M., and Wells, A. Q. Mucus secretion in the trachea. *Br. J. Exp. Pathol.* **13:**269–284, 1932.

93. Baker, A. P., Chakrin, L. W., Sawyer, J. L., Munro, J. R., Hillegass, L. M., and Giannone, E. Glycosyltransferases in canine respiratory tissue. Alterations in an experimentally induced hypersecretory state. *Biochem. Med.* **10:**387–399, 1974.

94. Park, S. S., Kikkawa, Y., Goldring, I. P., Daly, M. M., Zelefsky, M., Shim, C., Spierer, M., and Morita, T. An animal model of cigarette smoking in beagle dogs. Correlative evaluation of effects on pulmonary function, defense, and morphology. *Am. Rev. Respir. Dis.* **115:**971–979, 1977.

95. Evans, M. J., Gabrel-Anderson, L. J., and Freeman, G. Role of the Clara cell in renewal of the bronchiolar epithelium. *Lab. Invest.* **38:**648–653, 1978.

96. Freeman, G., and Haydon, G. B. Emphysema after low-level exposure to NO_2. *Arch. Environ. Health* **8:**125–128, 1964.

97. Jeffery, P. K., and Reid, L. The effect of tobacco smoke, with or without phenylmethyloxadiazole (PMO) on rat bronchial epithelium: A light and electron microscopic study. *J. Pathol.* **133:**341–359, 1981.

98. Jones, R., Bolduc, P., and Reid, L. Protection of rat bronchial epithelium against tobacco smoke. *Br. Med. J.* **2:**142–144, 1972.

99. Grieg, N., Ayers, M., and Jeffery, P. K. The effect of indomethacin on the response of bronchial epithelium to tobacco smoke. *J. Pathol.* **132:**1–9, 1980.

100. Schneyer, C. A., and Hall, H. D. Neurally mediated increase in mitosis and DNA of rat parotid with increase in bulk of diet. *Am. J. Physiol.* **230:**911–915, 1976.

101. Sturgess, J., and Reid, L. The effect of isoprenaline and pilocarpine on (a) bronchial mucus-secreting tissue and (b) pancreas, salivary glands, heart, thymus, liver and spleen. *Br. J. Exp. Pathol.* **54:**388–403, 1973.

102. Baker, A. P., Chakrin, L. W., and Wardell, J. R., Jr. Chronic cholinergic stimulation of canine respiratory tissue. Its effect on the activities of glycosyltransferases and release of macromolecules. *Am. Rev. Respir. Dis.* **111:**423–431, 1975.

103. Widdicombe, J. G., and Pack, R. J. The Clara cell. *Eur. J. Respir. Dis.* **63:**202–220, 1982.

104. Azzopardi, A., and Thurlbeck, W. M. The histochemistry of the nonciliated bronchiolar epithelial cell. *Am. Rev. Respir. Dis.* **99:**516–525, 1969.

105. Ebert, R. B., Kronenberg, R. S., and Terracio, M. J. Study of the surface secretion of the bronchiole using radioautography. *Am. Rev. Respir. Dis.* **114:**567–573, 1976.

106. Jeffery, P. K. Structure and function of mucus-secreting cells of cat and goose airway epithelium. *Ciba Found. Symp.* **54**(new ser.):5–20, 1978.

107. Lamb, D. The composition of tracheal mucus and the nervous control of its secretion in the cat. Appendix. *Proc. R. Soc. London, Ser. B* **192:**72–76, 1975.

108. Adler, K. B., Hardwick, B. S., and Craighead, J. E. Effect of cholera toxin on secretion of mucin by explants of guinea pig trachea. *Lab. Invest.* **45:**372–377, 1981.

109. Peatfield, A. C. The control of mucus secretion into the lumen of the trachea. Ph.D. Thesis, London University, London, 1980.

110. Gallagher, J. T., Hall, R. L., Jeffery, P. K., Phipps, R. J., and Richardson, P. S. The nature and origin of tracheal secretions released in response to pilocarpine and ammonia. *J. Physiol. (London)* **275:**36P–37P, 1978.

111. Oliver, R. E., Davis, B., Marin, M. G., and Nadel, J. A. Active transport of Na^+ and Cl^- across the canine tracheal epithelium in vitro. *Am. Rev. Respir. Dis.* **112:**811–815, 1975.

112. Widdicombe, J. H., and Welsh, M. J. Ion transport by dog tracheal epithelium. *Fed. Proc., Fed. Am. Soc. Exp. Biol.* **39:**3062–3066, 1980.

113. Boucher, R. C., Jr., Bromberg, P. A., and Gatzy, J. T. Airway transepithelial electric potential in vivo: Species and regional differences. *J. Appl. Physiol.* **48:**169–176, 1980.

114. Knowles, M. R., Murray, G. F., Shallal, J. A., Gatzy, J. T., and Boucher, R. C. Bioelectrical properties (BEP) and ion transport (IT) in excised human bronchi. *Physiologist* **23:**100, 1980.

115. Boucher, R. C., Stutts, M. J., Bromberg, P. A., and Gatzy, J. T. Regional differences in airway surface liquid composition. *J. Appl. Physiol.* **50:**613–620, 1981.

116. Welsh, M. J., Widdicombe, J. H., and Nadel, J. A. Fluid transport across the canine tracheal epithelium. *J. Appl. Physiol.* **49:**905–909, 1980.

117. Nathanson, I. T., Widdicombe, J. H., and Highland, E. Effect of MK-196 on ion transport by dog tracheal epithelium. *Fed. Proc., Fed. Am. Soc. Exp. Biol.* **40:**373, 1981.

118. Marin, M. G., Davis, B., and Nadel, J. A. Effect of acetylcholine on Cl^- and Na^+ fluxes across dog tracheal epithelium in vitro. *Am. J. Physiol.* **231:**1546–1549, 1976.

119. Davis, B., Marin, M. G., and Nadel, J. A. Adrenergic receptor in canine tracheal epithelium. *Am. Rev. Respir. Dis.* **111:**947, 1975.

120. Al-Bazzaz, F., Khan, A., and Cheng, E. Stimulation of chloride secretion across canine tracheal epithelia by theophylline and epinephrine. *Clin. Res.* **25:**414A, 1977.

121. Al-Bazzaz, F., and Al-Awqati, Q. Interaction between sodium and chloride transport in canine tracheal mucosa. *J. Appl. Physiol.* **46:**111–119, 1979.

122. Al-Bazzaz, F. J. Role of cyclic AMP in regulation of chloride secretion by canine tracheal mucosa. *Am. Rev. Respir. Dis.* **123:**295–298, 1981.

123. Nathanson, I., Widdicombe, J. H., and Barnes, P. J. Effect of vasoactive intestinal peptide on ion transport across the dog tracheal epithelium. *J. Appl. Physiol.* **55:**1844–1848, 1983.

124. Marin, M. G., Davis, B., and Nadel, J. A. Effect of histamine on electrical and ion transport properties of tracheal epithelium. *J. Appl. Physiol.* **42:**735–738, 1977.

125. Al-Bezzaz, F., and Yadava, V. P. Ion transport across tracheal epithelium: Effect of prostaglandins. *Clin. Res.* **26:**687A, 1978.

126. Erdos, E. G. Kininases. *Handb. Exp. Pharmakol.* **25** (Suppl.):427–487, 1979.

127. Piper, P. J., and Vane, J. R. The release of prostaglandins during anaphylaxis in guinea pig isolated lungs. *In* "Prostaglandins, Peptides and Amines" (P. Mantegazza and E. W. Horton, eds.), pp. 15–19. Academic Press, London, 1969.

128. Abe, K., Watanabe, N., Kumagai, N., Mouri, T., Seki, T., and Yoshinaga, K. Circulating plasma kinin in patients with bronchial asthma. *Experientia* **23:**626–627, 1967.

129. Dolovich, J., Back, N., and Arbesman, E. The presence of bradykinin-like activity in nasal secretions from allergic subjects. *J. Allergy* **41:**103 (abstr.), 1968.

130. Johasson, O., and Becker, E. L. Release of kallikrein from guinea pig lung during anaphylaxis. *J. Exp. Med.* **123:**509–522, 1966.

131. Hilding, A. C. The relation of ciliary insufficiency to death from asthma and other respiratory diseases. *Ann. Otol., Rhinol., Laryngol.* **52:**5–19, 1943.

132. Alexander, H. L. A historical account of death from asthma. *J. Allergy* **34:**305–322, 1963.

133. Dunnill, M. S. The pathology of asthma, with special reference to changes in the bronchial mucosa. *J. Clin. Pathol.* **13:**27–33, 1960.

134. Mossberg, B., Strandberg, L., and Philipson, K. Tracheobronchial clearance in bronchial asthma. Response to beta-adrenoreceptor stimulation. *Scand. J. Respir. Dis.* **57:**119–128, 1976.

135. Ahmed, T., Greenblatt, D. W., Birch, S., Marchette, B., and Wanner, A. Mucociliary transport in allergic patients with antigen-induced bronchospasm: Role of slow reacting substance of anaphylaxis (SRS-A). *Am. Rev. Respir. Dis.* **121:**106, 1980.

136. Wanner, A. The role of mucociliary dysfunction in bronchial asthma. *Am. J. Med.* **67:**477–485, 1979.

DISCUSSION

Kay: What is the evidence for the involvement of free radicals in your epithelial model?

Nadel: Certainly, ozone has effects in other systems via free radical generation. However, we do not know yet for sure whether the ozone effects that I described are caused by free radical effects. The use of free radical scavengers should help to answer this question.

Lewis: Is the availability of arachidonic acid alone sufficient to initiate epithelial LTB_4 production or is prior cell damage required? How much LTB_4 is produced per unit number of epithelial cells? In other words, is it an adequate quantity to theoretically stimulate neutrophil chemotaxis?

Also, which mast cells does 15-HETE stimulate to secrete? What are the mediator products that are released, and is 15-HETE over the same dose response sufficient for the effect or is it only effective as a coactivator?

Nadel: Our initial observation was that the addition of arachidonic acid to isolated canine epithelial cells resulted in the generation of LTB_4 and a concomitant loss of cell viability (M. J. Holtzman, H. Aizawa, J. A. Nadel, and E. J. Goetzl, *Biochem. Biophys. Res. Commun.* **114:**1071–1076, 1983). It is too early to state whether loss of viability is required for the generation of LTB_4. However, we showed that the quantities of LTB_4

generated by a small number of cells were capable of causing neutrophil chemotaxis *in vitro*. Thus, it is fascinating that cell damage produces a material (LTB_4) which, by causing neutrophil chemotaxis, contributes to the cellular response to the damage. Teleologically, such a mechanism could provide an important defence mechanism not only in the airway, but also in other organs such as the skin and gut

The experiments in which 15-HETE was shown to cause mast cells to secrete were performed by Dr. Gold and his associates (E. J. Goetzl, M. J. Phillips, and W. M. Gold, *J. Exp. Med.*, **158**:731–737, 1983). The cells were isolated and purified from canine mastocytomas, as described in M. J. Phillips, W. M. Gold, and E. J. Goetzl (*J. Immunol.* **131**:906, 1983). Dose–response curves with 15-HETE (0.1–3.0 mcg/ml) produced a dose-dependent release of leukotrienes, but did not evoke the release of histamine. One microgram per milliliter of 15-HETE generated 26.1 ng $LTC_4/10^6$ mastocytoma cells at 30 min. 15-HPETE (0.3–3.0 μg/ml) had no effect on LTC_4 generation, but 12-HETE (1 μg/ml) generated 4.9 ng $LTC_4/10^6$ cells at 30 min. These results were obtained with the HETEs alone; they might also potentiate the effects of other secretagogues, but this was not examined.

Hogg: Is the timing of the migration of PMNs and the onset of hyperreactivity the same? Do you think they are related, and if so, how?

Nadel: Neutrophil chemotaxis (as evidenced by airway biopsies and bronchopulmonary lavage) occurred within an hour after ozone exposure (2 hr of exposure) and correlated well with the development of increased bronchomotor responsiveness.

Oates: What is the EC50 for the activation of mast cells by 15-HETE?

Nadel: Approximately 0.3 μg/ml.

Schiffmann: Can the ozone damage to epithelial cells resulting in leukotriene production be explained by an influx of calcium into the cell?

Nadel: We have not yet demonstrated directly that ozone stimulates epithelial cells to generate LTB_4, but if it can be demonstrated, it will be important to examine the role of calcium influx.

Austen: Can you please give quantitative data on 15-HETE production per unit mass of epithelial cells and quantitative data on 15-HETE activation of dog mastocytoma?

Nadel: 320 ng/10^6 cells, 90 min at 200 μg/ml of arachidonic acid (M. J. Holtzman, H. Aizawa, J. A. Nadel, and E. J. Goetzl, *Biochem. Biophys. Res. Commun.*, **114**:1071–1076, 1983).

Barnes: Could you clarify the relationship between neutrophil depletion and change in bronchial reactivity? Is the effect of hydroxyurea specific to neutrophils or are other cells affected?

Nadel: Dr. O'Byrne in my laboratory has shown that depletion of neutrophils with hydroxyurea prevented ozone-induced hyperresponsiveness of airway smooth muscle. To be further convinced that depletion of neutrophils was responsible for hydroxyurea's effect, it is necessary to reinfuse neutrophils into the circulation and restore the response in the presence of hydroxyurea (P. O'Byrne, E. Walters, B. Gold, H. Aizawa, L. Fabbri, S. Alpert, J. Nadel, and M. Holtzman, *Physiologist* **26**:A35, 1983).

Kaliner: I would caution about species variations. Clearly data do not freely extrapolate from dog, cat, or ferret to man. Moreover, our experience indicates that even within humans, there is tissue variability. Thus nonsteroidal antiinflammatory drugs enhance human airway glycoprotein release but do not affect nasal mucosal glycoprotein release.

As to the 15-HETE experiments, we have tested this question in three models and failed to confirm your data. In collaboration with Dr. Jack Vanderhook, we have challenged rats *in vivo* with dose–responses of 15-HETE and analysed LTC_4 or LTD_4 generation by HPLC; none was formed. 15-HETE may modulate A23187-generated LTD_4 or LTD_4, but does not form LTC_4 or LTD_4 without additional stimuli. We have also challenged human airway and nasal mucosa with 1–10 nM of 15-HETE, and the challenge caused mucus glycoprotein release from airways (Z. Marom, F. Sun, J. F. Shelhamer, and M. Kaliner, *J. Clin. Invest.* **72:**122, 1983) but none from nasal mucosa, and in neither instance was histamine release or leukotriene generation seen. Thus, 15-HETE failed to activate mast cells or cause LTC_4 or LTD_4 generation in any of these three models.

Nadel: Dr. Kaliner's point about species variation is an important one. Our new observation is that *canine* epithelial cells can, upon provocation, generate potent lipoxygenase products and thereby participate in inflammatory responses. The extent and importance of these epithelial cell responses and the differences among species need to be investigated. Dr. Kaliner's studies in rats are interesting. Because their studies were not performed in isolated cells, they could not determine whether airway epithelial cells produced lipoxygenase products for the following reasons: first, released products might not be accessible for sampling in his animals. Second, other cells in the preparation could modify the effects of secretory products of epithelial cells. Dr. Kaliner also referred to his work on challenged human airway mucosa (Z. Marom, J. H. Shelhamer, F. Sun, and M. Kaliner, *J. Clin. Invest.* **72:**122, 1983). Again, this study was not performed with isolated epithelial cells, so unfortunately the studies cannot be compared with ours. Furthermore, the manuscript does not mention any data on histamine release by 15-HETE. Dr. Kaliner refers to a third study of nasal mucosa in the *J. Clin. Invest.* article. Review of this article does not reveal data on nasal mucosa. In summary, I would not be surprised if human airway epithelial cells generate lipoxygenase products that are different from those of dogs. Such studies may provide exciting new information.

Kerr: Can you transfer smooth muscle hyperresponsiveness to a nonozone-treated model by bronchial lavage material from the ozone-treated model?

Nadel: An interesting approach.

CHAPTER 10

The Potential Role of Alveolar Macrophages as a Source of Pathogenic Mediators in Allergic Asthma*

JOHN A. RANKIN

Pulmonary Disease Section
Department of Medicine
Yale University School of Medicine
New Haven, Connecticut, U.S.A.

PHILIP W. ASKENASE

Section of Clinical Immunology and Allergy
Department of Medicine
Yale University School of Medicine
New Haven, Connecticut, U.S.A.

INTRODUCTION

IgE-induced release of mediators from mast cells is a central event in immediate hypersensitivity reactions. Many mediators are potentially involved in these responses. Some of these include histamine, slow-reacting substances (SRS), platelet-activating factor (PAF), chemotactic factors, and kinin-generating substances (1,2). Over the past decade, evidence has accumulated suggesting that cells other than mast cells may also play important roles as sources of many of these mediators in IgE-dependent diseases such as allergic asthma. The macrophage is one such cell. This cell is part of a family of mononuclear phagocytic cells found in virtually every organ. The traditional classification of lung macrophages separates

* Supported in part by grants from the U.S. Public Health Service, National Institutes of Health, Nos. A1-12211, AI-11077, AI-17555 and AI-10497. J. A. R. is a recipient of the Charles E. Culpeper Award, Yale University School of Medicine and a Parker B. Francis Fellow of Puritan–Bennett Foundation.

157

them by their anatomic distribution into two types: alveolar and interstitial. Alveolar macrophages reside in the air spaces at the surface of the lung. Because of their location at the interface between the environment and lung tissue and because of their phagocytic capacity, alveolar macrophages are considered part of the first line of body defence (3,4). Indeed, their anatomic location makes them one of the first cells to encounter inhaled particles and solubilized constituents of particles that may be allergens.

Alveolar macrophages secrete numerous enzymes and mediators important in the initiation and regulation of inflammatory reactions (3,4), but a full understanding of their secretory capacity is far from complete. This is especially true in regard to the recently described release of mediators of immediate hypersensitivity by macrophages. In fact, it has been discovered only in the 1970s that macrophages can be activated by IgE-dependent mechanisms (5–11), and that macrophages can be stimulated by non-IgE-dependent mechanisms to release SRS (12–14) and PAF (15,16). In the past few years we have been interested in the alveolar macrophage as a potential source of mediators such as SRS, now known as leukotrienes LTC_4, LTD_4, and LTE_4 (2,17,18), and therefore in the potential involvement of this cell in immediate hypersensitivity reactions in the lung. In this chapter, we will focus on this cell as a source of SRS and PAF and show how release of these mediators from macrophages can be induced by immunologic mechanisms of relevance to asthma (11,19,19a). Leukotrienes and PAF are potent bronchoconstrictors (1,2,20) and leukotrienes and other macrophage-derived metabolites of arachidonic acid also can act to promote mucus secretion and mucosal edema (1,2,21–23). Thus, alveolar macrophages should be considered as potential participants in IgE-dependent allergic lung disease.

MACROPHAGE ACTIVATION BY AN IgE-DEPENDENT MECHANISM

In the early 1970s, Capron and co-workers first implicated IgE antibodies in macrophage-dependent cytotoxic damage to parasites (5). They demonstrated that incubation of *Schistosoma mansoni* schistosomules (larvae) with serum from rats immune to *S. mansoni* caused activation and adherence of peritoneal macrophages from normal rats and subsequent cytotoxic damage to the schistosomules (5,8). Further studies revealed that serum immune complexes composed of specific anti-schistosomal IgE and soluble parasite antigen induced this adherence and cytotoxicity (8). Thereafter, similar observations were made using normal human or baboon peripheral blood monocytes incubated with sera from humans or baboons with schistosomiasis (7), and with rat macrophages incubated with filaria and antifilarial IgE (24).

Dessaint and co-workers also observed that IgE–anti-IgE complexes caused rat peritoneal macrophages to release lysozomal enzymes and superoxide anion (6). Subsequently, these observations led to investigation of whether IgE activation of macrophages could have an important role in IgE-mediated diseases by examination of the ability of human alveolar macrophages to be activated by IgE-dependent mechanisms. When alveolar macrophages from normal individuals were incubated with IgE and then with anti-IgE, or with sera from atopic persons and with specific allergen, or with anti-IgE antibody alone, release of lysosomal enzymes such as neutral proteases and β-glucuronidase was observed (10,11). Alveolar macrophages from asthmatic individuals also release lysosomal enzymes in response to challenge with specific allergen or anti-IgE (11).

These observations argue strongly in favor of a role for alveolar macrophages in IgE-dependent pulmonary diseases.

EVIDENCE FOR IgE-Fc RECEPTORS IN MACROPHAGES

An important finding was that the activation of rat antischistosomal cytotoxicity of rat peritoneal macrophages occurred through the interaction of IgE immune complexes with an IgE-Fc receptor (FcR) on the macrophage surface (25). IgE-FcR exist on rat peritoneal and alveolar macrophages (26,27), and approximately 80% of rat lung lavage cells that adhere to glass (i.e., alveolar macrophages) possess IgE-FcR (26).

Specific receptors for IgE also have been found on the monocyte-like human cell line U937 (28), on human peripheral blood monocytes (29), and on about 10% of normal human alveolar macrophages (11,30). Interestingly, the number of IgE-FcR positive alveolar macrophages and peripheral blood monocytes is increased in atopic individuals compared to normals (10,11,30,31). IgE binding to IgE-FcR on various types of macrophages is of much lower affinity (about 100 times less) than IgE binding to FcR on mast cells (25,27,28,30). The lower affinity binding of IgE to monocytes and macrophages suggests that IgE immune complexes may be more important in activation of these cells, compared to mast cells and basophils that are sensitized by monomeric IgE, because of the greater strength of binding to FcR.

PERITONEAL MACROPHAGE RELEASE OF SRS

It has been established that rat peritoneal macrophages, when stimulated with the calcium ionophore A23187 *in vivo* or *in vitro,* release an SRS-like substance (12,13) that is a combination of LTC (32) and LTD (33). Several investigators have shown that peritoneal macrophages from mice, stimulated with either zymosan or A23187, also will release SRS (13,16,34,35).

RAT ALVEOLAR MACROPHAGE RELEASE OF SRS

We have shown that rat alveolar macrophages release easily quantifiable amounts of SRS when stimulated with A23187 and L-cysteine using conditions that optimize SRS release from these cells (Fig. 1A). We also wished to determine if rat alveolar macrophages could release SRS when incubated with IgE and antigen. For these studies, we used hapten affinity-purified mouse monoclonal anti-DNP IgE antibody and specific antigen (DNP-HSA). In 56 separate experiments performed over 3 years, we found repeatedly that rat alveolar macrophages release SRS in readily detectable quantities (Fig. 1B) when stimulated with this IgE and antigen. As the chemical nature of the SRS released by IgE and antigen was unknown initially, quantitative comparisons were made between the magnitude of the muscle contractions produced by our supernatants and those produced by a synthetic LTE. Therefore, our data are expressed as LTE equivalents. Subsequent analysis of our SRS using high-performance liquid chromatography (HPLC) has shown that LTC is the sole detectable SRS leukotriene produced by rat alveolar macrophages stimulated with IgE and antigen (19). These studies established for the first time that alveolar macrophages could be activated by an IgE-dependent mechanism to release a mediator of known importance in asthma.

Our next studies characterized the mechanism of LTC release by IgE and antigen. To study if LTC release by alveolar macrophages incubated with IgE and antigen was due to macrophage interaction with complexes of IgE and antigen, we performed three types of experiments. Our standard method of inducing release of LTC involved incubating alveolar macrophages with anti-DNP IgE for 20 min and then with DNP-HSA for an additional 20 min. In our experiments, LTC release from alveolar macrophages that were challenged in this fashion was greater than from alveolar macrophages that were washed after the 20-min incubation with IgE and before addition of antigen, but was equivalent to LTC release

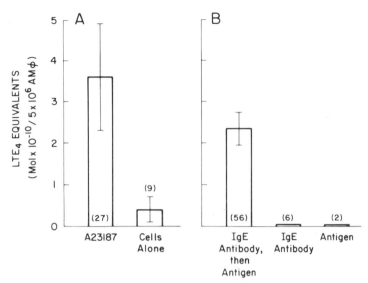

Fig. 1. Release of SRS from rat alveolar macrophages activated by A23187 (A) or IgE and antigen (B). The number of experiments is shown at the base of the columns, the height of which shows the mean ± SEM. (A) 5×10^6 viable alveolar macrophages were first incubated with 5×10^{-4} M L-cysteine for 150 sec and then for 18 min with 1 μM A23187 (left) or in media alone (right). After centrifugation, the supernatants were assayed on the guinea pig ileum, as described previously (19). Measured contractions were compared with a synthetic LTE_4 standard, and the amount of SRS released was expressed as LTE_4 equivalents, as shown on the ordinate. (B) Alveolar macrophages, 5×10^6 viable cells/ml, were incubated with hapten affinity-purified anti-DNP IgE (10 g) for 20 min at 37°C and for an additional 20 min with DNP-HSA (100 ng) (left), with IgE alone (middle) or with DNP-HSA alone (right).

from alveolar macrophages challenged with IgE and antigen that were first preincubated together for 30 min at room temperature before addition to the cell suspensions. These results strongly suggested that IgE immune complexes were responsible for eliciting LTC release.

A third set of experiments was performed to confirm this. DNP-HSA was labeled with ^{125}I, and immune complexes with anti-DNP IgE were isolated using Sephacyl S200 column chromatography. These complexes induced LTC release from rat alveolar macrophages in a dose-dependent fashion. LTC release was observed with IgE–antigen complexes containing as little as 2 ng/ml of antigen. These experiments confirmed that IgE immune complexes are responsible for eliciting LTC release from rat alveolar macrophages.

Other studies in our laboratory have determined that LTC release from rat alveolar macrophages can also be elicited by a phagocytic stimulus, such as zymosan, and by IgG-dependent mechanisms. Indeed, as little as

10 ng of aggregated IgG induces the release of SRS. The ability of alveolar macrophages to release SRS by IgG-dependent mechanisms is of clinical interest, since most human lung macrophages possess IgG receptors (3,4) that are crucial for the optimal phagocytic function of this cell, and because it has been demonstrated that IgG can mediate SRS release from guinea pig lung fragments *in vitro* (36) and from rat peritoneal cells *in vivo* (37). Recently, it has been proposed that IgG is involved in immediate hypersensitivity reactions in human asthma (38–40). Thus, it is possible that IgG–macrophage interactions may sometimes make an important contribution to asthmatic syndromes.

MACROPHAGE RELEASE OF PLATELET-ACTIVATING FACTOR

Platelet-activating factor (PAF) is a phospholipid mediator originally noted to be released via IgE activation of rabbit basophils. This naturally occurring PAF has been identified recently as acetyl glyceryl ether phosphorylcholine (AGEPC) (41). In addition to its ability to cause platelet aggregation and release of vasoactive amines, PAF is now known to induce bronchoconstriction (20,42). The precise mechanism by which PAF elicits bronchoconstriction is unclear but may be platelet dependent (20,42). Indeed, PAF stimulates rabbit platelets to release SRS (43), and the infusion of PAF into isolated perfused rat lungs causes vasoconstriction and edema that appear to be due to secondary release of LTC and LTD (44). These observations suggest that changes in lung mechanics induced by the infusion of PAF may be brought about indirectly through the action of other mediators, such as SRS.

Numerous cell types are capable of releasing PAF. Human neutrophils or monocytes release PAF in response to nonspecific stimuli, such as A23187, or to phagocytic stimuli (16,45). Rabbit, rat, and human alveolar macrophages incubated with A23187 also release PAF (15). Importantly, alveolar macrophages from asthmatic patients, when incubated with specific allergens, release PAF (11). Therefore, PAF release from antigen challenge of lung fragments sensitized with IgE (46) could be, in part, from alveolar macrophages.

DISCUSSION

Are human alveolar macrophages stimulated *in vivo* by IgE-dependent mechanisms and do they release SRS and/or PAF in response to this

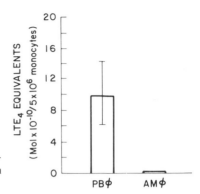

Fig. 2. A23187-induced release of SRS from human peripheral blood monocytes (left) and human alveolar macrophages (right).

stimulation? The answer to this important question is not yet known. Studies thus far have not convincingly shown that human alveolar macrophages can release SRS. However, the likelihood that this cell will be found to be a source of SRS is supported by several recent observations. Human peripheral blood monocytes have been shown to release SRS, probably LTC and LTD, when incubated with A23187, (47) and we have confirmed this (Fig. 2). This cell is a direct precursor of the alveolar macrophage (4). In addition, human alveolar macrophages when incubated with zymosan release prostaglandins PGE_2, PGF_2, PGA_2, and thromboxane B_2 (48), and monohydroxyeicosatetraenoic acids (HETE) 5- and 12-HETE (49), as well as leukotriene B (50). These latter findings establish that the human alveolar macrophage is a source of some products of the lipoxygenase pathway of arachadonic acid metabolism.

In addition to what has been just discussed, there are other reasons to consider that alveolar macrophages may play an important role in IgE-mediated diseases in the lung. The alveolar macrophage resides on top of the airway and alveolar epithelial surfaces where it is the first phagocytic cell of the lower respiratory tract to encounter inhaled particulate matter and allergens. In addition, it is by far the most numerous cell on the air–surface interface of the human lung (4,5). In contrast, almost all lung mast cells lie deep in the submucosa, protected from antigen in the air spaces by a triple layer consisting of mucus, a tightly joined mucosal epithelium, and a basement membrane (51). Thus, a substantial anatomic barrier exists in normal lungs between inhaled allergen and lung mast cells coated with IgE. The epithelial portion of this barrier does not appear to be abnormally porous in asthmatic subjects (52). It is widely held that immediate hypersensitivity reactions in the lung commence when antigen combines with IgE located on lung mast cells. However, <1.0% of monkey or human bronchial lumen cells are mast cells (53,54). Also, it is estimated that above the basement membrane in monkey airways there is only about 1 mast cell per 10^5 epithelial cells (55). Since alveolar macrophages constitute more than 90% of the cells in the airways and virtually all pulmonary mast cells are not in direct contact with the airway, initial activation of alveolar macrophages could be an early step in a cascade of events that eventually leads to antigen activation of submucosal mast cells.

Thus, immunologic events that culminate in the signs and symptoms of acute asthma may actually begin when inhaled allergen meets the alveolar macrophage. Specific IgE antibody is available to interact with the alveolar macrophage as it is present in the lung lining fluid of most normal individuals (3,4). It is, in part, synthesized locally as plasma cells secreting IgE have been detected in lung lining fluid (56). Furthermore, there is good reason to believe that levels of IgE in the lower respiratory tract are increased in people with allergic asthma. IgE levels are increased in the nasal secretions of patients with allergic rhinitis, and the nasal mucosa closely resembles that of the lower respiratory tract in many ways.

The precise sequence of events that may occur when allergen meets the alveolar macrophage remains to be determined. On the basis of what has been discussed in this review, one plausible scheme is depicted in Fig. 3. As theorized here, allergen interacting with IgE or IgG in the air spaces induces alveolar macrophages to release several mediators. These mediators initiate bronchoconstriction, chemotaxis of eosinophils to the airways, and alterations in mucosal permeability that permits the passage of allergen to the submucosa where interaction with IgE-coated mast cells occurs, augmenting the events begun by the alveolar macrophage. IgG, which with IgA constitutes most of the immunoglobulin in lung lining fluid, also could contribute to the proposed participation of alveolar macrophages in the early events that lead eventually to allergen-induced activation of IgE-sensitized submucosal lung mast cells and subsequent release of diverse mediators. Also, the well-known ability of irritants and infections to trigger asthma could be due, in part, to nonspecific activation of alveolar macrophages, leading to their release of mediators that initiate bronchoconstriction and inflammation and penetration of environmental allergens to submucosal tissues where mast cells are then activated via specific IgE antibodies.

In summary, substantial evidence supports the hypothesis that human alveolar macrophages can be activated by IgE-dependent mechanisms and also by IgG or nonspecifically. Activation of alveolar macrophages by these stimuli can potentially lead to the release of several mediators of known importance in allergic lung diseases. Research over the next few years should define more clearly the role that this cell plays in asthma.

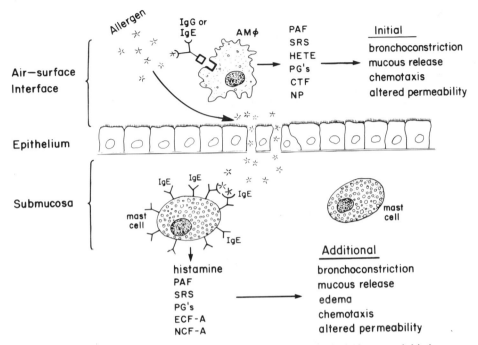

Fig. 3. Schematic representation of hypothesized immunological events initiating an immediate hypersensitivity reaction in the airways of the lungs. Abbreviations: PGs, prostaglandins; CTF, chemotactic factors; NP, neutral proteases: ECF-A, eosinophil chemotactic factor of anaphylaxis; NCF-A, neutrophil chemotactic factor of anaphylaxis.

REFERENCES

1. Bach, M. K. Mediators of anaphylaxis and inflammation. *Annu. Rev. Microbiol.* **36:**371–413, 1982.
2. Lewis, R. A., and Austen, K. F. Mediation of local homeostasis and inflammation by leukotrienes and other mast cell-dependent compounds. *Nature (London)* **293:**103–108, 1981.
3. Reynolds, H. Y., and Merrill, W. W. Lung immunology: the inflammatory response in lung parenchyma. *Curr. Pulmonol.* **1:**299–323, 1980.
4. Hocking, W. G., and Golde, D. W. The pulmonary-alveolar macrophage. *N. Engl. J. Med.* **301:**580–588, 639–645, 1979.
5. Capron, A., Dessaint, J.-P., Capron, M., and Bazin, H. Specific IgE antibodies in immune adherence of normal macrophages to *Schistosoma mansoni* schistosomules. *Nature (London)* **253:**474–475, 1975.
6. Dessaint, J.-P., Capron, A., Joseph, M., and Bazin, H. Cytophilic binding of IgE to the macrophage II. Immunologic release of lysozomal enzyme from macrophages by IgE

and anti-IgE in the rat. A new mechanism of macrophage activation. *Cell. Immunol.* **46:**24–34, 1979.

7. Joseph, M., Capron, A., Butterworth, A. E., Sturrock, R. F., and Houba, V. Cytotoxicity of human and baboon mononuclear phagocytes against schistosomula *in vitro:* Induction by immune complexes containing IgE and *Schistosoma mansoni* antigens. *Clin. Exp. Immunol.* **33:**48–56, 1978.

8. Capron, A., Dessasint, J.-P., Rousseau, R., Capron, M., and Bazin, H. Interaction between IgE complexes and macrophages in the rat: A new mechanism of macrophage activation. *Eur. J. Immunol.* **7:**315–322, 1977.

9. Joseph, M., Tonnel, A. B., Capron, A., and Voisin, C. Enzyme release and superoxide anion production by human alveolar macrophages stimulated with immunoglobulin E. *Clin. Exp. Immunol.* **40:**416–422, 1980.

10. Joseph, M., Tonnel, A. B., Capron, A., and Dessaint, J.-P. The interaction of IgE antibody with human alveolar macrophages and its participation in the inflammatory processes of lung allergy. *Agents Actions* **11:**619–622, 1981.

11. Joseph, M., Tonnel, A., Torpier, G., Capron, A., Arnoux, B., and Benveniste, J. Involvement of immunoglobulin E in the secretory processes of alveolar macrophages from asthmatic patients. *J. Clin. Invest.* **71:**221–230, 1983.

12. Bach, M. K., and Brashler, J. R. Ionophore A23187-induced production of slow reacting substance of anaphylaxis (SRS-A) by rat peritoneal cells *in vitro:* Evidence for production by mononuclear cells. *J. Immunol.* **120:**998–1005, 1978.

13. Orange, R. P., Moore, E. G., and Gelfand, E. W. The formation and release of slow reacting substance of anaphylaxis (SRS-A) by rat and mouse peritoneal mononuclear cells induced by ionophore A23187. *J. Immunol.* **124:**2264–2267, 1980.

14. Rouzer, C. A., Scott, W. A., Hamill, A. L., and Cohn, Z. A. Synthesis of leukotriene C and other arachidonic acid metabolites by mouse pulmonary macrophages. *J. Exp. Med.* **155:**720–733, 1982.

15. Arnoux, B., Duval, D., and Benveniste, J. Release of platelet activating factor (PAF-ACEther) from alveolar macrophages by the calcium ionophore A23187 and phagocytosis. *Eur. J. Clin. Invest.* **10:**437–441, 1980.

16. Roubin, R., Mencia-Huerta, J. M., and Benveniste, J. Release of platelet activating factor (PAF-acether) and leukotrienes C and D from inflammatory macrophages. *Eur. J. Immunol.* **12:**141–146, 1982.

17. Hammarström, S., Murphy, R. C., Samuelsson, B., Clark, D. A., Mioskowski, C., and Corey, E. J. Structure of leukotriene C: Identification of the amino acid part. *Biochem. Biophys. Res. Commun.* **91:**1266–1271, 1979.

18. Morris, H. R., Taylor, G. W., Piper, P. J., and Tippins, J. R. Structure of slow-reacting substances of anaphylaxis from guinea pig lung. *Nature (London)* **285:**104–106, 1980.

19. Rankin, J. A., Hitchcock, M., Merrill, W. W., Bach, M. K., Brasher, J. R., and Askenase, P. W. IgE-dependent release of leukotriene C$_4$ from alveolar macrophages. *Nature (London)* **297:**329–331, 1982.

19a. Rankin, J. A., Hitchcock, M., Merrill, W. W., Huang, S. S., Brashler, J. R., Bach, M. K., and Askenase, P. W. IgE immune complexes induce immediate and prolonged release of leukotriene C$_4$ (LTC$_4$) from rat alveolar macrophages. *J. Immunol.* **132:**1993–1999, 1984.

20. Vargaftig, B. B., Lefort, J., Chignard, M., and Benveniste, J. Platelet-activating factor induces a platelet-dependent bronchoconstriction unrelated to the formation of prostaglandin derivatives. *Eur. J. Pharmacol.* **65:**185–192, 1980.

21. Shelhamer, J. H., Marom, Z., and Kaliner, M. Immunologic and neuropharmacologic stimulation of mucous glycoprotein release from human airways *in vitro. J. Clin. Invest.* **66:**1400–1408, 1980.

22. Marom, Z., Shelhamer, J. H., and Kaliner, M. The effects of arachidonic acid, monohydroxyeicosatetraeonic acid, and prostaglandins on the release of mucous glycoprotein from human airways in vitro. J. Clin. Invest. 67:1695–1702, 1981.

23. Marom, Z., Shelhamer, J. H., Bach, M. K., Morton, D. R., and Kaliner, M. Slow-reacting substances, leukotrienes C_4 and D_4, increase the release of mucus from human airways in vitro. Am. Rev. Respir. Dis. 126:449–451, 1982.

24. Haque, A., Joseph, M., Ouaissi, M. A., Capron, M., and Capron, A. IgE antibody-mediated cytotoxicity of rat macrophages against microfilaria of Dipetalonema viteae in vitro. Clin. Exp. Immunol. 40:487–495, 1980.

25. Dessaint, J.-P., Torpier, G., Capron, M., Bazin, H., and Capron, A. Cytophilic binding of IgE to the macrophage I. Binding characteristics of IgE on the surface of macrophages in the rat. Cell. Immunol. 46:12–23, 1979.

26. Boltz-Nitulescu, G., and Spiegelberg, H. L. Receptors specific for IgE on rat alveolar macrophages. Cell. Immunol. 59:106–114, 1981.

27. Finbloom, D. S., and Metzger, H. Binding of immunoglobulin E to the receptor on rat peritoneal macrophages. J. Immunol. 129:2004–2008, 1982.

28. Anderson, C. L., and Spiegelberg, H. L. Macrophage receptors for IgE; binding of IgE to specific IgE Fc receptors on a human macrophage cell line, U937. J. Immunol. 126:2470–2473, 1981.

29. Melewicz, F. M., Plummer, J. M., and Spiegelberg, H. L. Comparison of the Fc receptors for IgE on human lymphocytes and monocytes. J. Immunol. 129:563–569, 1982.

30. Spiegelberg, H. L., Boltz-Nitulescu, G., Plummer, J. M., and Melewicz, F. M. Characterization of the IgE Fc receptors on monocytes and macrophages. Fed. Proc., Fed. Am. Soc. Exp. Biol. 42:124–128, 1983.

31. Melewicz, F. M., Zeiger, R. S., Mellon, M. H., O'Connor, R. D., and Spiegelberg, H. L. Increased peripheral blood monocytes with Fc receptors for IgE in patients with severe allergic disorders. J. Immunol. 126:1592–1595, 1981.

32. Bach, M. K., Brashler, J. R., Hammarström, S., and Samuelsson, B. Identification of leukotriene C-1 as a major component of slow-reacting substance from rat mononuclear cells. J. Immunol. 125:115–117, 1980.

33. Bach, M. K., Brashler, J. R., Hammarström, S., and Samuelsson, B. Identification of a component of rat mononuclear cell SRS as leukotriene D. Biochem. Biophys. Res. Commn. 93:1121–1126, 1980.

34. Rouzer, C. A., Scott, W. A., Hamill, A. L., and Cohn, Z. A. Dynamics of leukotriene C production by macrophages. J. Exp. Med. 152:1236–1247, 1980.

35. Humphray, H. P., Coote, J., Butchers, P. R., Wheeldon, A., Vardey, C. J., and Skidmore, I. F. The release of prostaglandin and slow reacting substance from mouse macrophages. Agents Actions 11:577–578, 1981.

36. Stechschulte, D. J., Austen, K. F., and Bloch, K. J. Antibodies involved in antigen-induced release of slow reacting substance of anaphylaxis (SRS-A) in the guinea pig and rat. J. Exp. Med. 125:127–147, 1967.

37. Baker, A. R., Bloch, K. J., and Austen, K. F. In vitro passive sensitization of chopped guinea pig lung by guinea pig 7S antibodies. J. Immunol. 93:525–531, 1964.

38. Bryant, D. H., Burhns, M. W., and Lazarus, L. Identification of IgG antibody as a carrier of reaginic activity in asthmatic patients. J. Allergy Clin. Immunol. 56:417–428, 1975.

39. Gwynn, C. M., Ingram, J., Almousawi, T., and Stanworth, D. R. Bronchial provocation tests in atopic patients with allergen-specific IgG antibodies. Lancet 1:1254–1256, 1982.

40. Perelmutter, L. L. The possible role of IgG_4 in allergic disease. Immunol. Allergy Proc. 4:51–54, 1982.

41. Hanahan, D. J., Demopoulos, C. A., Liehr, J., and Pinckard, R. N. Identification of

platelet activating factor isolated from rabbit basophils as acetyl glyceryl ether phosphorylcholine. *J. Biol. Chem.* **255:**5514–5516, 1980.

42. Halonen, M., Palmer, J. D., Lohman, I. G., McManus, L. M., and Pinckard, R. N. Differential effects of platelet depletion on the physiologic alterations of IgE anaphylaxis and acetyl glyceryl ether phosphorylcholine infusion in the rabbit. *Am. Rev. Respir. Dis.* **124:**416–421, 1981.

43. Mencia-Huerta, J. M., Hadji, L., and Benveniste, J. Release of a slow-reacting substance from rabbit platelets. *J. Clin. Invest.* **68:**1586–1591, 1981.

44. Voelkel, N. F., Worthen, S., Reeves, J. T., Henson, P. M., and Murphy, R. C. Nonimmunological production of leukotrienes induced by platelet activating factor. *Science* **218:**286–288, 1982.

45. Clark, P. O., Hanahan, D. J., and Pinckard, R. N. Physical and chemical properties of platelet-activating factor obtained from human neutrophils and monocytes and rabbit neutrophils and basophils. *Biochim. Biophys. Acta* **628:**69–75, 1980.

46. Kravis, T. C., and Henson, P. M. IgE-induced release of a platelet-activating factor from rabbit lung. *J. Immunol.* **115:**1677–1681, 1975.

47. Gunter, K., and Stechschulte, D. J. Generation of slow reacting substance (SRS) termed leukotriene C4 from human peripheral blood monocytes. *Clin. Res.* **28:**707A, 1980.

48. Laviolette, M., Chang, J., and Newcombe, D. S. Human alveolar macrophage: A lesion in arachidonic acid metabolism in cigarette smokers. *Am. Rev. Respir. Dis.* **124:**397–401, 1981.

49. Chang, J., Liu, M. C., and Newcombe, D. S. Identification of two monohydroxyeicosatetraeonic acids synthesized by human pulmonary macrophages. *Am. Rev. Respir. Dis.* **126:**457–459, 1982.

50. Fels, A. O., Pawlowski, N. A., Cramer, E. B., King, T. K. C., Cohn, Z. A., and Scott, W. A. Human alveolar macrophages produce leukotriene B4. *Proc. Natl. Acad. Sci. U.S.A.* **79:**7866–7870, 1982.

51. Hogg, J. C., Pare, P. D., Boucher, R., Michoud, M.-C., Guerzon, G., and Moroz, L. Pathologic abnormalities in asthma. *In* "Asthma: Physiology, Immunopharmacology, and Treatment" (L. M. Lichtenstein and K. F. Austen, eds.), pp. 1–19. Academic Press, New York, 1977.

52. Elwood, R. K., Belzberg, A., Hogg, J. C., and Pare, P. D. Bronchial mucosal permeability in asthma. *Am. Rev. Respir. Dis.* **125:**63, 1982.

53. Patterson, R., Tomita, Y., Oh, S. H., Suszko, I. M., and Pruzansky, J. J. Respiratory mast cells and basophiloid cells. I. Evidence that they are secreted into the bronchial lumen: Morphology, degranulation and histamine release. *Clin. Exp. Immunol.* **16:**223–234, 1974.

54. Patterson, R., McKenna, J. M., Suszko, I. M., Solliday, N. H., Prozansky, J. J., Roberts, M., and Kehoe, T. J. Living histamine-containing cells from the bronchial lumens of humans. *J. Clin. Invest.* **59:**217–225, 1971.

55. Guerzon, G. M., Pare, P. D., Michoud, M.-C., and Hogg, J. C. The number and distribution of mast cells in monkey lungs. *Am. Rev. Respir. Dis.* **119:**59–66, 1979.

56. Lawrence, E. C., Blaese, R. M., Martin, R. R., and Stevens, P. M. Immunoglobulin secreting cells in normal human bronchial lavage fluids. *J. Clin. Invest.* **62:**832–835, 1978.

DISCUSSION

Wasserman: Is the reason that human alveolar macrophages do not make bronchoconstrictive sulfidopeptide leukotrienes due to a lack of production or rather to their generation followed by a very rapid degradation, perhaps via oxygen metabolites: Can one recover such leukotrienes added directly to human alveolar macrophages?

Askenase: The human alveolar macrophage data suggest that there is a change in leukotriene pathways with differentiation from monocyte to macrophage, resulting in preferential LTB_4 formation relative to LTC_4. This could be from (a) decreased glutathione, (b) shunting from LTA_4 to LTB_4 (more enzyme?), (c) increased degradation of LTC_4, or (d) down-regulation of glutathione s-transferase. The big questions are (1) how does it happen, and (2) how do asthmatics compare to normals?

Holgate: Have you detected any preformed mediator release in your experiments with bronchoalveolar macrophages?

Askenase: Other groups (M. Joseph, A. Tonnel, G. Torpier, A. Capron, B. Arnoux, and J. Benveniste, *J. Clin. Invest.* **71:**221, 1983) have reported release of β-glucuronidase from alveolar macrophages activated by IgE. We have not managed to get that assay to work well enough to do those studies. Often our background release of β-glucuronidase is unpredictably high.

Schwartz: Were the mast cells removed from the preparations of rat alveolar macrophages prior to IgE-dependent activation? Would not all mast cells be activated in such experiments?

Askenase: The alveolar lavage cells (macrophages) had only 0.14% mast cell contamination. Most of this is eliminated by adherence to plastic at 37°C, but IgE-dependent release of SRS continues in the nonadherent cells. In addition, I think that if these few mast cells played a role, then passive IgE sensitization and washing would not result in decreased SRS release, as we have found.

Kaplan: What is the minimum size IgE aggregate that seems to trigger a rat alveolar macrophage?

Askenase: We do not know what size IgE–antigen complexes are optimal in LTC_4 release from rat alveolar macrophages.

Johansson: Could the differences in IgE-mediated reactivity of alveolar macrophages in rats and humans be explained by activation by parasite infestations in the rats? In our experience most rats are infested and have raised serum IgE concentrations. Did you measure serum IgE in your rats? Was there a relation between alveolar macrophage reactivity and serum IgE levels?

Askenase: We have not yet looked intentionally at infected rats, particularly those with parasites. I can say that, in collaboration with Dr. Alain Dessein at Harvard, who has produced IgE-suppressed rats, that alveolar macrophages uniformly form 80–85% rosettes with IgE-coated RBC. Those animals have no IgE, as judged by a failure of their peritoneal mast cells to release mediators following anti-IgE challenge.

Flenley: I believe that Benveniste and Arnoux have recently found PAF acether in lavage fluid obtained from young atopic asthmatics, and also that PAF acether is released from alveolar macrophages under appropriate stimulation. If this is so would the PAF acether cause contraction of the guinea pig ileum, which you failed to find? Does this mean that there was no release of PAF acether from alveolar macrophages?

Askenase: PAF is inactivated in biologic fluids and would not be detected adequately on our guinea pig ileum preparations. Dr. Pinkard has measured our IgE-activated rat alveolar macrophages and corresponding supernatants. He has demonstrated that IgE- and antigen-dependent activation results in generation of PAF in the cells, but not in the supernatants, as was shown for purified human mast cells by Dr. Lichtenstein.

Turner-Warwick: Have you tried to study your macrophage experiments *in vivo?* If so, do they develop inflammation responses in the acinar ("deep lung") or the airways?

Askenase: We have not yet challenged IgE-sensitized rats *in vivo* with aerosolized antigen.

Oates: Are there IgE-immune complexes in the airways of atopic individuals?

Askenase: There is just beginning to be data concerning the presence of IgE in airways secretions. If the situation is similar to that of the nose (as described by Dr. Platts-Mills) we could expect to find increased IgE in atopic asthmatics. IgE-immune complexes in this fluid have not yet been looked for.

Kay: We have found house dust mite-specific IgE in lung washings from asthmatics [P. Diaz, F. R. Galleguillos, M. C. Gonzalez, and A. B. Kay, *Thorax* **38:**702 (abstr.), 1983]. The concentrations fell following a course of disodium cromoglycate.

Platts-Mills: In thinking about what situations we would look for your antigen-specific T cell factor (P. W. Askenase, R. W. Rosenstein, and W. Ptak, *J. Exp. Med.* **157:**862, 1983) in humans, could you tell us whether you can detect skin sensitivity in actively immunized mice, or is the factor only demonstrable by passive transfer?

Askenase: Yes, we can detect T cell–dependent immediate hypersensitivity in actively sensitized mice (H. Van Lovenen, R. Meade, and P. W. Askenase, *J. Exp. Med.* **157:**1604, 1983). There are as yet no data concerning an antigen specific IgE-like T cell factor in humans.

Nadel: Do type II cells, abundant in lavage fluid, have IgE receptors?

Askenase: No IgE-Fc receptors have been detected on Type II alveolar cells by our rosetting techniques.

Gleich: I am interested in your findings of an intitial vasopermeability step in delayed-type contact sensitivity reactions, presumably mediated by the T-cell factor (with antigen specificity) that you have described. Do you have any evidence that such a reaction occurs in the human?

Askenase: I have no data on that.

Lewis: In collaboration with Philippe Godard of Montpelier, France, Frank Austen and I have been evaluating the generation of LTB_4 and of the sulfidopeptide leukotrienes by plated human alveolar macrophages from both normal subjects and asthmatics, in response to the calcium ionophore A23187 and to the phagocytic stimuli, opsonized and nonopsonized zymosan. Alveolar macrophages from both normal and asthmatic subjects responded in a dose-dependent basis to A23187 in generating LTB_4 as measured by radioimmunoassay, with or without prior HPLC. The maximal quantities generated were in the range of 200 to 400 $ng/10^6$ cells. Likewise, A23187 also stimulated dose-dependent generation of sulfido-peptide leukotrienes, but in much smaller quantities, with average maximal generation of 4–12 $ng/10^6$ cells by macrophages of various donors, as quantitated by a class-specific radioimmunoassay. Although we have not been able to measure the generation of sulfidopeptide leukotrienes from alveolar macrophages in response to zymosan or opsonized zymosan stimuli, phagocytosis of these particles was clearly associated with generation of net LTB_4, in several instances to as much as 150 $ng/10^6$ cells.

Askenase: Can you compare the amounts of sulfidoleukotriene released by human alveolar macrophages with ionophore to those reported by Dr. Lichtenstein's group to be released by human lung mast cells via IgE? It is my impression that mast cells release a little more, but that there are a lot of macrophages in the airways.

Schleimer: The human parenchymal mast cells produce approximately 200 ng of sulfido-peptide leukotriene per 10^6 cells. This is roughly 20 times the amount that Dr. Lewis is showing to be derived from A23187-stimulated human alveolar macrophages and 3 times the amount that the rat alveolar macrophages are producing.

Austen: The ratio of LTB_4 to LTC_4 production by alveolar macrophages is similar to that of peripheral monocytes with ionophore activation. The use of zymosan as well is central since ionophore is not a physiologic probe. In considering mechanisms for augmenting bronchial permeability, perhaps it relates to the combined action of PMNs and LTB$_4$ to release a PMN permeability factor.

Askenase: The idea that alveolar macrophages might be important as a source of LTB$_4$ to attract neutrophils which in turn release permeability factors is interesting; particularly if these factors act on bronchial epithelium as they do on the vasculature.

Clark: Alveolar lavage cannot identify the site from which cells were washed or the site of their activity. This must be borne in mind when interpreting your results.

CHAPTER 11

Phospholipid Metabolism and Regulation of Leukocyte Chemotaxis

ELLIOTT SCHIFFMANN, V. GEETHA, D. PENCEV, and J. MATO

National Institute of Dental Research
National Institutes of Health
Bethesda, Maryland, U.S.A.

I. GARCIA-CASTRO and P. K. CHIANG

Walter Reed Army Institute of Research
Washington, D.C., U.S.A.

R. MANJUNATH and A. MUKHERJEE

National Institute of Child Health and Human Development
National Institutes of Health
Bethesda, Maryland, U.S.A.

INTRODUCTION

One of the important responses of leukocytes to inflammatory stimuli is chemotaxis (1). These cells can be attracted to foci of allergic reactions, such as asthma, through the generation of complement-derived attractants at the site of the pathophysiologic event (2). In addition, leukocytes exposed to chemoattractants generate and release leukotrienes, some of which are themselves leukoattractants (3) and others that are potent bronchoconstrictors (4). It is obvious, then, that the arrival of activated leukocytes at a bronchial site could be a primary contribution to an asthmatic attack. If strategies are to be devised for controlling this problem, it would seem essential to understand some of the molecular events that may play a role in leukocyte chemotaxis. In fact, a considerable body of such information has been obtained. The basement membrane glycoprotein laminin has been shown to function as an attachment factor for neutro-

ASTHMA: Physiology,
Immunopharmacology,
and Treatment
THIRD INTERNATIONAL SYMPOSIUM

phils to type IV collagen (5). This finding may be quite relevant to the migration of these cells to extravascular sites, since cells must penetrate subendothelial basement membrane during this course. Chemotaxis appears to be a receptor-mediated process (1). The postreceptor reactions have not been clarified but may involve modulation of receptor affinity (6,7), "down-regulation" of receptors (8), and turnover of membrane phospholipids (9,10). Even less is known about the putative biochemical steps that link the transduction of the chemical signal to the cytoskeletal elements of the cell. Here we shall consider a model for chemical events in the membrane that may participate in the chemotactic response of leukocytes. The studies to be described deal principally with neutrophils, and many aspects of the scheme are quite speculative.

MOLECULAR EVENTS IN THE MEMBRANE

Reactions of phospholipids that may be involved in leukotaxis are outlined in Fig. 1. Binding of a chemoattractant (formyl peptide) to its receptor produces a signal that induces rapid Ca^{2+} fluxes and a redistribution of "bound" Ca^{2+} to the free cation (① and ⑤ in Fig. 1) (11). These latter findings were obtained using a tetracycline probe. It is possible that such a probe may have diverse effects upon the cell, complicating the interpretation that membrane-bound Ca^{2+} is released intracellularly. It has been reported that chemoattractants stimulate an increase in neutrophil phosphorylase *a* activity (12). Since this enzyme is Ca^{2+}-dependent, this observation may lead to a reliable, although indirect, assay for intracellular and membrane flux alterations of the divalent cation in stimulated neutrophils. Chemoattractants have been shown to stimulate phospholipase A_2 in neutrophils (② in Fig. 1) (9). We have indicated phosphatidylcholine (PC) as the principal substrate for phospholipase A_2. It has been shown that PC but not phosphoinositol (PI) was the major phospholipid labeled when cells were incubated with [^{14}C]arachidonic acid, and that it was this acid whose release was selectively stimulated when cells labeled with radioactive arachidonic, stearic, linoleic, or oleic acid were exposed to a formyl peptide chemoattractant (13). Since phospholipase A_2 requires Ca^{2+}, it is likely that the stimulated, increased levels of the divalent cation (① and ⑤ in Fig. 1) augment this enzymatic activity. The released arachidonic acid is converted to various hydroxyeicosatetraenoic acids (HETEs) (③ in Fig. 1) via the lipoxygenase pathway (4) and to prostaglandins and thromboxanes via the cyclooxygenase pathway (4). The HETEs may serve to increase Ca^{2+} fluxes (11) and also as leukoattrac-

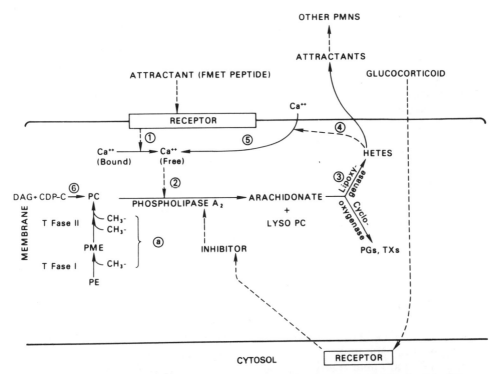

Fig. 1. Molecular events in the cell membrane postulated to play a role in leukotaxis. PE, phosphatidylethanolamine; PME, phosphatidylmonomethylethanolamine; PC, phosphatidylcholine; DAG, diacylglycerol; CDP-C, CDP-choline; TFase, methyl transferase; HETEs, hydroxyeicosatetraenoic acids; PGs, prostaglandins; TXs, thromboxanes. Reprinted with permission from Schiffman *et al.* (5).

tants on their release from the cell (3). This latter effect could lead to an amplification of the chemotactic response. In addition, the generation of leukotrienes C_4 and D_4 from a HETE derivative can occur (4), yielding compounds with potent effects on bronchial smooth muscle. The role (if any) of these compounds in normal physiological processes is not known.

The substrate for phospholipase A_2 (PC) may be generated by two pathways: by successive transmethylation of phosphotidylethanolamine (a) or by conjugation of CDP-choline with diacylglycerol ((6) in Fig. 1). The latter is the major pathway of PC synthesis in the neutrophil but is not affected by the presence of chemoattractants (9). However, attractants cause alterations in the "minor" transmethylation pathway of PC formation. In monocytes, the presence of formyl peptide attractants appears to inhibit transmethylation (14), and in neutrophils these attractants appear to cause a "demethylation" of prelabeled phospholipids (9). This observation may actually reflect the stimulated phospholipase reaction, because an increased release of arachidonic acid was found to parallel the decrease in methylated phospholipids (Fig. 2). In addition, there was a concomitant appearance of lysolecithin. However, the role of the transmethylation pathway in chemotaxis still is not clear. A study (13) has reported that exposure of neutrophils to pharmacological agents that generate methyltransferase inhibitors causes a parallel reduction in carboxymethylation of proteins, methylation of phospholipids, and chemotaxis (Fig. 3). The role of protein carboxymethylation in leukotaxis (15) is not nearly as well established as it is in bacterial chemotaxis (16). The inhibitors of methyltransferase also caused a partial inhibition of the increased, receptor-mediated $^{45}Ca^{2+}$ influx stimulated by formyl peptide attractants. Evidence for a linkage between phospholipid methylation and phospholipase A_2 activation by chemoattractants was provided by the finding that the stimulated release of arachidonic acid was inhibited in a concentration-dependent manner by methyltransferase inhibitors (Fig. 4). The activation of phospholipase A_2 by the Ca^{2+} ionophore A23187 was not blocked by methyltransferase inhibitors, suggesting that methylation played a role in only the receptor-mediated events. Yet even in this case, the putative methylation events may not directly be involved in the stimulated Ca^{2+} flux. They may principally be providing substrate (PC) for activated phospholipase A_2. This, in turn, would yield arachidonate derivatives that might themselves be direct mediators of Ca^{2+} flux (Fig. 1).

While it is likely that the transmethylation pathway contributes to the chemotactic response, it may not be obligatory. We have found that prior

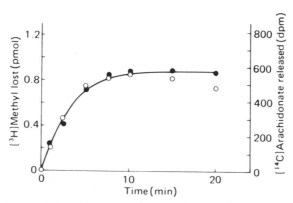

Fig. 2. Stimulatory effect of a formyl peptide attractant upon release of [^{14}C]arachidonic acid (○) and disappearance of [^{3}H]methyl (●) from phospholipids. Neutrophils were labeled with isotopic substrates prior to stimulation with the attractant. Reprinted with permission from Hirata *et al.* (9).

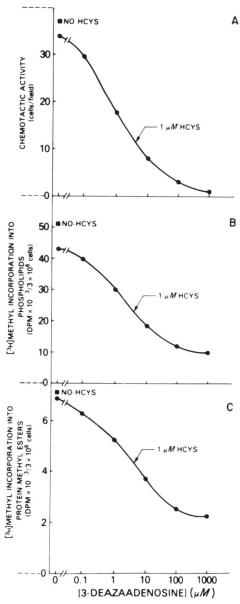

Fig. 3. Inhibition of formylpeptide attractant-stimulated chemotaxis (A), phospholipid methylation (B), and protein carboxylmethylation (C) by 3-deazaadenosine and homocysteine (Hcys). Neutrophils were preincubated with [³H]methylmethionine. Reprinted with permission from Bareis *et al.* (13).

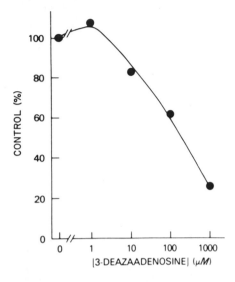

Fig. 4. Inhibition of attractant-stimulated release of [¹⁴C]arachidonic acid by 3-deazaadenosine. Neutrophils were prelabeled with [¹⁴C]arachidonic acid. Reprinted with permission from Bareis *et al.* (13).

addition of adenosine to cells subsequently treated with 3-deazaadenosine, an inhibitor of methylation, reverses the inhibition of chemotaxis by the latter compound (Table I) (17). It was determined that adenosine prevented the uptake of 3-[³H]deazaadenosine by the cells. This result could account for the failure of the drug to inhibit chemotaxis. However, the picture is more complicated, for adenosine alone inhibited phospholi-

TABLE I
Effects of Adenosine and 3-Deazaadenosine on Neutrophils[a]

Addition to cells	Chemotaxis[b]	Control phospholipid methylation (%)[c]	Protein carboxymethylation[c]
0.1 mM DZA[d]	9	61	29
1 mM Ado[e]	100	79	90
1 mM Ado[f]; 0.1 mM DZA	97	77	35
0.1 mM DZA; 1 mM Ado	35	58	34

[a] Reprinted with permission from Garcia-Castro *et al.* (17).
[b] Chemotaxis was determined by assay in the modified Boyden chamber.
[c] Cells were incubated with [³H]methylmethionine.
[d] DZA, 3-deazaadenosine.
[e] Ado, adenosine.
[f] Order of addition as indicated.

pid methylation to about the same extent as that produced by the drug, but did not affect chemotaxis. Also, adenosine alone, unlike the drug, did not inhibit protein carboxymethylation. The combination of adenosine (added first) and 3-deazaadenosine (added after the cells) did overcome the inhibition of chemotaxis by the drug but did not prevent the inhibition of carboxymethylation. The inhibition of methylation was determined for early time periods (15–30 min) of the chemotactic response (2 hr). It is possible that cellular S-adenosylhomocysteine, during later time periods, may have decreased as a result of deamination (17a), leading to decreased inhibition of chemotaxis. The synthesis of phospholipid by the CDP-choline pathway (Fig. 1) was not affected by addition of any combination of purine ribosides to the cells (not shown). However, in other systems, addition of 3-deazaadenosine produced a stimulation of PC synthesis via the CDP-choline pathway (18).

It appears from these results that chemotaxis may occur during the inhibition of methylation of lipid and protein substrates. This suggests both that the transmethylation pathway may not be obligatory for chemotaxis and that the actions of drugs such as 3-deazaadenosine may be at other sites in addition to those of the transmethylation pathway. There is evidence in other cells that agonists can stimulate arachidonate release from phosphoinositol and a subsequent cell function in the presence of methylation inhibitors, allowing a biochemical flexibility for the cell (18a). The complexity arising from the use of pharmacological agents is further underscored by our results with another inhibitor of methylation, 3-deazaaristeromycin (Table II). The extent of inhibition of chemotaxis produced by this drug (30%) was in this case increased (75–90%) by the

TABLE II

Effects of Adenosine (Ado) and 3-Deazaari on Neutrophil Chemotaxis

Additions to cells	Inhibition of chemotaxis (%)[a]
1 mM Ado	0
1 mM 3-deazaAri[b]	30
0.1 mM Ado; 1 mM 3-deazaAri[c]	75
1 mM 3-deazaAri; 0.1 mM Ado[c]	90

[a] Chemotaxis was assayed in the modified Boyden chamber.

[b] 3-deaza-(±)-aristeromycin.

[c] Order of addition as indicated.

presence of adenosine. The homocysteine conjugates, adenosylhomocysteine, 3-deazaadenosylhomocysteine and 3-deazaaristeromycinylhomocysteine can also inhibit chemotaxis. Since these compounds would not be expected to enter the cell, these results raise the possibility that novel types of adenosine receptors may be involved in the regulation of chemotaxis.

We have also considered the possible role in leukocyte chemotaxis of the CDP-choline pathway for PC synthesis (Fig. 1). Although chemoattractants did not cause changes in PC formation (9), we have found that a number of agents that inhibit endocytosis, such as dansylcadaverine, (19) blocked chemotaxis and PC formation via both the CDP-choline and the transmethylation pathways (20) (Table III). A given extent of inhibition of chemotaxis by an agent was associated with a greater degree of inhibition of PC formation through the "cholination" pathway than that which occurred through the methylation pathway. An unexpected result was that these agents produced an increase in the synthesis of phosphatidylinositol (PI), which was correlated with their abilities to inhibit both PC synthesis via cholination and chemotaxis. It is possible that diacylglycerol levels may be increased from the inhibition of PC synthesis (Fig. 1) and thus be available for PI synthesis. The inhibition of endocytosis of labeled chemoattractant by neutrophils was also observed in the presence of dansylcadaverine (not shown). Marked perturbation of phospholipid metabolism was occurring in the presence of these inhibitors of endocytosis. It appears then that a certain level of PC synthesis or rate of turnover may

TABLE III
Effects of Inhibitors of Endocytosis on Chemotaxis and Phospholipid Synthesis in Neutrophils

	Control (%)			
		Phosphatidyl choline synthesis[b] by		Phosphatidyl inositol synthesis[c]
Addition[a]	Chemotaxis	Methylation	Cholination	
Dansylcadaverine	33	50	9	356
Rimantidine	44	—	26	235
Amantadine	78	—	64	145

[a] Concentrations used were dansylcadaverine, 250 μM; rimantidine and amantadine, 500 μM each.

[b] Cells were labeled with [³H]methylmethionine or [³H]methylcholine.

[c] Cells were labeled with [2-³H]myoinositol.

be required for efficient chemotaxis. The significance of this is not clear. Local alterations in lipid metabolism could conceivably affect the cooperative interactions between receptors and facilitate changes in both ion fluxes and membrane potential (6). These events have been linked to the adaptation of neutrophils moving in a gradient of attractant.

MODULATION OF CHEMOTAXIS

Calcium as a Modulator of Chemotaxis

The role of Ca^{2+} as a "second messenger" in the expression of the chemotactic response has not been extensively treated here. Although it appears to be necessary for a number of the reactions outlined above as well as for the presumed "mechanochemical" coupling between molecular events in the membrane (11) and cytoskeletal elements of the cell, the chemical nature of such requirements is not yet clear. We shall, therefore, discuss Ca^{2+} when its participation in a reaction appears to be definitive, for example, as a cofactor for an enzyme (phospholipase A_2).

Inhibition of Phospholipase A_2

Phospholipase A_2 is probably a key enzyme in the membrane events that seem to be involved in chemotaxis (Fig. 1). As stated above, the arachidonate produced from PC by this enzyme is converted to compounds that profoundly affect the cell. Therefore, the regulation of phospholipase A_2 is of major importance. It has been found that glucocorticoids stimulated the formation of a phospholipase inhibitory protein, lipomodulin ($M_r \approx 40,000$), in leukocytes and other tissues (21,22). This may in part explain the antiinflammatory effects of glucocorticoids. In the absence of inflammatory stimuli such as chemoattractants, the leukocyte may be maintained in an inactive state by the presence of endogenous lipomodulin in the cell membrane. It was proposed that chemoattractants activate the cell by inactivating the endogenous lipomodulin, thus releasing the phospholipase A_2. A study of the mechanism by which the attractant inactivated this inhibitor indicated that lipomodulin was phosphorylated to produce an inactive compound (23) (Fig. 5). Dephosphorylation followed, indicating the reversibility of the reaction. Therefore, this endogenous inhibitor could be available for cycles of protein modification that might be related to adaptation of the cell in a gradient of chemoattractant. Concomitant with the phosphorylation of lipomodulin was the influx

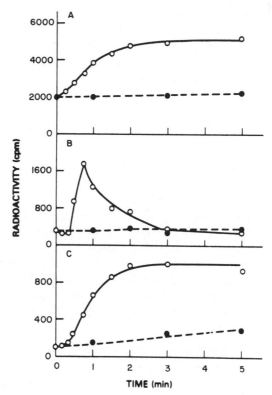

Fig. 5.   Time course in neutrophils of ^{45}Ca influx (A), phosphorylation of lipomodulin (B), and release of arachidonic acid (C) in presence (O——O) and absence (●----●) of peptide chemoattractant. Cells were labeled with isotopic substrates prior to stimulation. Reprinted with permission from Hirata (23).

of Ca^{2+}, which by itself would enhance phospholipase activity, and the release of arachidonic acid (Fig. 5). Similar results were obtained in a cell-free system in which a cAMP-dependent kinase was shown to produce inactive, phosphorylated lipomodulin.

Lipomodulin appears to be a cell-surface protein, as implied in the previous discussion. An appropriate level of lipomodulin in cells may be required to modulate leukocyte activation. Evidence to support this is in the finding that autoantibodies for this protein were present in the sera of patients with lupus and severe rheumatoid arthritis (24). It was demonstrated that such sera abolished the inhibitory effect *in vitro* of lipomodulin upon phospholipase A_2. However, sera from normal individuals did not affect this enzymatic activity. Therefore, some of the inflammatory consequences of these diseases might be the result of the binding of

TABLE IV
Effect of Lipomodulin on Neutrophil and Monocyte Chemotaxis

Additions to cells[a]	Control chemotaxis (%)[b]
To neutrophils	
Lipomodulin[c] (10^{-9} M)	52
Lipomodulin (10^{-8} M)	33
Lipomodulin (10^{-7} M)	26
To monocytes	
Lipomodulin (10^{-9} M)	58
Lipomodulin (10^{-8} M)	41
Lipomodulin (10^{-7} M)	27

[a] Cells were incubated 30 min with lipomodulin prior to chemotaxis assay.

[b] The cellular response to a formyl peptide was measured.

[c] These experiments were performed in collaboration with F. Hirata (National Institute of Mental Health, Bethesda, Maryland), who prepared and purified the lipomodulin.

antibodies for lipomodulin to this protein in phagocytic cells. It was conceivable that the antibodies in the sera of patients with inflammatory diseases might also be reacting to a normally occurring humoral form of lipomodulin released from cells responsive to glucocorticoids. An additional mechanism of *in situ* synthesis might then be available for lipomodulin to exert its antiinflammatory effect: its uptake by phagocytes. We tested this possibility by determining the effect of added lipomodulin[1] on phagocyte chemotaxis *in vitro*. It was found (Table IV) that lipomodulin did indeed inhibit chemotaxis in a concentration-dependent manner. The protein at a concentration of 0.1 μM inhibited both neutrophil and monocyte chemotaxis to a formylated peptide by about 75%. A similar effect upon chemotaxis to either leukotriene B4 or a C5-derived attractant was observed for lipomodulin (not shown). Therefore, the action of this inhibitor against a diverse selection of inflammatory mediators appears to be a general one that is directed at the cell and not on the attractant. Lipomodulin did not compete with a labeled formylated peptide for its receptor but did reduce the internalization of the peptide by neutrophils (not

[1] These experiments were performed in collaboration with F. Hirata, National Institute of Mental Health, Bethesda, Maryland.

shown). The extent of internalization may be a reflection of the degree of receptor down-regulation. The inhibition of internalization, however, was not well correlated with the inhibition of chemotaxis. It is likely, then, that the major antiinflammatory effects of lipomodulin can at present be ascribed to its action upon phospholipase A_2.

In addition to its antiinflammatory effects upon phagocyte functions, there is evidence to suggest that lipomodulin stimulates differentiation in lymphoma cells (25) and inhibits the normal killer and antibody-dependent cell cytotoxic activities of peripheral lymphocytes (26), presumably via the inhibition of phospholipase A_2. It may be anticipated that future studies will establish lipomodulin as a major immunological regulator as well as a role for it in developmental events.

Inhibition of Leukotaxis during Embryogenesis

Trophoblastic cells of the developing embryo normally proliferate *in utero,* even though they bear antigenic determinants foreign to the host. One mechanism whereby these cells evade the host's immune surveillance may be through a covalent link between the determinants on the cell's surface and a protein, uteroglobin ($M_r \approx 15,000$), synthesized *in utero* by the host during gestation (27). The "foreign" antigens would, therefore, be shielded from detection by the host's defense. When determining whether uteroglobin, in addition to interacting with the target cells, had any effect upon phagocytes, major components of the immune defense system, we found that uteroglobin inhibited both neutrophil and monocyte chemotaxis at micromolar concentrations (Table V). A marked

TABLE V
Effects of Uteroglobin on Phagocyte Functions

Concentration uteroglobin (μM)	Inhibition of chemotaxis (%)[a]		Inhibition of internalization[b] in neutrophils
	Neutrophils	Monocytes	
1.33	55	35	40
1.66	78	65	63
2.00	100	95	80

[a] Chemotaxis was determined by the modified Boyden chamber assay [Schiffman and Gallin (1)].

[b] Internalization of [^{3}H]formyl peptide was measured as the amount of peptide that was not displaced by the addition of unlabeled peptide [Schiffman *et al.* (5)].

inhibition of the internalization (80%) of labeled formyl peptide attractant was also observed at a concentration of uteroglobin that completely inhibited neutrophil chemotaxis. However, uteroglobin did not appreciably inhibit binding of peptide to cells at 4°C. These results suggested that uteroglobin might act at a step subsequent to binding of attractant to receptor that affected availability of receptors and was required for a chemotactic response. The inhibitory effects of this protein were reversible and were also observed when other attractants (leukotriene B_4- and C_5-derived attractant) were used to induce cell motility. Therefore, uteroglobin, like lipomodulin, apparently exerted its effect upon the cell and not upon the attractant. The biochemical reactions affected by uteroglobin have not yet been elucidated. However, they would appear to differ from those by which uteroglobin protects the trophoblast as the interaction between this protein and phagocytic cells is reversible.

We conclude that uteroglobin uniquely subverts the host's immune defense by two distinct mechanisms: it shields antigenic determinants on the "foreign" trophoblasts from recognition by the host's antibodies, and it directly impairs the motile response in phagocytes.

Inhibition of Chemotaxis by Tumor-Associated Substances

Factors from Fibrosarcomas

A number of studies (28,29) have shown that products of tumors have antileukotactic effects. The macrophage is more sensitive than is the neutrophil to these factors. This characteristic along with the capability to induce angiogenesis, and in some cases, fibrosis, may in large measure explain survival of the tumor in the host. We have partially purified an inhibitor of leukotaxis from extracts of murine fibrosarcomas (Table VI).

TABLE VI

Properties of Antileukotactic Factor from a Murine Fibrosarcoma

Characteristics
  Heterogeneous with an average $M_r = 500$
  Anionic at neutral pH; stable to heating
  Inactivated by acid hydrolysis and proteases; possible peptide nature
  Inhibitor of neutrophil and monocyte chemotaxis, but not fibroblast chemotaxis
Possible Mode of Action
  Inhibitor of hydrolysis of peptide attractants, cleavage of which may be required for chemotaxis
  Inhibitor of methylation of lipids and protein carboxyl groups

It is heterogeneous, as revealed by the results of high-performance liquid chromatography. The molecular weight is low ($M_r \approx 500$), as estimated from gel filtration. It may have a peptide character, since certain proteolytic enzymes inactivate it. Indeed, in early findings in collaboration with F. Hirata (personal communication), we have shown that synthetic peptides related to the middle T polyoma antigen (30) and the Src gene product (31) have antichemotactic activity. Our factor differs from others in that it inhibits both macrophages and neutrophils with equal efficacy. It also appears to act upon the cell directly, since it inhibits the chemotactic response induced by a number of chemically dissimilar attractants: complement-derived chemotaxin, formylated peptides, and a leukotriene. The mechanism by which this tumor-derived material exerts its inhibitory effect is still not determined. It may act at a postreceptor site since it does not compete with a formylated peptide for the latter's receptor in the neutrophil but does appear to inhibit both lipid and carboxymethylation in cells. These results are not definitive, since they were obtained with an incompletely characterized material. We did not find this type of antichemotactic activity in extracts from a quantity of normal tissue equivalent to an amount of "active" tumor tissue. However, in preliminary findings we did obtain evidence for such activity in a low molecular weight fraction isolated from human placenta. At early stages of development, the organism may benefit from the production of immunosuppressive substances *in utero* like uteroglobin (discussed above), which would prevent rejection by the host. After parturition, however, the synthesis of these factors is discontinued, as might be expected. A tumor, however, may constantly produce similar materials in order to ensure its survival in the host.

Antichemotactic Activity of Oligosaccharides Associated with Human Tumor Antigens

A cell-surface ganglioside that is an antigen of certain human tumor cells has been identified (32). The carbohydrate structure is likely to be:

$$\text{NeuNAc-}\alpha\text{-(2} \rightarrow \text{3)-Gal-}\beta\text{-(1} \rightarrow \text{3)-GlcNAc-}\beta\text{-(1} \rightarrow \text{3)-Gal-}\beta\text{-(1} \rightarrow \text{4)-Glc}$$
$$\overset{\displaystyle 4}{\underset{\displaystyle \text{Fuc-}\alpha\text{-1}}{|}}$$

This is identical to a sialylated Lewis *a* pentasaccharide, characteristic of a class of blood group antigens. We therefore tested a number of oligosaccharides isolated from the milk of a Lewis *a* positive individual for their efforts on chemotaxis (Table VII) (33). The oligosaccharides LNFII and LNDI were good inhibitors of chemotaxis. On the other hand, LNFI, a compositional isomer of LNFII, is inactive. The concentration was 1 mM

TABLE VII
Antileukotactic Activity of Oligosaccharides from Human Milk[a]

Trivial name	Activity[b]	Structure
2'-Fucosyllactose	−[c]	Fuc-α-(1 → 2)-Gal-β-(1 → 4)-Glc
3-Fucosyllactose	−	Gal-β-(1 → 4)} Fuc-α-(1 → 3)}Glc
Lactodifucotetraose	−	Fuc-α-(1 → 2)-Gal-β-(1 → 4)} Fuc-α-(1 → 3)}Glc
Lacto-N-tetraose	−	Gal-β-(1 → 3)-GlcNAc-β-(1 → 3)-Gal-β-(1 → 4)-Glc
Lacto-N-neotetraose	−	Gal-β-(1 → 4)-GlcNAc-β-(1 → 3)-Gal-β-(1 → 4)-Glc
Lacto-N-fucopentaose I	−	Fuc-α-(1 → 2)-Gal-β-(1 → 3)-GlcNAc-β-(1 → 3)-Gal-β-(1 → 4)-Glc
Lacto-N-fucopentaose II	+	Gal-β-(1 → 3)} Fuc-α-(1 → 4)}GlcNAc-β-(1 → 3)-Gal-β-(1 → 4)-Glc
Lacto-N-fucopentaose III		Gal-β-(1 → 4)} Fuc-α-(1 → 3)}GlcNAc-β-(1 → 3)-Gal-β-(1 → 4)-Glc
Lacto-N-difucohexaose I	+	Fuc-α-(1 → 2)-Gal-β-(1 → 3)} Fuc-α-(1 → 4)}GlcNAc-β-(1 → 3)-Gal-β-(1 → 4)-Glc
Lacto-N-difucohexaose II		Gal-β-(1 → 3)} Fuc-α-(1 → 4)}GlcNAc-β-(1 → 3)-Gal-β-(1 → 4)}Glc Fuc-α-(1 ← 3)}

[a] Taken with permission from Kobata (33).

[b] Chemotactic assays were performed in the Boyden chamber.

[c] Signs in parentheses refer to the absence of activity of a mixture of the three oligosaccharides.

for each compound. The feature that may be required for activity is the presence of a branched structure in which galactose and fucose are linked to N-acetyl glucosamine in (at least) a pentasaccharide. This conclusion must be tentative in view of the limited number of oligosaccharides tested. However, a mixture of oligosaccharides from a fraction of milk sugars containing many of the oligosaccharides that were not tested individually and did not possess the active structures did not contain anti-leukotactic activity. It is of interest that normal adult tissues do not make the complete ganglioside; at present, only the tumor and fetal tissue have been found to produce this antigen. This may be another example of a tumor utilizing, for its survival, biochemical reactions that occur during an early stage of normal development.

CONCLUDING REMARKS

Although the evidence is not conclusive, it would appear that phospholipid metabolism plays a role in the development of the chemotactic response in neutrophils. The generation of arachidonic acid may be a key step in this process. This lipid is converted to a host of products: some may be critical to the expression of the motile response; others can amplify this response (as attractants); and still others are known to have pathophysiologic effects (smooth muscle contraction). It is not known whether any of these reactions is linked to the contractile elements of the cell.

The sequence of reactions that may be involved in chemotaxis (Fig. 1) could be subject to regulation at a number of points. There are two pathways for the generation of the substrate PC for the phospholipase reaction, each of which may be subject to different controls. In addition, the inhibition of one may lead to an enhancement of the other, providing more versatility for the cell. Lipomodulin inhibits the release of arachidonic acid and is itself subject to regulation: it is inactivated by phosphorylation, and the phosphorylated product is reactivated by dephosphorylation. Since the neutrophil does not carry out protein synthesis on a scale comparable to that of replicating cells, the "recovery" of lipomodulin would be an obvious advantage to this leukocyte.

In addition to lipomodulin, a number of diverse compounds, generally of low molecular weight, have been found to inhibit chemotaxis: the protein uteroglobin, an incompletely characterized material derived from tumors, and a group of defined oligosaccharides that are related to well-characterized tumor products. In some cases these products are also found in embryonic tissue, suggesting that the tumor carries out reactions that are characteristic of early developmental stages of mammalian organisms. The sites at which these substances exert their antileukotactic effects are not yet known. However, the small molecular size of the defined products would make them amenable for the design of antiinflammatory agents as well as for probes in further studies on the mechanism and regulation of leukotaxis. Additionally, in the case of the incompletely characterized tumor factor, elucidation of its structure may lead to strategies whereby either the biosynthesis of the inhibitor can be blocked or the effect of the inhibitor can be antagonized. Presumably the leukocyte would then have a better opportunity to approach and kill the tumor cell. Finally, this "tumor factor" may be a natural regulator (like lipomodulin) of cell motility. Normal levels of this substance would then contribute to homeostasis by maintaining the leukocyte in a noninflammatory state.

REFERENCES

1. Schiffmann, E., and Gallin, J. I. Biochemistry of phagocyte chemotaxis. *Curr. Top. Cell. Regul.* **15**:203–261, 1979.
2. Wright, D. G., and Gallin, J. I. Functional differentiation of neutrophil granules. *J. Immunol.* **119**:1068–1076, 1977.
3. Goetzl, E. J., and Pickett, W. C. Human PMN leukocyte chemotactic activity of complex hydroxy-eicosatetraenoic acids (HETEs). *J. Immunol.* **125**:1789–1791, 1980.
4. Samuelsson, B. Oxidative products of arachidonate. In "Biochemistry of the Acute Allergic Reactions" (E. L. Becker, A. S. Simon, and K. F. Austen, eds.), pp. 1–11. Alan R. Liss, Inc., New York, 1981.
5. Schiffmann, E., Geetha, V., Pencev, D., Warabi, H., Mato, J., Hirata, F., Brownstein, M., Manjurath, R., Mukherjee, A., Liotta, L., and Terranova, V. P. Adherence and regulation of leukotaxis. In "Agents and Actions Supplements" (H. Keller and E. D. Till, eds.), Vol. 12, pp. 106–120. Birkhauser, Verlag, Basel, 1983.
6. Seligmann, B. E., Fletcher, M. P., and Gallin, J. I. Adaptation of human neutrophil responsiveness to the chemoattractant *N*-formylmethionyldansylphenylalanine. *J. Biol. Chem.* **257**:6280–6286, 1982.
7. Lohr, K. M., and Snyderman, R. Amphotericin B alters the affinity and functional activity of the oligopeptide chemotactic factor receptor on human PMNs. *J. Immunol.* **129**:1594–1599, 1982.
8. Donabedian, H., and Gallin, J. I. Deactivation of human neutrophil chemotaxis by chemoattractants. *J. Immunol.* **127**:839–844, 1981.
9. Hirata, F., Corcoran, B. A., Venkatasubramanian, K., Schiffmann, E., and Axelrod, J. Chemoattractants stimulate degradation of methylated phospholipids and release of arachidonic acid from rabbit leukocytes. *Proc. Natl. Acad. Sci. U.S.A.* **76**:2640–2643, 1979.
10. Homma, Y., Onozaki, K., Hashimoto, T., Nagai, Y., and Takenawa, T. Differential activation of phospholipid metabolism by formylated peptide and ionophore A23187 in guinea pig macrophages. *J. Immunol.* **129**:1619–1626, 1982.

11. Becker, E. L., and Stossel, T. P. Chemotaxis. *Fed. Proc., Fed. Am. Soc. Exp. Biol.* **39:**2949–2952, 1980.
12. Slonczeuoski, J. L., and Zigmond, S. H. Phosphorylase a activity may reflect calcium flux during neutrophil chemotaxis. *J. Cell Biol.* **95:**326a, 1982.
13. Bareis, D. L., Hirata, F., Schiffmann, E., and Axelrod, J. Phospholipid metabolism, calcium flux, and receptor-mediated induction of chemotaxis in rabbit neutrophils. *J. Cell Biol.* **93:**690–697, 1982.
14. Pike, M. C., Kredich, N. M., and Snyderman, R. Phospholipid methylation in macrophages is inhibited by chemotactic factors. *Proc. Natl. Acad. Sci. U.S.A.* **76:**2922–2926, 1979.
15. O'Dea, R. F., Viveros, O. H., Axelrod, J., Aswanikumar, S., Schiffmann, E., and Corcoran, B. A. Rapid stimulation of a protein carboxymethylation in leukocytes by a chemotactic peptide. *Nature (London)* **272:**462–464, 1978.
16. Kort, E. N., Goy, M. F., Larson, S. H., and Adler, J. Methylation of a membrane protein involved in bacterial chemotaxis. *Proc. Natl. Acad. Sci. U.S.A.* **72:**3939–3943, 1975.
17. Garcia-Castro, I., Mato, J. M., Vasanthakumar, G., Wiesmann, W. P., Schiffmann, E., and Chiang, P. K. Paradoxical effects of adenosine upon neutrophil chemotaxis. *J. Biol. Chem.* **258:**4345–4349, 1983.
17a. Schanche, J.-S., Schanche, T., and Ueland, P. M. Inhibition of phospholipid methylation by analogs of adenosine. *Biochim. Biophys. Acta* **721:**399–407, 1982.
18. Pritchard, T. H., Chiang, P. K., Cantoni, G. L., and Vance, D. E. Inhibition of phosphatidylethanolamine methylation and stimulation of phosphatidylcholine synthesis via the CDP-choline pathway in the presence of 3-deazaadenosine. *J. Biol. Chem.* **257:**6362–6367, 1982.
18a. Bareis, D. L., Manganiello, V. C., Hirata, F., Vaughan, M., and Axelrod, J. Bradykinin stimulates phospholipid methylation, Ca influx, prostaglandin formation and cAMP in fibroblasts. *Proc. Natl. Acad. Sci. U.S.A.* **80:**2514–2518, 1983.
19. Pastan, I. H., and Willingham, M. C. Receptor-mediated endocytosis of hormones in cultured cells. *Annu. Rev. Physiol.* **43:**239–250, 1981.
20. Mato, J. M., Pencev, D., Vasanthakumar, G., Schiffmann, E., and Pastan, I. Inhibition of endocytosis perturb phospholipid metabolism in rabbit neutrophils and other cells. *Proc. Natl. Acad. Sci. U.S.A.* **80:**1929–1932, 1983.
21. Blackwell, G. J., and Flower, R. J. Anti-inflammatory steroids induce biosynthesis of a phospholipase A_2 inhibitor which prevents prostaglandin generation. *Nature (London)* **278:**456–459, 1979.
22. Hirata, F., Schiffmann, E., Venkatasubramanian, K., Saloman, D., and Axelrod, J. A phospholipase A_2 inhibitory protein induced in rabbit neutrophils by glucocorticoids. *Proc. Natl. Acad. Sci. U.S.A.* **77:**2533–2536, 1980.
23. Hirata, F. Regulation of lipomodulin, a phospholipase inhibitory protein, in rabbit neutrophils by phosphorylation. *J. Biol. Chem.* **256:**7730–7733, 1981.
24. Hirata, F., del Carmine, R., Nelson, C., Axelrod, J., Schiffmann, E., Warabi, H., DeBlas, A. L., Nirenberg, M., Manganiello, V., Vaughan, M., Kumagai, S., Green, I., Decker, J. L., and Steinberg, A. D. Presence of autoantibody for phospholipase inhibitory protein, lipomodulin, in patients with rheumatic diseases. *Proc. Natl. Acad. Sci. U.S.A.* **78:**3190–3194, 1981.
25. Hattori, T., Hoffman, T., and Hirata, F. Differentiation of a histocytic lymphoma cell line by lipomodulin, a phospholipase inhibitory protein. *Biochem. Biophys. Res. Commun.* **111:**551–559, 1983.

26. Hattori, T., Hirata, F., Hoffman, T., Hizuta, A., and Herberman, R. Inhibition of human natural killer activity and antibody-dependent cellular cytotoxicity by lipomodulin, a phospholipase inhibitory protein. *J. Immunol.* **131:**662–665, 1983.
27. Mukherjee, A. B., Ulane, R. E., and Agrawal, A. K. Role of uteroglobin in masking the antigenicity of implanted rabbit embryos. *Am. J. Reprod. Immunol.* **2:**35–40, 1982.
28. Cianciolo, G. J., Mathews, T. J., Bolognesi, D. P., and Snyderman, R. Macrophage accumulation in mice is inhibited by low molecular weight products from murine leukemia viruses. *J. Immunol.* **124:**2900–2905, 1980.
29. Dvorak, H. F., Orenstein, N. S., and Dvorak, A. M. Tumor-secreted mediators and the tumor neuroenvironment: Immunological surveillance. *Lymphokines* **2:**203–233, 1981.
30. Schaffhausen, B., Benjamin, T. L., Pike, L., Casnellie, J., and Krebs, E. Antibody to a nonapeptide is specific for polyoma middle T antigen and inhibits *in vitro* kinase activity. *J. Biol. Chem.* **257:**12467–12470, 1982.
31. Wong, T. W., and Goldberg, A. R. Synthetic peptide fragment of src gene product inhibits src protein kinase. *Proc. Natl. Acad. Sci. U.S.A.* **78:**7412–7416, 1981.
32. Magnani, J. L., Nilsson, B., Brockhaus, M., Zopf, D., Steplewski, Z., Koprowski, H., and Ginsburg, V. A monoclonal antibody-defined antigen associated with gastrointestinal cancer is a ganglioside containing sialylative lacto-N-fucopentaose II. *J. Biol. Chem.* **257:**14365–14369, 1982.
33. Kobata, A. Isolation of oligosaccharides from human milk. *In* "Methods in Enzymology" (V. Ginsburg, ed.), Vol. 28, Part B, pp. 262–271. Academic Press, New York, 1972.

DISCUSSION

Kay: Would you care to speculate how important lipomodulation is in the beneficial effects of corticosteroids in asthma?

Schiffmann: The formation of lipomodulin may be a significant feature in the effect of the long-term glucocorticoid regulation of inflammation. It may also be an important immunologic modulator, in that Hattori *et al.* (T. Hattori, T. Hoffman, and F. Hirata, *Biochem. Biophys. Res. Commun.* **111:**551, 1983) have shown that it stimulates differentiation of lymphoma cells and exercises a suppressing effect upon normal killer lymphocytes.

Lewis: Was it appreciated that the actual intracellular phosphatidyl inositol concentration rose when FMLP-mediated chemotaxis was inhibited by the chemical probes, such as dansyl cadaverine, that you used?

Schiffmann: The evidence we have suggests that dansyl cadaverine stimulates the turnover of phosphatidyl inositol, not its accumulation.

Schleimer: The role of lipomodulin in cell activation is an interesting question. We have noted, based on data available in the literature, that the interaction of lipomodulin, phospholipases, and the diglyceride-activated, calcium-dependent protein kinase may allow for a model of cell activation which is amplifying in nature and explains the observation that in mast cells, for example, only a few receptors need be crosslinked to produce cell activation. We envision that a small amount of diglyceride, produced by receptor crosslinking, may activate the kinase, which in turn, can activate phospholipase C (by phosphorylating the inhibitor of phospholipase C, lipomodulin) and induce further production of diglyceride, etc.

In response to Dr. Kay's question to Dr. Schiffmann, for almost a decade now it has been known that steroids inhibit arachidonate release from many different tissues. As Dr. Lichtenstein reported, we have found that steroids inhibit the release of arachidonate products from cells other than the mast cell in human lung. Although we have not yet proven that this is the result of a lipomodulin-mediated mechanism, it seems likely to be, and leaves open the possibility that steroid inhibition of arachidonate release may play a role in the antiinflammatory action of steroids in human lung.

Schiffmann: I would agree that if phospholipase C is also inhibited by lipomodulin, the level of diacylycerol may decrease, leading to a fall in the activity of protein kinase C, which conceivably could be involved in the phosphorylation and consequent inactivation of lipomodulin. In this sense lipomodulin might inhibit its own inactivation by exerting its antiphospholipase effect, amplifying in this manner its action upon cell motility.

Ishizaka: In collaboration with Dr. Tim Sullivan, we are now studying a possible interrelationship between IgE-mediated activation of phospholipid diacylglycerol (DAG) cycle and stimulation of phospholipid methylation in rat mast cells. Our results revealed that inhibitors of proteolytic enzymes and those of methyl transferases inhibited both phospholipid methylation and phosphatidylinosotol (PI) turnover induced by anti-IgE in an identical dose response fashion. The results suggest an essential involvement of proteolytic enzyme(s) and methyl transferases in early triggering events and demonstrate a close linkage between the two activation pathways for mediator release.

Schiffmann: I would agree that the effects of methyl transferase inhibition in both mast cells and neutrophils have many common features. The methyl transferase pathway in leucocytes may not be the only one, and the sequence of events will probably become clear when we are able to study a more simplified system, that is, perform complementation experiments similar to those of McGivney *et al.* (A. McGivney, F. T. Crews, F. Hirata, J. Axelrod, and R. Siraganian, *Proc. Natl. Acad. Sci. U.S.A.* **78:**6176, 1981.) We also feel that protease activity may be an early event in leukotaxis in agreement with your results on histamine release from mast cells.

Holgate: You mentioned that adenosine blocked the inhibitory effect of 3-deazaadenosine on neutrophil chemotaxis. Does the adenosine-facilitated uptake blocker dipyridamole have a similar effect?

Schiffmann: Dipyramidole did not have an effect on deazaadenosine inhibition precisely similar to that of adenosine. The results were variable, and in some instances the drug (dipyramidole) actually inhibited chemotaxis. Conceivably, the latter phenomenon might have been the result of its not being metabolized by the cell.

Bach: U-60257, which was mentioned here yesterday, was shown to be a potent inhibitor of LTB_4 production, β-glucuronidase release and superoxide radical production in f-met-leu-phe or ionophore-stimulated human PMNs (R. J. Smith, F. F. Sun, B. J. Bowman, S. S. Iden, H. W. Smith, and J. C. McGuire, *Biochem. Biophys. Res. Commun.* **109:**943, 1982). These three events do not follow parallel dose–response relationships, however, as LTB_4 production is the most susceptible to inhibition and superoxide production the least. This has obvious implications in the interpretation of the role of arachidonate metabolism in PMN activation. I wonder if the inhibitors you have just described have parallel dose-dependent inhibition for methylation or phosphatidylcholine synthesis compared with chemotaxis?

Schiffmann: We have not looked at the inhibition of LTB_4 production in PMNs as a function of lipomodulin concentration. Therefore we cannot answer whether or not there is parallel inhibition of chemotaxis and production of this mediator.

Austen: Would you comment on the dose–response characteristics of the effect of exogenous lipomodulin on PMN chemotaxis? Would you speculate on how antibody to lipomodulin might be clinically significant?

Schiffmann: The dose response of lipomodulin inhibitor of chemotaxis does appear to be narrow. The data may actually be insufficient to give a more conclusive picture. That is, even at 10^{-9} M the inhibitor effect may already be leveling off. Also, with a relatively high molecular weight protein presumably entering the membrane, there may be complex permeability or negatively cooperative phenomena that may yield this result.

The antibody to lipomodulin may be binding to, and inactivating, circulating lipomodulin as well as binding to membrane-bound protein of the cell surface, presumably causing an "activated" phospholipase in the neutrophil. It is however, as you point out, still not easy to understand why there would not be a massive generalized inflammation in the instance of a marked reduction of active lipomodulin.

CHAPTER 12

Eosinophils and Bronchial Inflammation*

G. J. GLEICH, E. FRIGAS, W. V. FILLEY, and D. A. LOEGERING

Departments of Immunology and Medicine
Allergic Diseases Research Laboratory
Mayo Medical School
and Mayo Clinic and Foundation
Rochester, Minnesota, U.S.A.

INTRODUCTION

Peripheral blood and tissue eosinophilia are hallmarks of both allergic and nonallergic asthma (1–3). In addition, the pathology of asthma includes eosinophil infiltration of bronchial tissues and mucus plugs, denudation of the respiratory epithelial cells in clusters (Creola bodies), the presence of Charcot–Leyden crystals in the bronchial lumen, a thickened basement membrane zone, bronchial smooth muscle hypertrophy, and edema of the peribronchial tissues (4–9).

The role of the eosinophil in asthma is not understood. Eosinophils possess enzymes capable of neutralizing certain mast cell mediators, and the possibility that the eosinophil modulates immediate-type hypersensitivity inflammatory reactions has been suggested (10). Some studies show, however, that eosinophils can kill parasites *in vitro* (11) and that ablation of eosinophils by specific antisera abolishes immunity to the parasites (11–14). Thus, eosinophils could be regarded as helpful in asthma by dampening inflammation or as inimical by damaging tissue through the mechanisms with which they kill parasites.

* Supported by grants from the National Institutes of Health, AI 09728 and AI 15231, and from the Mayo Foundation.

THE EFFECT OF EOSINOPHIL GRANULE MAJOR BASIC PROTEIN ON RESPIRATORY EPITHELIUM

We have investigated the materials composing the eosinophil granule and have identified a major basic protein (MBP) in the granule. In the guinea pig, MBP accounts for >50% of the granule protein and thus ~25% of the total cellular protein (15–18). MBP has a molecular weight of 11,000 and contains 13% arginine; it possesses two sulfhydryl groups and readily self-aggregrates to form disulfide-linked polymers (16). Human and rat eosinophil granules contain a comparable molecule (17,19). In the guinea pig, MBP makes up the core of the granule (19). MBP kills parasites including schistosomula of *Schistosoma mansoni* (20), newborn larvae of *Trichinella spiralis* (21), and trypomastigotes of *Trypanosoma cruzi* (22). MBP is toxic to a number of mammalian cells, including those from organs whose dysfunction is associated with eosinophil infiltration (23).

Because preliminary experiments indicated that MBP was toxic to respiratory epithelium (23), we investigated in detail the changes produced by MBP (24). In these experiments guinea pig tracheal rings were placed in tissue culture, MBP was added, and the effect of MBP on the tissue was analyzed by microscopy. MBP concentrations as low as 10 μg/ml produced ciliostasis at 48 hr; 100 μg/ml caused slowing of ciliary beating within 3 hr and cessation of ciliary motion within 23 hr. Examination of fixed tissue showed varying degrees of epithelial damage, which were related to the dose and the length of exposure to MBP. With the lowest concentration of MBP tested (10 μg/ml), the epithelium was disrupted and damaged cells were free in the lumen. With MBP levels of 50 and 100 μg/ml, the epithelium was extensively damaged, showing detachment of ciliated and brush cells and destruction of individual cells leaving behind only basal cells. With MBP levels from 250 to 900 μg/ml, the entire mucosal layer was sloughed down to the level of the lamina propria. The exfoliated cells were severely damaged, with lysis of the cellular membrane and liberation of the cell contents. Cilia were stripped from cells. The lamina propria appeared edematous with separation of the collagen fibrils.

The experiments described above showed that guinea pig MBP damaged guinea pig tracheal epithelium; therefore, we tested the effect of human and guinea pig MBP on human bronchial ring organ cultures (25). Both human and guinea pig MBP caused pronounced exfoliation of cells, a moth-eaten appearance of the epithelial surfaces, and alteration of ciliary beating. By microscopic examination, the changes in the human bronchial epithelium appeared essentially the same as those described above for the guinea pig tracheal epithelium. Thus, human MBP was toxic to human respiratory epithelium.

LEVELS OF MBP IN THE SPUTUM OF PATIENTS WITH BRONCHIAL ASTHMA

We next tested whether MBP was detectable in human sputum by radioimmunoassay (RIA). Figure 1 shows the sputum MBP levels in 100 patients with various respiratory diseases (25). In 73 patients, the MBP levels were below the sensitivity of the RIA, while in the remaining 27 patients with measurable MBP 12 had bronchial asthma. Figure 1 also shows that 11 of 13 patients with sputum MBP levels greater than 0.1 μg/ ml had asthma. Among the 73 patients without detectable sputum MBP, only 1 had asthma. The sputum MBP levels in the 13 patients with asthma ranged from <0.04 to 7.4 μg/ml (geometric mean, 0.34 μg/ml). The levels of MBP in the patients without asthma ranged from <0.04 to 0.7 μg/ml

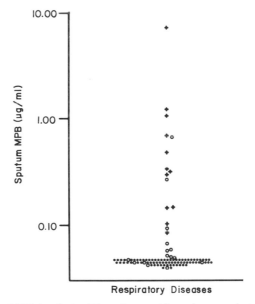

Fig. 1. Sputum MBP levels in 100 patients with various respiratory diseases. Each symbol represents 1 patient: patients whose sputa contained MBP and also had asthma (+); those whose sputa contained measurable MBP, but who did not have asthma (○); and those whose sputa did not contain measurable MBP (●). These sputa were assigned the lowest detectable MBP level. Reproduced from Frigas *et al.* (25), with permission.

(geometric mean, 0.05 μg/ml) for sputum MBP. The sputa MBP values in patients with and without asthma differed significantly ($p < .001$; rank sum test). In a second test of 96 sputa, all 14 patients with asthma had a sputum MBP >0.1 μg/ml (range, 0.01–3.0 μg/ml) (26).

Finding elevated MBP levels in the sputum of asthmatics led us to determine the MBP levels in the sputum of patients hospitalized with asthma. Fifteen consecutive patients with asthma were admitted for treatment of acute exacerbations. Their sputum MBP levels were measured serially, and peak values ranged from 0.3 to 92.9 μg/ml with a geometric mean of 7.1 μg/ml. Seven of the 15 patients had MBP sputum levels >10 μg/ml (1.1×10^{-6} M), the lowest level previously found toxic *in vitro* (24).

LOCALIZATION OF MBP IN THE LUNG TISSUES OF PATIENTS WITH BRONCHIAL ASTHMA

The observations summarized above indicated that MBP damaged respiratory epithelium and was present in sputa of patients with asthma in concentrations approximating those showing toxicity *in vitro*. We next determined whether MBP is present at the site of damage to epithelium in patients dying of asthma. To accomplish this we developed an immunofluorescence procedure for tissue localization of MBP and showed in the guinea pig that MBP could be detected in formalin-fixed, paraffin-embedded tissues (27). Using this technique, we studied formalin-fixed, paraffin-embedded lung tissue obtained postmortem from patients with asthma and from control patients dying of other diseases (28). The specificity of the antiserum for MBP was shown by staining of eosinophils in peripheral blood, by removal of staining by absorption with solid-phase MBP, and by failure of preimmunization serum from the same rabbits to stain eosinophils.

Lung tissues were studied from 22 autopsy cases between 1967 and 1979. The criteria for selection of the 11 patients with asthma were Group I, death associated with status asthmaticus, and typical pathology of severe asthma; Group II, death from other causes associated with severe asthma, and the typical pathology of asthma; Group III, death from other causes, and asthma adequately treated or in remission at the time of death and the absence of the typical pathology of asthma. All patients with asthma had a clinical history of asthma as defined by the American Thoracic Society (29). The 11 controls were age- and sex-matched with the patients with asthma and had died from causes other than asthma or primary pulmonary diseases.

Examination of sections stained with hematoxylin and eosin (H & E)

TABLE I
Pathologic Findings by Hematoxylin and Eosin Staining

	Asthma			Disease controls (11 patients)
	Group I (6 patients)	Group II (3 patients)	Group III (2 patients)	
Damaged respiratory epithelium[a]	6	1	0	0
Squamous metaplasia	4	2	0	0
Mucus plugs	6	2	1	0
Creola bodies	6	1	0	1
Eosinophils	6	3	2	3

[a] Denudation of the epithelial cells.

showed that all patients with asthma had a thickened basement membrane zone, goblet cell hyperplasia, and peribronchial inflammatory infiltrates with eosinophils in the lamina propria. Smooth muscle hypertrophy was seen in all but one of the patients and mucus gland hyperplasia was seen in seven. Table I shows that squamous metaplasia, mucus plugs, Creola bodies, epithelial damage, and frank denudation of respiratory epithelium occurred with a more variable frequency.

Examination of sections by immunofluorescence showed MBP staining that was cell associated as well as extracellular. The sites at which MBP was localized and the frequency of staining at these sites differed among the patients (Table II). Striking abnormalities were seen in patients dying

TABLE II
Localization of MBP by Immunofluorescence

Site	Asthma			Disease controls (11 patients)
	Group I (6 patients)	Group II (3 patients)	Group III (2 patients)	
Mucus plugs				
Cell-associated	6	2	0	0
Extracellular	6	1	0	0
Damaged epithelium[a]	3	1	0	0
Epithelial surface[a]	3	0	0	0
Necrotic area below[a] basement membrane	4	0	0	0
Macrophages	4	2	1	6
Eosinophils	6	3	2	11

[a] Both extracellular and cell-associated MBP localization.

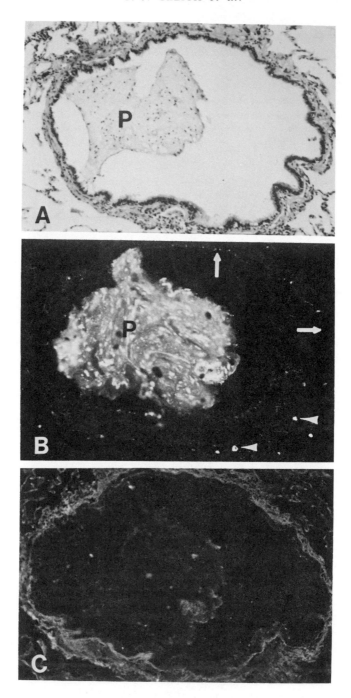

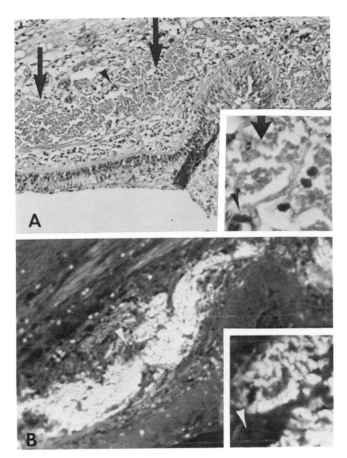

Fig. 3. Serial sections of a bronchus from another patient with asthma. (A) H & E staining reveals an inflammatory cell infiltrate in the lamina propria with large patches of amorphous necrotic eosinophilic material (arrows). (B) When stained for MBP, these areas below the basement membrane in the lamina propria glow intensely for extracellular MBP. Scattered discrete eosinophils can be seen. ×100. Inserts on right show the detail of this tissue at ×400 magnification. Although some discrete cells are present when stained by H & E (insert A), the entire area glows diffusely when stained with anti-MBP (insert B). For orientation, the arrowhead points toward a vessel in area of higher magnification. Reproduced from Filley *et al.* (28), with permission.

◄ **Fig. 2.** Serial sections of a bronchiole with mucus plug (P) from a patient with asthma. (A) Section stained with H & E. (B) Section stained with anti-MBP. Note the diffuse staining of the plug (P) with brilliant swirls as well as the patchy, scalloped, less intense glowing of the luminal surface of the respiratory epithelium (arrows). There are also discrete eosinophils in the peribronchiolar area (arrowheads). (C) Normal rabbit serum (NRS) control. ×100. Reproduced from Filley *et al.* (28), with permission.

with status asthmaticus, which patients dying of other causes with associated severe asthma showed to a lesser degree. Patients with death not due to asthma showed neither epithelial damage nor extracellular MBP immunofluorescence.

Examples of certain patterns of MBP immunofluorescence are shown in Figs. 2 and 3. Figure 2 shows diffuse staining of a mucus plug with streaks and whirls that glow brilliantly. In addition, the epithelial surface of this bronchiole is stained in a patchy, scalloped manner. Figure 3 shows diffuse extracellular MBP immunofluorescence in the lamina propria. This area of intense glowing corresponds to the presence of necrotic, amorphous, eosinophilic material on the H & E-stained section (Fig. 3A). Another striking abnormality was intense extracellular MBP staining of damaged epithelium, which was associated with eosinophil infiltration in the lamina propria and frank destruction of the basement membrane zone. Finally, some alveolar macrophages showed MBP immunofluorescence while others in the same field failed to stain.

DISCUSSION

Asthma is an inflammatory disease of the respiratory mucosa associated with a specific pathology (4–9,30–34). The pathology is characterized by infiltration of eosinophils into the bronchial wall and lumen, damage to respiratory epithelium, a thickened basement membrane zone due to collagen proliferation (35), smooth muscle hypertrophy, and edema of peribronchial tissue. Excessive shedding and desquamation of the bronchial epithelium down to the level of the lamina propria are reported as constant findings in bronchial asthma (8,9,30,33). The superficial columnar cells undergo detachment, leaving behind them a layer of basal cells; from these, regeneration of the mucosa takes place. Because of the prominence of the eosinophil in this pathology and because MBP damaged respiratory epithelium in a manner remarkably similar to that described in asthma (24), we investigated the hypothesis that eosinophils, through MBP, might damage bronchial epithelium in patients with asthma.

Measurement of MBP in the sputa of 100 patients with various respiratory diseases (Fig. 1) showed that an elevated MBP level is a good marker for asthma. Of the 13 patients with asthma, all but 2 had MBP levels >0.1 μg/ml. Although the numbers of eosinophils in the blood of the 13 patients with asthma were greater than in the patients without asthma, the twofold difference was considerably less than the sevenfold difference between sputum MBP levels in the patients with asthma and without asthma. Actually, the sevenfold difference is a minimum estimate because in most patients without asthma sputum MBP was undetectable. Thus, the sputum MBP level appears better than the number of blood eosinophils as a marker for asthma. In patients hospitalized with asthma the average peak sputum MBP level, 7 μg/ml, approximated the concentration of MBP that damaged respiratory epithelium in vitro.

Comparison of MBP immunofluorescence in the patients with asthma and controls showed marked differences. In the control patients, only eosinophils and occasional alveolar macrophages stained; this staining was entirely cell associated. Patients with asthma showed the same cell-associated staining of eosinophils and macrophages and, in addition, a marked eosinophil infiltration. The eosinophil infiltration in the lamina propria was readily appreciated by immunofluorescence in comparison to staining with H & E where the nature of the infiltrating cells was more difficult to define. Moreover, patients with asthma showed apparent extracellular MBP immunofluorescence. We considered MBP immunofluorescence as cell associated when it conformed to the size and shape of cells, whereas extracellular MBP was not confined to cellular structures. Mucus plugs showed striking extracellular MBP deposition. For example, Fig. 2A shows a paucity of cells in the mucus plug whereas Figure 2B shows diffuse MBP immunofluorescence throughout the entire mucus plug. Perhaps the most dramatic example of extracellular MBP immunofluorescence is the apparently necrotic areas in the lamina propria of patients dying of status asthmaticus (Fig. 3). These areas show few intact eosinophils in a sea of eosinophilic granular debris that stains intensely with anti-MBP. Taken together these results strongly suggest that eosinophils release their granule contents into bronchial tissues in severe asthma.

Our results confirm previous descriptions of tissue damage in asthma, including shedding and destruction of respiratory epithelial cells and the presence of Creola bodies in sputa (4–9,30–34). In the damaged tissues, MBP extracellular immunofluorescence was often seen. When MBP was found in extracellular sites, we regularly noted that these areas showed evidence of epithelial damage. However, not all damaged areas showed extracellular MBP immunofluorescence. For example, one section from a patient with asthma showed extensive epithelial damage in the absence of eosinophils and of extracellular MBP at these sites. The postmortem examination in this patient showed bilateral bronchopneumonia in addition to bronchial asthma. Another possibility for failure to find MBP deposition at all sites of damage is the denudation of this damaged tissue into the bronchial lumen. In several cases we observed bright glowing of cellular debris in the mucus plug, while most of the epithelium had been lost from the basement membrane.

As noted earlier, considerable evidence exists indicating that the eosin-

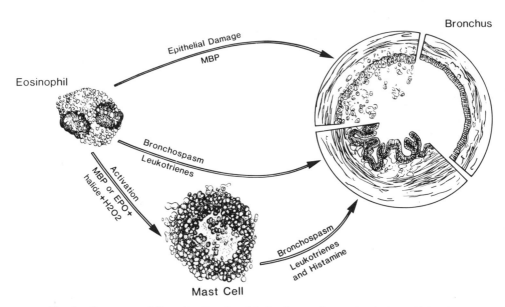

Fig. 4. Summary of the role of eosinophils in airway obstruction in bronchial asthma. The effects on the bronchus are shown comparing a section of normal bronchus (upper right) to a section damaged by MBP (upper left), which shows epithelial desquamation, and to a section (bottom), which shows smooth muscle hypertrophy and edema of the lamina propria resulting in a reduction in the caliber of the airway (EPO, eosinophil peroxidase).

ophil is able to kill helminths *in vitro* (11), and this damage is effected by release of granule contents onto the surface of the parasite (36). The granule contents evidently disrupt the parasite's external membrane, and in the case of schistosomula of *Schistosoma mansoni* eosinophils actually invade the body of the parasite through the breach in the wall. The ability of the eosinophil to disrupt the external membrane of the parasite implies the existence of powerful membrane active effector systems, many or all of which are brought into play by granule disruption. In fact, MBP (20), the eosinophil cationic protein (37), and the eosinophil peroxidase (EPO) system (38) are able to damage schistosomula of *S. mansoni*. In asthma the occurrence of striking blood and tissue eosinophilia (1–9), the relationship of eosinophilia to severity (3), and the release of granule contents into the damaged tissues and bronchial lumen point to the possibility that eosinophils damage respiratory tissues.

In the studies discussed above, we were concerned with the possibility that the eosinophil causes epithelial damage in asthma. Recent information suggests mechanisms by which the eosinophil might cause bronchospasm, either directly or indirectly. For example, leukotriene C4 and D4 can be produced by the horse and human eosinophil (39,40). Mast cells and basophils can be activated to secrete mediators either by EPO plus halide and hydrogen peroxidase (41) or directly by MBP (42). Thus, the eosinophil possesses the capability not only to damage epithelium, but also to produce bronchospasm by production of leukotrienes or by activation of mast cells (Fig. 4).

SUMMARY

The role of the eosinophil in bronchial asthma has been investigated. Peripheral blood and tissue eosinophilia are hallmarks of both allergic and nonallergic asthma. Analysis of the activities of the eosinophil granule major basic protein (MBP) revealed that the molecule was toxic both to helminthic parasites and to mammalian cells, including respiratory epithelium. The damage to respiratory epithelium consisted of desquamation and frank destruction of cells. Because these changes mimicked in part the pathology of bronchial asthma, we tested sputum for its content of MBP. Analyses of 100 random sputum samples for MBP showed that 13 were >0.1 μg/ml and 11 of the 13 patients had asthma. Patients treated for asthma have high levels of MBP in their sputum, and these levels decreased during treatment. To determine whether MBP was actually present in the lesions of bronchial asthma, MBP was localized by immunofluorescence in tissues of patients who had died of asthma. MBP was present outside of the eosinophil and in association with damaged bronchial epithelium. Overall, these results are in keeping with the hypothesis that in asthma the eosinophil damages respiratory tissues.

REFERENCES

1. Lowell, F. C. Clinical aspects of eosinophilia in atopic disease. *JAMA, J. Am. Med. Assoc.* **202:**875–878, 1967.
2. Franklin, W. Treatment of severe asthma. *N. Engl. J. Med.* **290:**1469–1472, 1974.
3. Horn, B. R., Robin, E. D., Theodore, J., and Van Kessel, A. Total eosinophil counts in the management of bronchial asthma. *N. Engl. J. Med.* **292:**1152–1155, 1975.
4. Ellis, A. G. The pathological anatomy of bronchial asthma. *Am. J. Med. Sci.* **136:**407–429, 1908.
5. Huber, H. L., and Koessler, K. K. The pathology of bronchial asthma. *Arch. Intern. Med.* **30:**689–760, 1922.
6. Thomson, J. G. Fatal bronchial asthma showing the asthmatic reaction in an ovarian teratoma. *J. Pathol.* **57:**213–219, 1945.

7. Houston, J. C., Navasquez, S. D., and Trounce, J. R. A clinical and pathological study of fatal cases of status asthmaticus. *Thorax* **8**:207–214, 1953.

8. Naylor, B. The shedding of the mucosa of the bronchial tree in asthma. *Thorax* **17**:69–72, 1972.

9. Dunnill, M. S. The pathology of asthma. *In* "Allergy: Principles and Practices" (E. Middleton, Jr., C. E. Reed, and E. F. Ellis, eds.), pp. 678–686. Mosby, St. Louis, Missouri, 1978.

10. Goetzl, E. J., Wasserman, S. I., and Austen, K. F. Eosinophil polymorphonuclear leukocyte function in immediate hypersensitivity. *Arch. Pathol.* **99**:1–4, 1975.

11. Kazura, J. W. Protective role of eosinophils. *In* "The Eosinophil in Health and Disease" (A. A. F. Mahmoud and K. F. Austen, eds.), pp. 231–251. Grune & Stratton, New York, 1980.

12. Mahmoud, A. A. F., Warren, K. S., and Peters, P. A. A role for the eosinophil in acquired resistance to *Schistosoma mansoni* infection as detected by anti-eosinophil serum. *J. Exp. Med.* **142**:805–813, 1975.

13. Grove, D. I., Mahmoud, A. A. F., and Warren, K. S. Eosinophils and resistance to *Trichinella spiralis*. *J. Exp. Med.* **145**:755–759, 1977.

14. Gleich, G. J., Olson, G. M., and Herlich, H. The effect of antiserum to eosinophils on susceptibility and acquired immunity of the guinea pig to *Trichostrongylus colubriformis*. *Immunology* **37**:873–880, 1979.

15. Gleich, G. J., Loegering, D. A., and Maldonado, J. E. Identification of a major basic protein in guinea pig eosinophil granules. *J. Exp. Med.* **137**:1459–1471, 1973.

16. Gleich, G. J., Loegering, D. A., Kueppers, F., Bajaj, S. P., and Mann, K. G. Physiochemical and biological activities of the major basic protein from protein guinea pig eosinophil granules. *J. Exp. Med.* **140**:313–332, 1974.

17. Gleich, G. J., Loegering, D. A., Mann, K. G., and Maldonado, J. E. Comparative properties of the Charcot–Leyden crystal protein and the major basic protein from human eosinophils. *J. Clin. Invest.* **57**:633–640, 1976.

18. Archer, G. T., and Hirsch, J. G. Isolation of granules from eosinophil leukocytes and study of their enzyme content. *J. Exp. Med.* **118**:277–286, 1963.

19. Lewis, D. M., Lewis, J. C., Loegering, D. A., and Gleich, G. J. Localization of the guinea pig eosinophil major basic protein to the core of the granule. *J. Cell Biol.* **77**:702–713, 1978.

20. Butterworth, A. E., Wassom, D. L., Gleich, G. J., Loegering, D. A., and David, J. R. Damage to schistosomula of *Schistosoma mansoni* induced directly by eosinophil major basic protein. *J. Immunol.* **122**:221–229, 1979.

21. Wassom, D. L., and Gleich, G. J. Damage to *Trichinella spiralis* newborn larvae by eosinophil major basic protein. *Am. J. Trop. Med. Hyg.* **28**:860–863, 1979.

22. Kierszenbaum, F., Ackerman, S. J., and Gleich, G. J. Destruction of bloodstream forms of *Trypanosoma cruzi* by eosinophil granule major basic protein. *Am. J. Trop. Med. Hyg.* **30**:775–779, 1981.

23. Gleich, G. J., Frigas, E., Loegering, D. A., Wassom, D. L., and Steinmuller, D. Cytotoxic properties of the eosinophil major basic protein. *J. Immunol.* **123**:2925–2927, 1979.

24. Frigas, E., Loegering, D. A., and Gleich, G. J. Cytotoxic effects of the guinea pig eosinophil major basic protein on tracheal epithelium. *Lab. Invest.* **42**:35–43, 1980.

25. Frigas, E., Loegering, D. A., Solley, G. O., Farrow, G. M., and Gleich, G. J. Elevated levels of the eosinophil granule major basic protein in the sputum of patients with bronchial asthma. *Mayo Clin. Proc.* **56**:345–353, 1981.

26. Dor, P. J., Ackerman, S. J., and Gleich, G. J. Charcot–Leyden crystal protein and eosinophil granule major basic protein in sputum of patients with respiratory diseases. *J. Allergy Clin. Immunol.* **71**(Pt.2):112 (abstr.), 1983.

27. Filley, W. V., Ackerman, S. J., and Gleich, G. J. An immunofluorescent method for specific staining of eosinophil granule major basic protein. *J. Immunol. Methods* **47:**227–238, 1981.
28. Filley, W. V., Holley, K. E., Kephart, G. M., and Gleich, G. J. Identification by immunofluorescence of eosinophil granule major basic protein in lung tissues of patients with bronchial asthma. *Lancet* **2:**11–16, 1982.
29. American Thoracic Society Chronic bronchitis, asthma, and pulmonary emphysema: A statement by the Committee on Diagnostic Standards for Nontuberculous Respiratory Diseases. *Am. Rev. Respir. Dis.* **85:**762–768, 1962.
30. Cardell, B. S., and Pearson, R. S. B. Death in asthmatics. *Thorax* **14:**341–352, 1959.
31. Cutz, E., Levison, H., and Cooper, D. M. Ultrastructure of airways in children with asthma. *Histopathology* **2:**407–421, 1978.
32. Dunnill, M. S. The pathology of asthma, with special reference to changes in the bronchial mucosa. *J. Clin. Pathol.* **13:**27–33, 1960.
33. Dunnill, M. S., Massarella, G. R., and Anderson, J. A. A comparison of the quantitative anatomy of the bronchi in normal subjects, in status asthmaticus, in chronic bronchitis, and in emphysema. *Thorax* **24:**176–179, 1969.
34. Glynn, A. A., and Michaels, L. Bronchial biopsy in chronic bronchitis and asthma. *Thorax* **15:**142–153, 1960.
35. McCarter, J. H., and Vasquez, J. J. The bronchial basement membrane in asthma. *Arch. Pathol.* **82:**328–335, 1966.
36. McLaren, D. J. M., Ramalho-Pinto, F. J., and Smithers, S. R. Ultrastructural evidence for complement and antibody-dependent damage to schistosomula of *Schistosoma mansoni* by rat eosinophils in vitro. *Parasitology* **77:**313–324, 1978.
37. McLaren, D. J., McKean, J. R., Olsson, I., Venge, P., and Kay, A. B. Morphological studies on the killing of schistosomula of *Schistosoma mansoni* by human eosinophil and neutrophil cationic proteins *in vitro. Parasite Immunol.* **3:**359–373, 1981.
38. Jong, E. C., Mahmoud, A. A. F., and Klebanoff, S. J. Peroxidase-mediated toxicity to schistosomules of *Schistosoma mansoni. J. Immunol.* **126:**468–471, 1981.
39. Jorg, A., Henderson, W. R., Murphy, R. C., and Klebanoff, S. J. Leukotriene generation by eosinophils. *J. Exp. Med.* **155:**390–402, 1982.
40. Henderson, W. R., Harley, J. B., Fauci, A. S., and Klebanoff, S. J. Leukotriene B4, C4 and D4 generation by human eosinophils. *J. Allergy Clin. Immunol.* **71:**138 (abstr.), 1983.
41. Henderson, W. R., Chi, E. Y., and Klebanoff, S. J. Eosinophil peroxidase-induced mast cell secretion. *J. Exp. Med.* **152:**265–279, 1980.
42. O'Donnell, M. C., Ackerman, S. J., Gleich, G. J., and Thomas, L. L. Activation of basophil and mast cell histamine release by eosinophil granule major basic protein. *J. Exp. Med.* **157:**1981–1991, 1983.

DISCUSSION

Kay: McLaren *et al.* (D. J. McLaren, J. R. McKean, I. Olsson, P. Venge, and A. B. Kay, *Parasite Immunol.* **3:**359, 1981) found that ECP has a very potent cytotoxic agent for schistosomula *in vitro* and that neutrophil-derived cationic proteins (NCP) appeared to be equipotent. Perhaps NCP should also be reckoned with in asthma. Is there antigenic cross-reactivity between MBP and NCP? Incidentally, do you still find the term "intrinsic asthma" useful?

Gleich: The relative potencies of MBP and the eosinophil cationic protein (ECP) in the killing of schistosomules of *Schistosoma mansoni* have recently been tested in collaboration with Dr. Anthony Butterworth (S. J. Ackerman, G. J. Gleich, D. A. Loegering, and A. E. Butterworth, *Fed. Proc., Fed. Am. Soc. Exp. Biol.* **42:**1247, 1983) and the findings were consistent with both prior studies (A. E. Butterworth, D. L. Wassom, G. J. Gleich, D. A. Loegering, and J. R. David, *J. Immunol.* **122:**221, 1979; D. J. McLaren *et al., Parasite Immunol.* **3:**359, 1981). ECP was about 10-fold more potent than MBP in killing schistosomules. Concerning the presence of MBP in neutrophils, we did not detect immunofluorescent staining of polymorphonuclear neutrophils with guinea pig (W. V. Filley, S. J. Ackerman, and G. J. Gleich, *J. Immunol. Methods* **47:**227, 1981) and human cells (W. V. Filley, K. E. Holley, G. M. Kephart, and G. J. Gleich, *Lancet* **2:**11, 1982). Therefore, MBP does not appear to be similar to the neutrophil cationic proteins. Finally, we use the term intrinsic asthma in the same sense as Rackemann did (F. M. Rackemann, *Arch. Intern. Med.* **41:**346, 1928) to denote a form of asthma that does not have an evident allergen trigger. This form of asthma is quite prevalent in the practice at our institution and may indeed be the major variety of asthma we treat. The term "idiopathic" might well be used to describe this form of asthma, in that we have little information about its pathogenesis.

Lessof: One of the many interesting questions concerns the diagnostic value of the MBP level in sputum, especially in patients with asthma who also have obstructive airways disease. When the case records of your original 100 control subjects were looked at again, some of them were rediagnosed. Was the rediagnosis carried out by somebody who did not know the result of the MBP assay, in which case the correlation is impressive, or was the diagnosis reviewed by somebody who knew the MBP results, because in that case it needs more work before it can be validated?

Gleich: In the first analysis (E. Frigas, D. A. Loegering, G. O. Solley, G. M. Farrow, and G. J. Gleich, *Mayo Clin. Proc.* **56:**345, 1981), the results of sputum MBP were compared to the diagnosis and patients with asthma had elevated levels. However, other patients also had elevated levels and review of their records showed that they had reversible bronchospasm and eosinophilia and were being treated with bronchodilators and glucocorticoids. Because of this we classified these latter patients as asthma, although their physicians often termed the disease chronic obstructive lung disease. Thus this study was not entirely without bias and the diagnostic value of sputum MBP, although promising, warrants further study.

Platt-Mills: Could you comment on the mechanism that leads to granule release from eosinophils in the lung?

Gleich: There are several factors that activate eosinophils, some produced by monocytes (M. C. Veith and A. E. Butterworth, *J. Exp. Med.* **157:**828, 1983) and others by eosinophil colony-stimulating factors (A. J. Dessein, M. A. Vadas, N. A. Nicola, D. Metcalf, and J. R. David, *J. Exp. Med.* **156:**90, 1982). One presumes that such factors might be operative in the lung, but this is not known at the present time.

Turner-Warwick: In the context of your talk, I am in a dilemma because many clinical syndromes associated with an intense eosinophil infiltrate of tissues do not appear to develop *permanent* tissue damage, while under other circumstances (e.g., hypereosinophilic syndrome and some eosinophil vasculitic syndromes) they do develop irreversible damage. First, do you agree that there is such variability, and second, have you any speculation why this is?

Gleich: I agree that many clinical syndromes associated with eosinophilia do not show permanent damage, an exception being the subendocardial fibrosis seen in the hypereosinophilic syndrome. In addition, one sees patients with asthma who do not show full reversibility; that is, their FEV_1, although improved, does not return to the expected normal. Thus in some situations there may be organ dysfunction in diseases associated with eosinophilia. The reason for the variability in permanent damage is not known.

Flenley: Do sputum concentrations of MBP, measured sequentially in the same patient, vary from day to day and do they correlate with FEV_1? Also, what are the appearances of MBP staining at autopsy in chronic bronchitis?

Gleich: In answer to your first question, there is a general relationship between MBP levels and the FEV_1 in the patients we have studied. However, these patients were receiving glucocorticoids, and as you know these affect many cellular processes. We have not examined the tissues of patients dying of chronic bronchitis for MBP.

Grant: If it is assumed the eosinophils cause epithelial damage in so-called intrinsic asthma, why do steroids not prevent it? Does MBP disappear when asthma is controlled by steroids? When it does not, could the patients be "steroid resistant"?

Gleich: In the series of 15 patients hospitalized for treatment of asthma we found that the concentration of sputum MBP initially went up and then fell as the patients improved following treatment with bronchodilators and glucocorticoids (E. Frigas, D. A. Loegering, G. O. Solley, G. M. Farrow, and G. J. Gleich, *Mayo Clin. Proc.* **56**:345, 1981). Therefore it seemed that asthma severity correlated roughly with sputum MBP and that treatment led to a decrease in the concentration of sputum MBP. However, certain patients who were receiving up to 30–40 mg prednisone daily still had elevated sputum MBP, suggesting that this dose of glucocorticoid was not adequate to control bronchial inflammation. I presume that glucocorticoids would prevent epithelial damage by eosinophils in asthma when they are given in sufficient dosage to ablate eosinophils from tissues.

McFadden: Following on from the previous question, why, in asthma, do the eosinophils attack the airways? In diseases such as eosinophilic pneumonia, etc., the lung is loaded with eosinophils, yet clinically there are no airway symptoms or airway pathology. Can you speculate why this might be?

Gleich: The eosinophil could home to bronchi because of chemotaxis by factors derived from mast cells or basophils, or possibly due to T lymphocytes. The latter suggestion is based on the observations of W. E. Parish [*Clin. Allergy* 12(Suppl. 47): 1982] who has claimed that sputum T cells produce a factor which stimulates eosinophils.

Kaplan: I noted that fewer eosinophils were present in the lung relative to the huge amount of MBP seen. Is it possible that lung mast cells might have MBP as do basophils?

Gleich: We have tested by immunofluorescence for the presence of MBP in other cells and have found it only in basophils (S. J. Ackerman, G. M. Kephart, T. M. Habermann, P. R. Greipp, and G. J. Gleich, *J. Exp. Med.* **157**:1981, 1983). In one collaborative experiment with Dr. Lichtenstein we were not able to detect MBP in lung mast cells, but further studies are needed.

Lichtenstein: Did your pictures show eosinophils predominating over neutrophils in those pulmonary lesions? If so, what scenario do you suggest accounts for this?

Gleich: It is rather difficult to be definite about the numbers of cells in the bronchial inflammation of the patients. In fact, our studies have alerted me to the need for careful, modern, quantitative light and electron microscopic studies of the pathology of asthma. However, the lesions we have studied (with haemotoxylin and eosin staining) clearly show, as have prior studies, a very marked eosinophil infiltration and an apparent paucity of neutrophils.

Austen: The eosinophil may also have some beneficial functions such as inhibition of 5-lipoxygenase in mast cells by 15-HETE release. Also, eosinophil production of hypochlorous acid (HOCL) would rapidly inactivate the sulfidopeptide leukotrienes.

Gleich: It seems clear that eosinophils could function to down-regulate the inflammatory reaction in asthma. Our studies have focused on their possible deleterious effects because of the number of eosinophils in asthma and because we were stimulated by the finding that the eosinophil as well as its granule proteins, such as MBP, ECP, and eosinophil peroxidase, plus H_2O_2 and halide, damage parasites.

Schiffmann: Since fibrosis and thickening of basement membrane occur, is there any evidence that the major basic protein acts as a growth factor or chemoattractant?

Gleich: This is an interesting question, but one to which, at the present time, there is no answer.

Lewis: Since you have shown that alveolar macrophages ingest MBP *in situ,* do you know of any macrophage biochemical processes that are "turned on" by MBP? This would be particularly interesting with respect to scarring and fibrosis, since macrophages generate macrophage-derived growth factor, which stimulates fibroblast proliferation and collagen synthesis.

Gleich: At the present time we do not know whether eosinophils or their granule constituents can stimulate macrophages. It seems likely that alveolar macrophages ingest MBP as judged by immunofluorescent staining of the macrophages for MBP. This was evident both in the lungs of patients with asthma and in the lungs of control patients.

Morley: The converse, that is eosinophil stimulation by macrophages, is also likely. Human alveolar macrophages produce PAF-acether in response to a variety of stimuli (B. Arnoux, D. Duval, and J. Benveniste, *Eur. J. Clin. Invest.* **10:**437, 1980; B. Arnoux, M. H. Simoes-Caeioro, A. Lands, M. Mathieu, P. Duroux, and J. Benveniste, *Am. Rev. Respir. Dis.* **125:**70abs., 1982); PAF-acether activates eosinophils *in vitro,* and PAF-acether inhalation in the baboon produces a pronounced eosinophil accumulation in the airways.

Schwartz: It appears that eosinophils are incapable of releasing major basic protein without consequent suicide. Release of arachidonate metabolites also occurs. Is the expression of these events related to the concentration of agonist or to different agonists?

Gleich: At the present time, we have not studied eosinophil activation in any degree, and specifically we do not know what percentage of cells undergo dissolution with granule release. Nor do we know whether leukotriene secretion occurs in concert with eosinophil dissolution.

CHAPTER 13

Mediators of Hypersensitivity and Inflammatory Cells in Early- and Late-Phase Asthmatic Reactions

A. B. KAY, T. H. LEE, S. R. DURHAM, T. NAGAKURA, O. CROMWELL,
MARY CARROLL, NIKI PAPAGEORGIOU, and R. J. SHAW

Department of Allergy and Clinical Immunology
Cardiothoracic Institute, Bromptom Hospital
London, U.K.

INTRODUCTION

Several hours following the early response to an antigen-inhalation challenge, many asthmatic patients have a further, often more severe, increase in airflow obstruction (the late or late-phase reaction) (1). Early and late reactions differ in many respects (Table I). The early reactions are rapid in onset, that is, they peak 10–15 min following the appropriate challenge and readily reverse either spontaneously or following the administration of inhaled bronchodilators (2–4). In contrast, late-phase reactions develop more gradually and have a more sustained duration (2). Thus, late-phase asthmatic reactions occur over hours rather than minutes and are associated with considerably more lung hyperinflation (5). Unlike the early (or "early, spasmogenic") reactions, late sustained increases in airflow obstruction are more difficult to reverse with inhaled bronchodilators such as β-2-sympathomimetics (2,5), and in a proportion of individuals there is an increase in the degree of bronchial hyperreactivity for several days following the challenge (6). There was no significant difference in the site of airflow obstruction, as determined by helium–oxygen flow volume curves, between the early and late reactions (7).

The precise mechanism of the early- and late-phase asthmatic responses remains unclear. In general, late-phase reactions do not usually

ASTHMA: Physiology,
Immunopharmacology,
and Treatment
THIRD INTERNATIONAL SYMPOSIUM

211

TABLE I
Phases of the Asthmatic Response[a]

Early (Rapid, Spasmogenic) Phase

    Occurs 10–15 min following allergen or exercise challenge
    Involves mast cell/mediator cell activation (histamine, NCA)
    Largely histamine-mediated (directly, or by reflexes)
    Reversed by prior administration of DSCG, histamine H1- and H2-antagonists
    Not affected by corticosteroids (given immediately prior to challenge)
    Characterized by bronchial smooth muscle contraction

Late (Sustained) Phase

    Occurs 6–8 hr following allergen challenge or exercise
    More prolonged than rapid phase
    More hyperinflation
    More difficult to reverse with bronchodilators
    Sometimes takes several days to resolve
    Associated with enhanced bronchial hyperreactivity
    Associated with mast cell/mediator cell activation (histamine, NCA)
    Involvement of inflammatory cells (neutrophils, eosinophils, mononuclear cells)
    Reversed by prior administration of corticosteroids
    Possible involvement of leukotrienes, prostaglandins, thromboxanes
    Bronchial smooth muscle contraction and submucosal oedema are probably involved

Subacute/Chronic Inflammatory Phase

    The hallmark of continuing, day-to-day asthma
    Bronchial hyperreactivity a marked feature
    Eosinophils and mononuclear cell infiltrate prominent
    Lysosomal enzyme release and eosinophil basic proteins involved
    Bronchial smooth muscle contraction, submucosal oedema, plugging of lumen and
        denudation of epithelium are typical autopsy findings
    Often (but not always) responsive to corticosteroids

[a] From Kay (1a,1b).

occur in the absence of an early response, although isolated late asthmatic reactions are well documented, especially in association with exposure to occupational agents (8). It is possible that in these instances an early subclinical immunological event might have occurred that did not result in an alteration in airways calibre. Thus, with allergen-inhalation challenge, there is strong evidence for believing that the initial immunological trigger, that is, antigen and mast cell-bound IgE, leads to the manifestations of both the early and late-phase responses. For instance, the ability of anti-IgE to evoke late-phase cutaneous responses via the "reverse-phase reaction" was an important observation, as it demonstrated that other antibody classes such as IgG were not an essential prerequisite for the manifestations of the late-phase response (9,10).

Histological studies of cutaneous late-phase reactions have revealed the presence of numerous inflammatory cells, that is, neutrophils and mononuclear cells, as well as occasional basophils (10). These observations have suggested that late reactions might be caused, in part, by tissue injury resulting from the recruitment of secondary inflammatory cells mobilized as a result of the release of mast cell-derived chemotactic factors. Furthermore, as discussed below, it is likely that both inflammatory cells and mediators of hypersensitivity contribute to the late sustained response as well as to the subsequent subacute/chronic inflammatory phase, which is probably a central feature of continuing, day-to-day asthma in the untreated subject.

THE INCEPTION OF THE LATE-PHASE RESPONSE

Late-phase reactions have been described in the skin (9,10), nose (11,12), and bronchi (1) and can be elicited by a variety of allergens in appropriately sensitized individuals. Because of the growing appreciation that mast cells/mediator cells can be activated by several nonimmunologic triggers, that is, cold (13), cholinergic (14), solar (15), and heat (16) urticaria, and exercise-induced asthma (EIA), we attempted to determine whether a stimulus such as a treadmill exercise task would produce a late-phase as well as an early asthmatic reaction. We demonstrated that 2 adults and 13 children with exercise-induced asthma (EIA) gave nonimmediate, in addition to immediate, reductions in FEV_1 following treadmill exercise (17).

The late reactions developed 4–10 hr after exercise and in each instance were associated with wheezing and/or chest tightness. The exact prevalence of exercise-induced late-phase reactions is unknown, although it is our impression that this phenomenon is probably more common in children. The observation that late asthmatic reactions occur following exercise might have practical clinical implications. For instance, spontaneous exacerbation of asthma, especially at night, might be related to exercise undertaken several hours earlier. Furthermore, a late episode of asthma after exercise might be erroneously attributed to provocation by allergen.

In general, the factors predisposing to the development of late-phase reactions, whether initiated immunologically or nonspecifically, are still incompletely understood. Individuals with more hyperreactive airways and/or high baseline levels of the neutrophil chemotactic factor (18) (see below) might be more likely to develop late-phase responses, but this is yet to be shown conclusively.

MEDIATORS OF HYPERSENSITIVITY

At the present time, much of the information on mast cell/mediator cell activation in asthma, urticaria, and related disorders is derived from measurements of a high molecular weight neutrophil chemotactic factor (or activity) of anaphylaxis, variously termed NCF, NCF-A, NCA, or HMW-NCF. Atkins *et al.* described a high molecular weight, heat-stable neutrophil chemotactic factor (NCF), which was released into the circulation of patients with bronchial asthma during the early-phase response that followed inhalation of specific antigen (19). The same investigators demonstrated that prior administration of disodium cromoglycate (DSCG, cromolyn) inhibited the release of NCA indicating that the agent(s) might be derived from the mast cell (20,21). The observation that the changes in NCA concentrations accompany histamine release supported this view (19,22), as do *in vitro* experiments using immunologically sensitized lung fragments. Human lung fragments challenged with anti-IgE released an NCA that had identical physicochemical properties to the NCA obtained from the serum of asthmatic subjects and had a time course of release that paralleled the elaboration of histamine (23).

We have established that NCA is also released in late asthmatic reactions following antigen inhalation in sensitized individuals (18). Nine patients with bronchial asthma, who had early and late falls in FEV_1 (10 min and 6 hr, respectively) after inhalational challenge with specific antigens, were studied. NCA was detected during both the early and the late asthmatic response and the time course of appearance in the circulation paralleled that of the fall in FEV_1. In contrast, five patients with asthma who had early reactions only had a single early peak of NCA with no further rise up to 24 hr. Similarly, an NCA was also identified in the 2 adults and 13 children with exercise-induced late-phase reactions. As with allergen-induced reactions, there were both early and late rises in NCA, and these paralleled the changes in FEV_1.

Some physicochemical characteristics of the NCA released in early reactions and the NCA of late-phase exercise-induced asthma are shown in Fig. 1. They appeared to be identical, since (a) following gel filtration on Sephacryl S-400, both were associated with molecules of approximately 600,000 daltons, (b) both eluted as single peaks of activity follow-

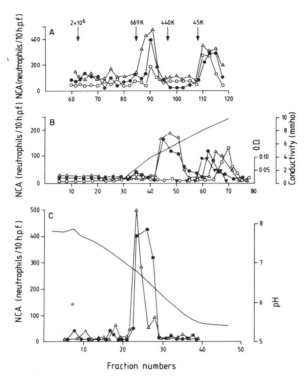

Fig. 1. Chromatographic properties of the neutrophil chemotactic activity (NCA) associated with early and late-phase exercise-induced asthma. The symbols represent the prechallenge (○), postchallenge (early phase) (●), and postchallenge (late phase) (△) serum samples. Characterization was performed by Sephacryl S-400 gel filtration (A), anion-exchange chromatography on DEAE-Sephacel (B), and chromatofocusing on polybuffer exchanger 94 (PBE 94) (C). The data shown are from sera of one patient, which have been subjected consecutively to the various chromatographic procedures. Sera from two further patients were also examined and gave virtually identical results. The elution profile of the molecular markers [Blue Dextran (2000 K), Thyroglobulin (669 K), Ferritin (440 K), and Albumin (45 K)] is indicated. Measurements of OD (optical density, ▲) in fraction numbers 0 to 50 were zero. Solid lines in (B) and (C) are conductivity and pH, respectively. With permission from the New England Journal of Medicine.

ing anion-exchange chromatography on DEAE-Sephacel (0.15 *M* NaCl, pH 8.1), and (c) both had an isoelectric point of 6.5, as determined by chromatofocusing on polybuffer exchanger 94 (17). We have now established that NCA obtained from asthmatic sera during early and late *allergen*- and *exercise*-induced asthma had virtually identical chromatographic characteristics (24). Furthermore, these properties were shared by the NCA released from human lung fragments challenged with anti-IgE (23).

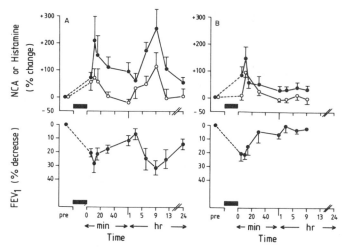

Fig. 2. Changes in serum NCA (●) and plasma histamine (○) in early- and late-phase dual (A) and single early (B) asthmatic reactions. The points represent the mean ± 1 SEM of ten patients who gave dual reactions following challenge with an extract of *D. pteronyssinus* (seven) or grass pollen (three), and seven patients with a single early reaction (*D. pteronyssinus*, two; grass pollen, five). With the Wilcoxon rank test, it was shown that with dual responders there was a significant increase in NCA (when compared to prechallenge values) at each of the time points indicated up to 9 hr (all giving $p < .01$). With single early reactions, there was a significant rise in NCA at 10 min only ($p < .05$). With histamine, the significant changes were dual responders, 10 min ($p < .05$) and 9 hr ($p < .01$); single early, 10 min ($p < .05$). With the Mann Whitney U test, NCA at 6–9 hr ($p < .01$) was significantly higher in dual responders compared to the corresponding values in patients with single early reactions. For histamine, this was $p < .05$ at 6–9 hr. The mean (± SEM) prechallenge values were NCA, 94.4 (±17.4) cells/10 hpf (dual) and 57.7 (±16.3) (single); histamine, 0.14 (±0.02) ng/ml (dual) and 0.17 (±0.04) (single).

Measurements of plasma histamine have also been undertaken in early- and late-phase allergen-induced asthma. Until recently, assays of histamine in the blood lacked the necessary specificity, reproducibility, and reliability (25). Many of these problems have been overcome with a modification of the double-isotope radioenzymatic method (26). Using this procedure, we have been able to identify a rise in plasma histamine during late-phase as well as early reactions, and these paralleled the rise in serum NCA and fall in FEV_1 (24) (Fig. 2). Patients who experienced isolated early reactions had a single rise only in NCA and histamine with no further elevation up to 9 hr. These studies suggest that mast cells are involved in late-phase asthmatic reactions, since at the present time there are no other recognized sources of lung histamine. On the other hand, the role of basophils in asthma has still to be clarified since this cell type may form part of the inflammatory infiltrate in and around the bronchi.

It is also possible that arachidonic acid metabolites (leukotrienes, prostaglandins, and thromboxanes) play a role in late reactions, since these lipid mediators tend to have a number of sustained biological effects *in vitro*. For example, prolonged contraction of bronchial smooth muscle is characteristic of LTC_4 and LTD_4, whereas LTB_4 (27) causes delayed induration when injected into the skin and so may contribute to oedema of the bronchial submucosa. Furthermore, late reactions are inhibited by prior administration of corticosteroids (28). As discussed elsewhere in this volume (Chapters 11 and 23), corticosteroids generate proteins (lipomodulin/macrocortin) that inhibit the action of phospholipase A_2 and so prevent the release of free arachidonic acid. It has also been reported that allergen-induced late-phase asthmatic reactions were blocked by the combination of indomethacin (a cyclooxygenase inhibitor) and benoxaprofen (a putative lipoxygenase pathway inhibitor) (29).

INFLAMMATORY CELLS AND THE ASTHMATIC RESPONSE

As mentioned above, the histological picture of late-phase reactions, at least in the skin, is characterized by an infiltrate of inflammatory cells, especially neutrophils, mononuclear phagocytes, and occasional eosinophils and basophils (10). This suggests that mediators released from mast cells/mediator cells might recruit these secondary inflammatory cells in addition to having a direct effect on smooth muscle and the vasculature. Accordingly we looked for evidence of neutrophil and monocyte "activation" in the peripheral blood following the release of mast cell mediators associated with exercise-induced asthma. It is known that chemotactic factors "activate" leucocytes *in vitro* as is shown, for example, by increased expression of surface membrane markers (30) and release of lysosomal enzymes. For this reason, we chose the "rosette" technique for measuring changes in the expression of complement (C) receptors on neutrophils and monocytes following EIA and compared these with the changes in circulating NCA. A time-dependent increase in the expression of neutrophil and monocyte complement (C3b) receptors was observed in asthmatic subjects who wheezed following a treadmill exercise task (Fig. 3) (31). NCA peaked at 15 min, whereas the increase in the percentage of C3b and neutrophil and monocyte rosettes continued for up to 60 min, at which time the study was discontinued. In contrast, documented asthmatic subjects who did not develop EIA following the same exercise task had no significant increase in rosette formation, elevation of NCA, or fall in peak flow. Furthermore, the enhancement of C3b rosettes following

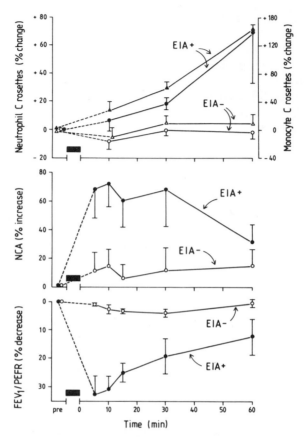

Fig. 3. Changes in neutrophil and monocyte complement rosettes following exercise-induced asthma (EIA). The points represent the mean (±SEM) of five patients (with EIA+) and five documented asthmatics who did not wheeze following an identical treadmill exercise task (EIA−) (31a). Complement (C) rosettes were measured using sheep erythrocytes (E) sensitized with rabbit IgM anti-E (EA$_M$) and a human R3 reagent stabilized with suramin (EA$_M$C) (32). NCA was assayed as described (31a). Neutrophil C rosettes were significantly higher in EIA+ patients, compared to EIA−, at 10, 30, and 60 min ($p < .05$, $p < .05$, and $p < .001$, respectively). Monocyte C rosettes were significantly higher in EIA+ patients compared with EIA− at 30 and 60 min ($p < .001$ and $p < .005$, respectively). NCA was significantly higher in EIA+ patients compared with EIA− at 5 and 10 min ($p < .05$ and $p < .02$, respectively). The solid bars represent the period of exercise and the data were analysed using the Student's t test. The percentage of neutrophil C rosettes prior to exercise (baseline values) was 24.7% (range, 18.5–30%) for EIA+ and 23% (range, 19–27%) for EIA−. For monocyte C rosettes, these were 29.6% (range, 20.8–38.5%) for EIA+ and 27% (range, 20–38.5%) for EIA−. NCA values (neutrophils/10 hpf) were 164.4 (range, 24–393) for EIA+ and 104.4 (range, 46–155) for EIA−.

EIA was inhibited by prior administration of DSCG. Thus, these studies suggest that leucocytes are "activated" during EIA, and that they may migrate to the site of degranulated mast cells to initiate the inflammatory events associated with airway narrowing. Although we have no direct evidence that neutrophils and monocytes infiltrate in and around the bronchi during the late-phase responses, it is of interest that in animal models of late asthmatic reactions, neutrophils disappear from the circulation following allergen challenge and accumulate in pulmonary tissues during this late response (Chapter 15, this volume).

The role of eosinophils in bronchial asthma continues to be the subject of some speculation and debate. Some doubt has been cast on the view that the principal role of eosinophils is to inactivate mediators of hypersensitivity, (33) since there is firm circumstantial evidence that eosinophil-derived products contribute markedly to the tissue damage characteristic of bronchial asthma (34). It is of particular interest that bronchoalveolar lavage (BAL) fluid from patients who experienced late asthmatic reactions contained larger numbers of eosinophils than that from those individuals who had a single early response (J. de Monchy, personal communication). Furthermore, patients with late reactions have a small but significantly greater rise in blood eosinophils during late reactions when compared with blood eosinophils from patients having single early response (35). Finally, in a study of BAL and bronchial mucus in asthma, it was shown that DSCG inhibited the local accumulation of eosinophils as well as the concentration of house dust mite-specific IgE (36).

CONCLUSIONS

In Fig. 4, an attempt has been made to summarize some of the observations relating to mediators of hypersensitivity and inflammatory cells in early- and late-phase asthmatic reactions. As already stated, it is reasonable to assume that mast cells, or other mediator cells, initiate the sequence of events that leads to carly- (rapid spasmogenic) and late-phase (late sustained) asthmatic reactions. It is well known that many agents can trigger mast cells *in vitro*. Similarly, in asthma it is recognized that in addition to IgE and allergen, nonspecific manoeuvres such as the respiratory heat exchange associated with treadmill exercise induce mediator release (37). The rapid spasmogenic phase is probably dependent on the abrupt release of mediators that act either directly on bronchial smooth muscle or indirectly through reflexes. Of the many mast cell mediators so

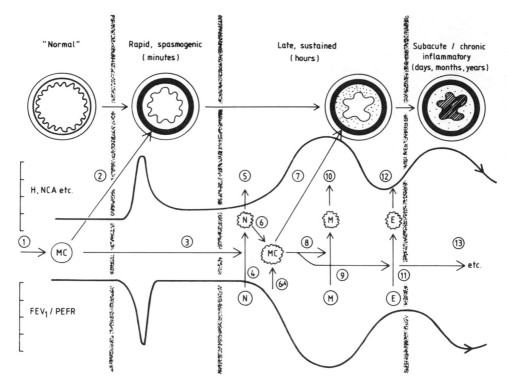

Fig. 4. A diagrammatic representation of events that follow mast cell/mediator cell activation (MC) in bronchial asthma. ① Activation of MC, i.e., the respiratory heat exchange of exercise or IgE/allergen interaction. ② MC-derived mediators causing the rapid spasmogenic phase. ③ Mediators that recruit and activate leucocytes. ④ Infiltration and activation of neutrophils. ⑤ The release of neutrophil products. ⑥ Neutrophil products inducing the second rise of mediators from "activated" MC. ⑥A Other unexplained MC stimuli in the late-phase response. ⑦ The release of mediators of the late-phase reaction. ⑧ Further release of mediators that activate and recruit cells. ⑨ Infiltrate and activation of mononuclear cells. ⑩ The release of mononuclear cell products. ⑪ Activation of eosinophils. ⑫ Release of eosinophil-associated agents. ⑬ Further amplification of the inflammatory response.

far recognized, there are several that have potential to recruit and activate inflammatory cells. These include leukotriene B_4 (38), the peptides of the eosinophil chemotactic factor of anaphylaxis (39), and NCA (40). These chemical agents, acting either alone or in combination, might account for the "activation" of peripheral blood leucocytes.

The second rise in plasma mediators, which corresponds to the late-phase fall in FEV_1/PEFR, is not clearly explainable at the present time. Perhaps lung mast cells themselves are "activated" as a result of the initial trigger, and that this renders them susceptible to a second release of mediators, which is in turn regulated by a distinct biochemical mechanism and initiated by the infiltrating inflammatory cells. In support of this suggestion are the findings that factors derived from the granules of stimulated neutrophils released histamine from tissue mast cells *in vitro* (41–44). Furthermore, other factors may be involved in mediator release observed during late-phase reactions. Persistence of antigen is possible but unlikely, as is a second spontaneous release from mast cells, since after approximately 15 min lung fragments challenged with anti-IgE had no further release of histamine and NCA for up to 12 hr (23). Nevertheless, whatever the mechanism, it appears that in late-phase reactions either the same mast cell responds a second time or a different population of mast cells participates in a delayed form of mediator release.

In any event, the persistent release of these chemical agents from mediator cells during late and subsequent rections will serve to amplify the inflammatory response and lead to further infiltration of inflammatory cells, including eosinophils, which in turn (in the context of day-to-day asthma) lead to subacute/chronic inflammatory bronchial reaction that is the hallmark of the disease of bronchial asthma. These events can be modulated, at least at the early stages, by compounds such as DSCG that stabilize mast cells, but at the later stages corticosteroids remain the mainstay of therapy. The precise mode of action of corticosteroids in late reactions and ongoing asthma is incompletely understood but may involve "lipomodulation" of arachidonic acid release, eosinophilopoiesis, inhibition of eosinophil and neutrophil chemotaxis, and the prevention of the release of lysosomal enzymes from "activated" cells.

REFERENCES

1. Pepys, J., Hargreave, F. E., Chan, M., and McCarthy, D. S. Inhibitory effects of disodium cromoglycate on allergen-inhalation tests. *Lancet* **2**:134–137, 1968.
1a. Kay, A. B. Basic mechanisms in allergic asthma. *Eur. J. Respir. Dis.* **63**(Suppl. 122):9–16, 1982.
1b. Kay, A. B. The immunological basis of asthma. *In* "Steroids in Asthma" (T. J. H. Clark, ed.), Chapter IV, pp. 46–60. ADIS Press Limited, Auckland, New Zealand, 1983.
2. Pepys, J., and Hutchcroft, B. J. Bronchial provocation tests in etiologic diagnosis and analysis of asthma. *Am. Rev. Respir. Dis.* **112**:829–859, 1975.
3. Olive, J. T., and Hyatt, R. E. Maximal expiratory flow and total respiratory resistance during induced bronchoconstriction in asthmatic subjects. *Am. Rev. Respir. Dis.* **106**:366–376, 1972.
4. Mansell, A., Dubrawsky, C., Levison, H., Bryan, A. C., Langer, H., Collins-Williams, C., and Orange, R. P. Lung mechanics in antigen-induced asthma. *J. Appl. Physiol.* **37**:297–301, 1974.

5. Warner, J. O. Significance of late reactions after bronchial challenge with house dust mite. *Arch. Dis. Child.* **51**:905–911, 1976.

6. Cockcroft, D. W., Ruffin, R. E., Dolovich, J., and Hargreave, F. E. Allergen-induced increase in nonallergic (nonspecific) bronchial reactivity: Its relation to the late asthmatic response. *J. Allergy Clin. Immunol.* **61**:175 (abstr.), 1978.

7. Macintyre, D., and Boyd, G. Site of airflow obstruction in immediate and late reactions to bronchial challenge with *Dermatophagoides pteronyssinus. Clin. Allergy* **13**:213–218, 1983.

8. Pepys, J. Clinical and therapeutic significance of patterns of allergic reactions of the lungs to extrinsic agents. *Am. Rev. Respir. Dis.* **116**:573–588, 1977.

9. Dolovich, J., Hargreave, F. E., Chalmers, R., Shier, K. J., Gauldie, J., and Bienenstock, J. Late cutaneous allergic responses in isolated IgE-dependent reactions. *J. Allergy Clin. Immunol.* **52**:38–46, 1973.

10. Solley, G. O., Gleich, G. J., Jordan, R. E., and Schroeter, A. L. The late phase of the immediate wheal and flare skin reaction: Its dependence upon IgE antibodies. *J. Clin. Invest.* **58**:408–420, 1976.

11. Taylor, G., and Shivalkar, P. R. 'Arthus-type' reactivity in the nasal airways and skin in pollen sensitivity subjects. *Clin. Allergy* **1**:407–414, 1971.

12. Price, J. F., Hey, E. N., and Soothill, J. F. Antigen provocation to the skin, nose and lung, in children, with asthma; immediate and dual hypersensitivity reactions. *Clin. Exp. Immunol.* **47**:587–594, 1982.

13. Wasserman, S. I., Soter, N. A., Center, D. M., and Austen, K. F. Cold urticaria. Recognition and characterisation of a neutrophil chemotactic factor, which appears in serum during experimental cold challenge. *J. Clin. Invest.* **60**:180–196, 1977.

14. Soter, N. A., Wasserman, S. I., Austen, K. F., and McFadden, E. R. Release of mast cell mediators and alterations in lung function in patients with cholinergic urticaria. *N. Engl. J. Med.* **302**:604–608, 1980.

15. Soter, N. A., Wasserman, S. I., Pathak, M. A., Parrish, J. A., and Austen, K. F. Solar urticaria: Release of mast cell mediators into the circulation after experimental challenge. *J. Invest. Dermatol.* **72**:282 (abstr.), 1979.

16. Atkins, P. C., and Zweiman, B. Mediator release in local heat urticaria. *J. Allergy Clin. Immunol.* **68**:286–289, 1981.

17. Lee, T. H., Nagakura, T., Papageorgiou, N., Iikura, Y., and Kay, A. B. Exercise-induced late asthmatic reactions with neutrophil chemotactic activity. *N. Engl. J. Med.* **308**:1502–1505, 1983.

18. Nagy, L., Lee, T. H., and Kay, A. B. Neutrophil chemotactic activity in antigen-induced late asthmatic reactions. *N. Engl. J. Med.* **306**:497–501, 1982.

19. Atkins, P. C., Norman, M., Weiner, M., and Zweiman, B. Release of neutrophil chemotactic activity during immediate hypersensitivity reactions in humans. *Ann. Intern. Med.* **86**:415–418, 1977.

20. Atkins, P. C., Norman, M., and Zweiman, B. Antigen-induced chemotactic activity in man: Correlation with bronchospasm and inhibition by disodium cromoglycate. *J. Allergy Clin. Immunol.* **62**:149–155, 1978.

21. Atkins, P. C., Norman, M., Zweiman, B., and Rosenblum, F. Further characterization and biologic activity of ragweed antigen-induced neutrophil chemotactic activity in man. *J. Allergy Clin. Immunol.* **64**:251–258, 1979.

22. Lee, T. H., Brown, M. J., Nagy, L., Causon, R., Walport, M. J., and Kay, A. B. Exercise-induced release of histamine and neutrophil chemotactic factor in atopic asthmatics. *J. Allergy Clin. Immunol.* **70**:73–81, 1982.

23. O'Driscoll, B. R., Lee, T. H., Cromwell, O., and Kay, A. B. Immunologic release of

neutrophil chemotactic activity from human lung tissue. *J. Allergy Clin. Immunol.* **72**:695–701, 1983.

24. Durham, S. R., Lee, T. H., Cromwell, O., Shaw, R. J., Merrett, T. G., Merrett, J., Brown, M. J., Causon, R., Cooper, P., and Kay, A. B. Immunologic studies of allergen-induced late phase asthmatic reactions. *J. Allergy Clin. Immunol.* **74**, 1984 (in press).

25. Gleich, G. J., and Hull, W. M. Measurement of histamine: A quality control study. *J. Allergy Clin. Immunol.* **66**:295–298, 1980.

26. Brown, M. J., Ind, P. W., Causon, R., and Lee, T. H. A novel double-isotope technique for the enzymatic assay of plasma histamine. Application to estimation of mast cell activation assessed by antigen challenge in asthmatics. *J. Allergy Clin. Immunol.* **69**:20–24, 1982.

27. Camp, R. D. R., Coutts, A. A., Greaves, M. W., Kay, A. B., and Walport, M. J. Responses of human skin to intradermal injection of leukotrienes C_4, D_4 and B_4. *Br. J. Pharmacol.* **75**:168P, 1982.

28. Booij-Nord, H., Orie, N. G. M., and de Vries, K. Immediate and late bronchial obstructive reactions to inhalation of house dust and protective effects of disodium cromoglycate and prednisolone. *J. Allergy Clin. Immunol.* **48**:344–354, 1971.

29. Morley, J., Fairfax, A. J., and Hanson, J. M. The role of phospholipid metabolites in airway hyperreactivity. *In* "Bronchial Hyperreactivity" (J. Morley, ed.), pp. 219–234. Academic Press, London, 1982.

30. Kay, A. B., Glass, E. J., and Salter, D. McG. Leucoattractants enhance complement receptors on human phagocytic cells. *Clin. Exp. Immunol.* **38**:294–299, 1979.

31. Papageorgiou, N., Carroll, M., Durham, S. R., Lee, T. H., Walsh, G. M., and Kay, A. B. Complement receptor enhancement of neutrophil activation after exercise-induced asthma. *Lancet* **2**:1220–1223, 1983.

31a. Lee, T. H., Nagy, L., Nagakura, T., Walport, M. J., and Kay, A. B. Identification and partial characterization of an exercise-induced neutrophil chemotactic factor in bronchial asthma. *J. Clin. Invest.* **69**:889–899, 1982.

32. Carroll, M., Lukacs, K., Hodson, M., and Kay, A. B. Defective chemotactic factor-induced monocyte complement receptor enhancement in lung cancer. *Clin. Exp. Immunol.* **54**:785–792, 1983.

33. Goetzl, E. J., Wasserman, S. I., and Austen, K. F. Eosinophil polymorphonuclear leukocyte function in immediate hypersensitivity. *Arch. Pathol.* **99**:1–4, 1975.

34. Filley, W. V., Holley, K. E., Kephart, G. M., and Gleich, G. J. Identification by immunofluorescence of eosinophil granule major basic protein in lung tissues of patients with bronchial asthma. *Lancet* **2**:11–16, 1982.

35. Booij-Nord, H., de Vries, K., Sluiter, H. J., and Orie, N. G. M. Late bronchial obstructive reaction to experimental inhalation of house dust extract. *Clin. Allergy* **2**:43–61, 1972.

36. Diaz, P., Galleguillos, F. R., Gonzalez, M. C., Pantin, C., and Kay, A. B. Bronchoalveolar lavage in asthma: the effect of disodium cromoglycate on leucocyte counts, immunoglobulins and complement. *J. Allergy Clin. Immunol.* **74**, 1984 (in press).

37. Lee, T. H., Assoufi, B. K., and Kay, A. B. The link between exercise, respiratory heat exchange, and the mast cell in bronchial asthma. *Lancet* **1**:520–522, 1983.

38. Nagy, L., Lee, T. H., Goetzl, E. J., Pickett, W. C., and Kay, A. B. Complement receptor enhancement and chemotaxis of human neutrophils and eosinophils by leukotrienes and other lipoxygenase products. *Clin. Exp. Immunol.* **47**:541–547, 1982.

39. Anwar, A. R. E., and Kay, A. B. The ECF-A tetrapeptides and histamine selectively enhance human eosinophil complement receptors. *Nature (London)* **269**:522–524, 1977.

40. Lee, T. H., Nagy, L., Nagakura, T., Walport, M. J., and Kay, A. B. Physicochemical

and biological properties of an exercise-induced, asthma-associated neutrophil chemotactic factor. *Fed. Proc., Fed. Am. Soc. Exp. Biol.* **41**:734 (abstr.), 1982.
41. Janoff, A., Shaefer, S. , Scherer, J., and Bean, M. A. Mediators of inflammation in leukocyte lysosomes. II. Mechanism of action of lysosomal cationic protein upon vascular permeability in the rat. *J. Exp. Med.* **722**:841–851, 1965.
42. Kelly, M. T., Martin, R. R., and White, A. Mediators of histamine release from human platelets, lymphocytes, and granulocytes. *J. Clin. Invest.* **50**:1040–1049, 1971.
43. Ranadive, N. S., and Cochrane, C. G. Isolation and characterization of permeability factors from rabbit neutrophils. *J. Exp. Med.* **128**:605–622, 1968.
44. Scherer, J., and Janoff, A. Mediators of inflammation in leukocyte lysosomes. VII. Observations on mast cell disrupting agents in different species. *Lab. Invest.* **18**:196–202, 1968.

DISCUSSION

Kaplan: Have you ever tried partially purified NCA or even sera of positive patients and tested exogenous neutrophils *in vitro* as you did with f-Met-Leu-Phe? Do you have antibody to NCA? It would certainly be of interest to do *in vitro* experiments and be able to antagonize NCA in some way. At present the neutrophil changes in receptor content you see *in vivo* which you infer could be due to NCA are based on *in vitro* experiments using other stimulators.

Kay: We have shown that partially purified NCA enhances the expression of C3b receptors on human neutrophils [T. H. Lee, L. Nagy, T. Nagakura, M. J. Walport, and A. B. Kay, *Fed. Proc., Fed. Am. Soc. Exp. Biol.* **41**:734 (abstr.), 1982]. When NCA is better characterized we can answer your other questions more precisely.

McFadden: Could you tell me what types of stimuli cause an increase in rosette formation?

Kay: We have found that agents that are chemotactic or chemokinetic enhance complement receptors on neutrophils, eosinophils, and monocytes [A. B. Kay, E. J. Glass, and D. McG. Salter, *Clin. Exp. Immunol.* **38**:294, 1979; A. B. Kay, A. J. Duncan, E. J. Glass, and J. Stewart, *in* "Biochemistry of Acute Allergic Reactions" (K. F. Austen and E. L. Becker, eds.), p. 197. Alan R. Liss, Inc., New York, 1981]. There seems to be a direct parallel between the ability of an agent to evoke chemotaxis/chemokinesis and enhancement of complement receptors. The list of substances that do this is quite formidable and includes the formyl methionyl peptides, LTB_4, PGD_2, the ECF-A tetrapeptides, histamine, casein, and supernatants from sensitized T cells challenged with antigen.

Platts-Mills: Could you give us more details on the children who showed late reactions after exercise? What were their baseline FEV_1 values and were they on treatment?

Kay: As far as we can ascertain, there was nothing particularly unusual about the children who developed exercise-induced late-phase asthmatic reactions. All medication was withdrawn for 24 hr prior to the study, and their FEV_1s were between 60 and 85% of predicted. Our impression is that exercise-induced late-phase reactions are probably quite common in children, but we do not know the exact prevalence.

Gleich: Can you tell us whether NCF is present in the basophil? Have you studied isolated basophils and mast cells to determine whether they will release NCF after allergen challenge?

Kay: We have undertaken a limited number of experiments with enriched basophil suspensions and dispersed pulmonary mast cells of ~20% purity. These experiments have been undertaken in association with Dr. Stephen Holgate and his colleagues. So far we have been unable to show that NCA is derived from these cell types, whereas we have identified this activity from human lung fragments challenged with anti-IgE (B. R. O'Driscoll, T. H. Lee, O. Cromwell, and A. B. Kay, *J. Allergy Clin. Immunol.* **72**:695, 1983). Another line of evidence against the basophil is the finding that there was no correlation between the peripheral blood basophil count and circulating levels of NCA following exercise-induced asthma (T. Nagakura, T. H. Lee, B. K. Assoufi, A. J. Newman Taylor, D. M. Denison, and A. B. Kay, *Am. Rev. Respir. Dis.* **128**:294, 1983).

Warner: I, like many others, have in the past looked for a late-phase reaction after exercise challenge and have failed to find it. Recently, in collaboration with an Italian colleague (Dr. Attilio Boner) I analysed the response to exercise of a group of asthmatic children resident in a special school in the mountains. These children had severe asthma in their home environment, but most at the school were weaned from their prophylactic therapy. Thirty-six percent had an unequivocal late reaction after exercise. During a control day without exercise there was no such change in lung function (spirometry). However, it must be added that the challenge was more potent than that usually employed in exercise tests; because the study was done at high altitude (1756 m), the humidity was low (30–35%). I suspect that this greater stimulus is more likely to produce a late response. Was there any difference in the severity of the immediate reaction in those of your patients who had a dual response compared with those who had an immediate reaction only?

Kay: The early-phase reaction, as judged by the fall in FEV_1, was not substantially different in the children who experienced a single early reaction as compared to those who had a dual, that is, an early- and late-phase, reaction.

Piper: Can you explain the actions of steroids (glucocorticoids) in the late phase of asthma? Do steroids inhibit the generation of NCA?

Kay: Corticosteroids, given immediately prior to challenge, will inhibit antigen-induced late-phase reactions. They seem to have little or no effect on the immediate response. On the other hand, the immediate response is blunted by corticosteroids when these are administered for several days prior to antigen challenge [P. S. Burge, *Eur. J. Respir. Dis.* **63** (Suppl. 122):163, 1982]. We have not undertaken comparable studies with exercise-induced late-phase reactions.

Austen: Does the late reaction also lead to an increase in cellular C3b receptors, that is, is the receptor increase also biphasic just like the mediators?

Kay: Preliminary data suggest that increased C3b receptor expression, like mediator release, is biphasic.

Lichtenstein: In the nasal system we also find an early rise in histamine, a fall to zero and an increase at 6–8 hr. We find PGD (a mast cell mediator) early but not late. We might speculate that basophils are involved in the late reaction.

The NCA in late reactions stays up significantly above controls for 10 hr. Is the mast cell secreting all that time?

Kaplan: How long does it take NCA to return to normal in asthmatics with an immediate reaction but no late phase?

Kay: As you point out NCA values do not return completely to baseline values and the explanation for this is not entirely clear. Of course, there could be some background release after the "initial burst." On the other hand I think it is difficult to arrive at firm conclusions about fluctuations in NCA levels following these challenge procedures because of the inherent problems of measurements by bioassay.

Lichtenstein: As we discussed before, the basophilia which occurs on exercise could account for the small increase in histamine. If 1% of the blood histamine is released on handling the blood, it would be more than enough.

Kay: The question regarding basophils and NCA in the context of exercise-induced asthma will be discussed by Dr. Lee (Chapter 17).

Lessof: Could you give us a little more detail and comment on the fall in mite-specific IgE that you found in your bronchoalveolar lavage/DSCG study?

Kay: The decrease in the concentrations of eosinophils and house dust mite-specific IgE in bronchoalveolar lavage fluid of asthmatics taking DSCG was an unexpected finding. We assumed that DSCG is somehow influencing the local concentration of eosinophils and IgE, although the precise mechanism is unclear. This could be an effect on local capillary permeability, although it is conceivable that DSCG effects local antibody formation.

Holgate: Could you summarize the data that might suggest that NCF is a preformed mediator of the mast cell granule?

Kay: The source of NCA is unknown and we also do not know if it is preformed or newly generated. It is reasonable to assume that it is mast cell-associated, since NCA was generated from human lung fragments stimulated with anti-IgE and in asthmatic subjects this mediator was released in exercise- and antigen-induced bronchospasm with a time course similar to that of histamine. In addition, the release of NCA and histamine in these situations was blocked by prior administration of DSCG by inhalation. This sort of evidence is still circumstantial and it may well turn out that NCA is released from some other cell type, but at the present time we have not got the methodology tools to answer this question precisely.

McFadden: Are you using the word "wheezing" as synonymous with airway obstruction measured by FEV_1?

Kay: The asthmatics who did not get (EIA−) had a small rise in NCA and a very small fall in PEFR but they did not wheeze.

McFadden: In the children with late reactions to exercise (mentioned by Dr. Warner), could we know the altitude and duration of their stay there?

Warner: The study on late-phase EIA was conducted in the Dolomites (altitude 1756 m) after the children had been resident there for 6 months.

Gleich: I would like to follow up on the question Dr. Lichtenstein posed a moment ago, namely the role of the basophil in the late-phase reaction. In the skin one sees a clear-cut basophil infiltration in the late-phase reaction, which can be recognized by performing a skin window. Therefore, it seems, if there is a parallel between the human skin and the lung, one should look carefully for basophils in the pulmonary late-phase reaction.

Kay: As you say, basophils are occasionally observed in late-phase cutaneous reactions and this cell could well be implicated in late-phase reactions in the lung. On the other hand, as already stated, we feel that the basophil is unlikely to be a major source of NCA. If basophils are the explanation for the second wave of mediators then how are they triggered? Does antigen persist for up to 9 hr, and what is the mechanism in exercise-induced late-phase reactions? The hypothesis I favour is that infiltrating neutrophils "activated" by NCA or other agents, release factors that trigger already primed mast cells for a second release of mediators.

Askenase: I like your hypothesis and would like to suggest experiments to test it such as (i) give DSCG just prior to the LPR; (ii) give steroids just prior to the LPR; (iii) infuse NCA to neutralize chemotactic gradient for leucocytes and then maybe block the LPR.

Kay: I believe that a limited number of studies have been undertaken in which DSCG was given immediately after the early phase and that this dampened the late phase. As far as I remember, these studies were not conclusive and many of these individuals had precipitating antibodies against the allergen in question, and in that sense it was not a totally IgE-dependent system. I agree that it would be interesting to repeat these DSCG studies given at various time intervals after antigen challenge, especially perhaps in those with exercise-induced late-phase reactions.

Regarding your second point, I agree that it would be interesting to reinfuse NCA, but on the other hand I do not necessarily imply a cause-and-effect relationship since NCA may only be a marker of mediator cell activation and have no direct bearing on the aetiology of the activation process.

Hogg: It is well known that white cell numbers increase with exercise. Is there a difference between those who develop an asthmatic response following exercise and those who do not (with respect to the level that the white cell count reaches in peripheral blood)? Is there any evidence that polymorphonuclear cells stick in the lung in patients with exercise-induced asthma?

Kay: The total white cell and neutrophil counts in individuals with late-phase reactions were higher than those with isolated early-phase reactions. In addition, the asthmatics with late reactions had a small but significant rise in peripheral blood eosinophil counts (S. R. Durham, unpublished observations).

Hargreave: Is there a difference in the quantities of histamine or NCA released or in the relative quantities of one mediator to the other in people with isolated early or dual asthmatic responses after allergen exposure or exercise?

Kay: The percentage increase in NCA and histamine during the early reaction did not appear to be appreciably higher in patients with dual responses compared with those who had a single early wheeze.

Wasserman: The association of early- and late-phase reactions is made somewhat more tenuous by the fact that there are occasional patients who manifest late-phase reactions in the absence of discernible early-phase responses.

Kay: Individuals who experience isolated late reactions may have subclinical early responses with local mediator release.

Kaplan: Have you ever observed a second peak of NCA activity when fractionating the gel filtered material by ion exchange chromatography. If so, have you ever recycled the other peak on gel filtration. Since NCA is >600,000 MW, I have wondered whether it might represent a smaller molecule that is bound to a carrier protein and perhaps dissociable by conditions of high ionic strength.

Kay: We sometimes observe minor peaks of chemotactic activity following DEAE-Sephacel anion exchange chromatography of material prepared on Sephacryl S-400. We have not gone back and sized these, and I think this would be an interesting thing to do, although compared to the main peak eluting at 0.15 M, there was far less activity in these other peaks.

To answer your other point, NCA may be a small molecule bound to a large carrier. On the other hand, attempts to dissociate it using high salt concentrations, for instance, have so far been unsuccessful.

CHAPTER 14

Mast Cell–Derived Inflammatory Factors and Late-Phase Allergic Reactions

MICHAEL KALINER

Allergic Diseases Section
Laboratory of Clinical Investigation
National Institute of Allergy and Infectious Diseases
National Institutes of Health
Bethesda, Maryland, U.S.A.

ROBERT LEMANSKE, JR.

Departments of Medicine and Pediatrics
University of Wisconsin Medical School
Madison, Wisconsin, U.S.A.

INTRODUCTION

Asthma is an inflammatory disease affecting airways of all sizes with characteristic pathologic features including mucosal edema, inflammatory cell (neutrophil and eosinophil) infiltrates, basement membrane thickening, mucosal denudation, and goblet cell and submucosal gland hyperplasia. These inflammatory changes contribute to the airflow obstruction along with bronchial muscle contraction and airway luminal congestion caused by excessive mucus, desquamated cells, and trapped secretions (1,2).

Antigen challenge of sensitive humans elicits clinical manifestations after cutaneous, nasal, gastrointestinal, and bronchial exposures that cause symptoms consistent with allergic rhinitis, urticaria, food allergy, or asthma, respectively. Thus, antigen-induced mast cell degranulation in these organs is thought to be an initial event in the pathogenesis of these diseases. While there is general acceptance that mast cell-derived mediators may contribute to allergic asthma, there has only been indirect (albeit

ASTHMA: Physiology,
Immunopharmacology,
and Treatment
THIRD INTERNATIONAL SYMPOSIUM

ISBN 0-12-402750-4

compelling) evidence for mast cell involvement in other variants of asthma (reviewed in refs. 3–5). Recent analyses of plasma mediators after antigen (6,7) and exercise (8) challenge of asthmatics has directly demonstrated mast cell activation and thereby support the possibility that respiratory mast cells may contribute to other forms of asthma as well (3).

For many years, allergic reactions have been considered acute and short lived, capable of causing ephemeral clinical problems with few chronic features. There have always been peculiar clinical features that failed to fit within this concept, however. Moreover, it became clear in the laboratory assessment of mast cell mediators that this cell could elicit intense, prolonged inflammatory reactions. Since the early 1970s, there has been a growing clinical and experimental appreciation of the capacity of allergic reactions to evolve into a subacute, inflammatory response, initially noted 4–8 hr after the initial mast cell degranulation, which has been termed the *late-phase reaction* (LPR). It is the purpose of this manuscript to review the experimental studies that provide part of the basis for our current comprehension of LPR.

RAT LATE-PHASE REACTIONS

In order to evaluate mechanisms by which mast cells can elicit a prolonged inflammatory reaction, an animal model employing rat cutaneous cellular infiltration was developed (9). Rodent skin is richly endowed with perivascular mast cells surrounding both the superficial and deeper blood vessels. Degranulation of cutaneous mast cells with either monospecific anti-rat IgE or compound 48/80 causes a dose-related cellular invasion appearing in two phases. The first phase, consisting of polymorphonuclear leukocytes, peaks 2–6 hr after skin testing. The second phase consists primarily of mononuclear cells and peaks at 24 hr. There is a close correlation between the intensity of the immediate reaction as reflected in blueing responses and these inflammatory reactions. Thus, mast cell degranulation in rat skin causes cellular infiltrates to accumulate over time, and the full development of the infiltration persists through at least 24 hr. Human allergic reactions involving skin, nasal, and respiratory tissues also manifest prolonged cellular infiltrates associated with clinical signs of inflammation (reviewed in refs. 10,11).

The rodent model of LPR was employed in order to uncover the underlying mechanisms as well as to pharmacologically manipulate the response. Studies of human LPR suggested that mast cell-derived mediators might be responsible for causing the reaction. However, it was only after observing that purified secretory granules obtained from mast cells were capable of reproducing the inflammation that the relationship was confirmed (9).

The ability of isolated mast cell granules (MCG) to elicit LPR prompted further investigation into the identification of the granular constituent(s) that is responsible, at least in part, for the generation of these reactions. Rat peritoneal MCG contain a number of biologically active compounds, which are bound in varying degrees to the proteoglycan matrix. Some mediators, such as histamine, are rapidly eluted from the MCG whereas others, such as chymotrypsin/trypsin, are more tightly bound under physiologic conditions to the granule matrix. The chemical bonds of the granule matrix involve very tight, noncovalent linkages between heparin and a number of enzymes. These bonds do not dissociate until they are exposed to 1–3 M NaCl in which they dissolve. In order to determine when the granule fractions containing LPR-inducing factors would dissociate, MCG were exposed to increasing concentrations of NaCl.

Mast cells were isolated and then exposed to graded sonication and differential centrifugation in order to isolate MCG that were encased within their limiting perigranular membranes. These "intact" granules were sequentially washed in 1.0 ml H_2O (three times) followed by 1 ml each of 0.01, 0.05, 0.1, 0.5, 1.0, and 3.0 M NaCl. The supernatants from these washings were analyzed for histamine, the granule matrix constituent, peroxidase, and protein. In addition, each eluant was dialyzed and injected in the dorsal skin of rats. The resultant skin test sites were analyzed histologically for cellular infiltration (9) (Table I).

The initial washes in water resulted in considerable loss of both dissociable mediators (as reflected in histamine release) and granule matrix material (as reflected in protein and peroxidase). Nonetheless, after three sequential water washes, the residual histamine and matrix materials appeared to stabilize and act in a more predictable fashion. Thus, exposure to dilute salt solution (0.05 M NaCl) eluted histamine from the matrix unaccompanied by the inflammatory-provoking factor(s), whereas dissolution of the granule in 1 to 3 M NaCl liberated peroxidase and factors capable of inducing cutaneous cellular infiltrates. The inflammatory-provoking factors were released from the granules during the initial washes and when the granule was dissolved, but not when histamine was dissociated (Table I). These data indicated that a constituent or constituents of the MCG matrix had inflammatory-provoking activity.

Accordingly, MCG were isolated, solubilized, and fractionated by ultramembrane filtration into high (>10,000) and low (500–10,000) molecular weight (HMW and LMW) components (12). When the HMW and LMW components and intact MCG were compared for their capacity to elicit rat

TABLE I
Elution of Factors from Membrane-Intact Rat Peritoneal MCG[a,b]

Eluant	Histamine (ng)	Peroxidase (ng)	Protein (μg)	PMN/HPF[c] (8 hr)	Monos/HPF[c] (24 hr)
H₂O-1	110,000	2,400	1,700	125.0 ± 12.6	106.0 ± 10.8
H₂O-2	52,000	80	950	110.0 ± 20.8	52.4 ± 6.8
H₂O-3	7,500	20	30	60.6 ± 8.2	90.4 ± 11.4
0.01 M NaCl	1,000	10	0	38.2 ± 8.2	40.3 ± 6.2
0.05 M NaCl	75,000	0	0	5.8 ± 1.6	20.4 ± 0.8
0.1 M NaCl	4,000	0	0	2.6 ± 0.8	18.6 ± 1.6
0.5 M NaCl	500	0	0	10.8 ± 1.9	55.6 ± 3.4
1.0 M NaCl	<100	0	300	60.7 ± 10.2	106.8 ± 22.4
3.0 M NaCl	<100	90	700	96.8 ± 10.4	158.0 ± 18.8
Phosphate-buffered saline	—	—	—	1.6 ± 1.0	20.6 ± 1.4

[a] Reprinted with permission from Tannenbaum et al. (9).

[b] MCG, isolated with intact perigranular membranes (I-granules), were sequentially washed in 1.0 ml H₂O (three washes) followed by 0.01, 0.05, 0.1, 0.5, 1.0, and 3.0 M NaCl. The supernatant from each wash was analyzed for histamine, peroxidase, and protein content, and then dialyzed against PBS for 48 hr. The dialyzed supernatant (100 μl) was then injected into the dorsal skin of rats. Histologic changes after 8 and 24 hr were analyzed.

[c] Polymorphonuclear or mononuclear cells per high-power field in rat skin at 8 or 24 hr after injection of the MCG fractions.

LPR, each was active, but the LMW component was the most potent on a weight basis (Table II). When solubilized MCG were filtered on Sephadex G-25, two peaks of inflammatory-provoking activity were noted; one filtered in the void fraction and the other with the 1,200-dalton marker (12). The fractions appeared to correspond to the HMW and LMW factors, and purification of the LMW factor was attempted initially. The LMW fraction was sequentially chromatographed by gel filtration (Sephadex G-25) (Fig. 1), ion-exchange (DE-52 cellulose followed by CM-52 cellulose), and thin layer chromatography followed by amino acid analysis (Table III) (12). The resultant *inflammatory factor of anaphylaxis* (IF-A) has a molecular weight of 1400, consists of 12 amino acids, is active *in vivo* in provoking inflammation in submicrogram quantities, and reproduces the precise sequence of cellular infiltrates *in vivo* in rat skin as is seen after mast cell degranulation.

The HMW fraction is currently under investigation, and preliminary data suggest that it chromatographs in the void fraction of a Sepharose 2B column, indicating its large molecular size. It should be noted that no prostaglandin or leukotriene activity was observed in the active fractions

TABLE II
The Capacity of MCG Fractions to Elicit Cellular Infiltrates in Rat Skin[a]

Preparation	Injected (μg)				
	0.5	2.5	5	15	20
MCG	30.4 ± 1.7[b]	83.3 ± 3.8	133.0 ± 17.1	>200	>200
	(1+)	(2+)	(3+)	(5+)	(5+)
HMW	83.6 ± 4.6	131.3 ± 11.3	181.4 ± 7.2	>200	>200
	(2+)	(3+)	(4+)	(5+)	(5+)
LMW	185.7 ± 4.5	>200	>200	>200	>200
	(4+)	(5+)	(5+)	5+)	(5+)

[a] 0.5–20 μg (protein) of the test substances were injected into rat skin. Biopsies were taken at 24 hr, and the cellular infiltrates were quantitated. The results represent the mean ± SEM of two experiments, each run on duplicate animals. Reprinted with permission from Oertel and Kaliner (12).

[b] The results are presented as both actual cells/HPF (mean of 10 HPF ± SEM) and in parentheses in a semiquantitative fashion. 1+ = <50 cells/HPF; 2+ = 50–100 cells/HPF; 3+ = 100–150 cells/HPF; 4+ = 150–200 cells/HPF; 5+ = >200 cells/HPF. Animals injected with buffer had 1+ infiltrates at 24 hr, which do not differ from uninjected control sites.

TABLE III
Amino Acid Analysis of IF-A[a]

Amino acid[b]	Residues per molecule[c]	Mean ± SEM of 3 analyses[d]
Aspartic acid	2	1.62 ± 0.08
Threonine	1	0.81 ± 0.09
Serine	1	1.05 ± 0.28
Glutamic acid	2	2.11 ± 0.06
Glycine	1	0.92 ± 0.37
Alanine	1	0.90 ± 0.15
Valine	1	0.84 ± 0.22
Isoleucine	1	1.16 ± 0.30
Leucine	1	0.76 ± 0.14
Phenylalanine	1	0.69 ± 0.08

[a] Reprinted with permission from Oertel and Kaliner (12).

[b] Estimated MW: 1407.

[c] Results represent the closest integer determined after combining three separate amino acid analyses of LMW components sequentially fractionated through Sephadex G-25, DE 52, and CM 52.

[d] Results present the actual mean ± SEM of the three analyses from which the closest integer was derived.

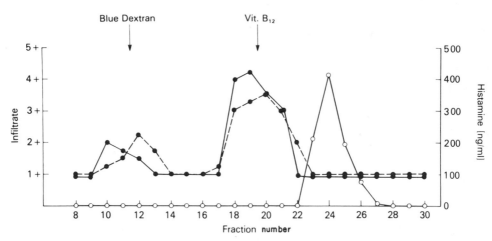

Fig. 1. Sephadex G-25 filtration of LMW. The LMW was obtained after YM10 and UM05 filtration of solubilized MCG and had been lyophilized and dissolved in 0.05 M NH$_4$HCO$_3$, pH 7.9, before filtration on a 1.8 × 30 cm column. Each column fraction was lyophilized, resuspended in saline, and injected into rat skin. The filtrates ensuing after 8 (●———●) or 24 (●---●) hr were graded 1 to 5+. Residual histamine contained in the LMW preparation (○———○) was also determined. Reprinted with permission from Oertel and Kaliner (12).

of the LMW IF-A. Therefore, MCG contain at least two preformed factors capable of eliciting LPR *in vivo* in rats.

MECHANISMS BY WHICH LPR ARE GENERATED

Immunofluorescent staining of biopsies taken from human LPR fails to consistently show complement deposition (13). However, because complement activation has the potential to induce LPR-like inflammatory reactions, it was important to critically examine the possible role of complement in LPR. To this end, rats were effectively decomplemented employing cobra venom factor (250 units/kg iv, single dose), which resulted in >99% depletion of both CH$_{50}$ and C$_3$ titers (14). Cobra venom factor-treated animals produced a normal cutaneous LPR in response to either anti-IgE or isolated MCG despite the extensive depletion of complement components, indicating no requirement for complement activation in the generation of rodent LPR.

The early phase of human LPR may include many eosinophils, but rodent LPR has been noted to be lacking in eosinophil. It seemed possible that the eosinophilia of human LPR might simply be a reflection of the increased numbers of tissue eosinophils seen in atopic humans. Therefore, rodents were made eosinophilic in response to the intravenous injection of Sephadex G-200 beads (15). Animals treated with Sephadex increased their peripheral eosinophil counts by five- to sixfold within 6 days. The LPR that was induced in eosinophilic rats contained significantly more eosinophils in the skin lesions than noted in reactions induced in normal animals, but neither the intensity nor kinetics of the LPR was affected by the presence of eosinophils. It was concluded that (1) rat LPR can be induced to include increased numbers of eosinophils simply by making the animals eosinophilic, (2) the eosinophilia of human LPR may reflect the inherent tissue eosinophilia in atopic humans, and (3) the eosinophils infiltrating LPR sites do not exert any significant modulatory functions on the LPR itself (15).

Both human and rat LPR are characterized by neutrophil infiltrates. In order to investigate what role the neutrophil infiltrate plays in rodent LPR, rats were made neutropenic by the injection of vinblastine sulfate (16). Rats treated with vinblastine sulfate (0.75 mg/kg) develop profound neutropenia within 4–6 days (Fig. 2). It was found that reversed anaphylaxis with anti-IgE, isolated MCG, or purified HMW and LMW mast cell granular components, when injected intracutaneously into neutropenic rats, was unable to evoke either the initial neutrophil-rich or the second mononuclear-rich phase of LPR. These data strongly suggested that infiltration of skin sites with neutrophils was required to elicit the mononuclear phase of rat LPR.

To further evaluate the importance of the neutrophil to the development of LPR, neutrophil reconstitution was attempted. Neutrophil reconstitution experiments involved the administration of exogenous neutrophils to neutropenic animals after treatment with vinblastine sulfate. Following the intravenous administration of 3×10^8 neutrophils, neutrophil counts increased in peripheral blood for up to 2 hr (16). Attempts to induce LPR in neutropenic animals that were subsequently reconstituted included both intravenous and intraperitoneal reconstitution. After either route, the LPR that was elicited 24 hr after the intracutaneous injection of MCG was intermediate in intensity in neutrophil-reconstituted animals in comparison to the LPR observed in control animals or mock-reconstituted animals treated with vinblastine and reconstituted with saline. These data were compared by paired sample t testing, and the reconstituted rats were significantly more responsive than nonreconstituted animals ($p < .01$). Thus, there was a tendency for neutrophil reconstitution to increase the inflammatory intensity of LPR in neutropenic animals, thereby strengthening the suggestion that the neutrophil was required for the full expression of LPR.

In subsequent experiments (17) rats have been made neutropenic by employing rabbit anti-rat neutrophil antibodies. The neutropenia that was

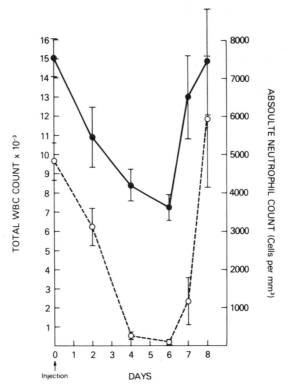

Fig. 2. Sprague Dawley rats were given vinblastine sulfate (0.75 mg/kg iv), and the effects of this treatment on total white blood cell counts (●——●) and absolute neutrophil counts (○---○) were determined at various times following injection. This treatment regimen was found to reproducibly induce selective neutropenia while having minimal effects on other white blood cell populations. Reprinted with permission from Lemanske and Kaliner (11).

induced immunologically was as profound as that caused pharmacologically, and the capacity of the immunologically induced neutropenia to suppress LPR was equivalent to the pharmacologic neutropenia. Thus, induction of LPR requires an influx of neutrophils in order to generate a second infiltration with mononuclear cells.

PROPOSED PATHOGENESIS OF LPR

Although it is recognized that the mast cell plays a primary role in the development of LPR, the precise sequence of events is still being unrav-

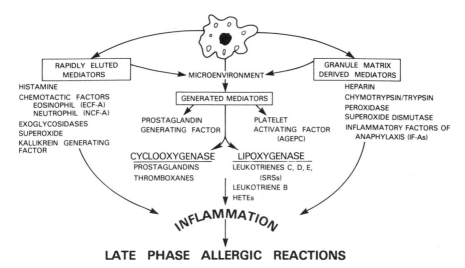

Fig. 3. Mediators that are released or formed in response to mast cell degranulation. The diverse biologic activities of these mediators produce multiple tissue effects that may contribute to late-phase allergic reactions. Reprinted with permission from Lemanske and Kaliner (11).

eled. The diverse chemical mediators (Fig. 3) of the MCG afford it the capability of orchestrating numerous tissue effects over a prolonged time period, including such actions as smooth muscle constriction, vascular contraction or dilation, increased vascular permeability, chemotaxis of eosinophils and neutrophils, promotion of fibrinolysis, and generation of kallikrein activity, among others. The physicochemical nature of the dissolution of the MCG matrix provides a temporal sequence of mediator release from the granule. Preformed mediators that are loosely bound to the granule, such as histamine, are released into the tissue fluid immediately after degranulation. Several of the secondarily formed mediators are generated immediately (prostaglandins) or within minutes (slow-reacting substances). The granule matrix and its constituent mediators may remain in the tissue for hours until they are phagocytosed or degraded.

Histamine is undoubtedly the best known mediator contained within the MCG. When injected intradermally, it reproduces the classic wheal and flare reaction and has multiple other actions including chemotactic properties. Despite these capabilities, however, studies both in man (18) and in rodents (9) have demonstrated that histamine when injected alone or in combination with antigen does not produce LPR. These data, further supported by the observation that LPR cannot be induced by cutaneous injections of bradykinin and prostaglandin E_1 (9), strongly suggest that alterations in vascular permeability are not by themselves primary factors in the induction of LPR.

A number of discrete factors that are released or generated as a result of mast cell degranulation have been shown to be chemotactic for various cell types. Eosinophil chemotactic factors of anaphylaxis are preformed peptides (Val-Gly-Ser-Glu and Ala-Gly-Ser-Glu) that demonstrate selective chemotactic properties for eosinophils when assayed in Boyden chambers (19). Further, neutrophil chemotactic factors have been described in postchallenge serum samples of patients with antigen-induced bronchospasm (5,20,21) and cold urticaria (22). Although the importance of these factors in the expression of LPR is unknown, their biologic activities suggest that they may contribute to the genesis of this reaction. Moreover, the initial description of rat mast cell IF-A suggests that this factor markedly resembles the HMW NCF (23). Thus, it is possible that NCF is an inflammatory factor.

The release of arachidonic acid from membrane phospholipids as a consequence of mast cell degranulation results in the generation of numerous oxidative derivatives capable of producing local tissue effects (24). Arachidonic acid release is the pivotal point for two important enzymatic pathways, the cyclooxygenase and lipoxygenase enzymes. Cyclooxygenase products include prostaglandins, prostacyclin, and thromboxanes with the specific types and amounts formed being dependent on the nature of the tissue being stimulated. Prostaglandins D_2, E_2, I_2, and $F_{2\alpha}$ are generated by allergic inflammation and may influence vascular tone and permeability, among other actions. Activation of the lipoxygenase pathway leads to the formation of diverse monohydroxyeicosatetraenoic acids (mono-HETE) and leukotrienes (LT). Both 5-HETE and 5,12-diHETE (LTB_4) are capable of regulating neutrophil and eosinophil function through chemotactic and chemokinetic effects, enhancement of expression of C3b receptors, stimulation of guanylate and adenylate cyclase, and the release of modest amounts of neutrophil lysosomal enzymes (24,25). Leukotrienes C_4, D_4, and E_4 (slow-reacting substances of anaphylaxis) are capable of contracting smooth muscles, constricting peripheral pulmonary airways and trachea, and altering vascular permeability. While no data implicate these molecules in the generation of LPR, their obvious ability to influence inflammatory pathways introduces the possibility that they may also participate.

Fibrin deposition has been reported by some (18) but not all (13) investigators as a characteristics feature of clinical LPR, suggesting a possible role for the coagulation system in LPR. Mast cells and basophils possess a preformed mediator with kallikrein-like activity [basophil kallikrein factor

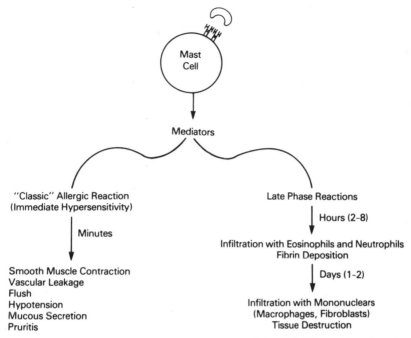

Fig. 4. Consequence of mediator release. Antigen-induced IgE-dependent secretion of MCG leads to classic allergic reactions or immediate hypersensitivity. Late-phase allergic reactions are initially appreciable at 2 to 8 hr and are characterized by polymorphonuclear leukocyte infiltrations. A second infiltration consisting of mononuclear cells is apparent after 24 to 72 hr. Reprinted with permission from Oertel and Kaliner (12).

of anaphylaxis (BK-A)] (26,27). Through the activation of Hageman factors, BK-A might have the potential of initiating the coagulation sequence, which in turn might influence both subacute and chronic cell-mediated inflammatory lesions. In addition, the formation of bradykinin might relate to the burning discomfort that accompanies cutaneous LPR.

Based upon these observations, it is possible to suggest the following pathogenesis for LPR (Fig. 4). Mast cell degranulation leads to the rapid appearance of many mediators including histamine, eicosinoids, bradykinin, and chemotactic factors that combine to cause the cutaneous vasodilation, vascular permeability, pruritus, and the initial attraction of polymorphonuclear leukocytes that are so characteristic of immediate hypersensitivity in the ''classic'' allergic sense. It can be anticipated that the effects of this group of primary and secondary mediators will be largely dissipated within minutes to hours. The macromolecular nature of the MCG matrix, however, provides an additional continuing source of mediators appearing over hours. Of these granule-associated mediators, HMW and LMW IF-A continue to induce the characteristic cellular infiltrates of LPR, presumably facilitated by the actions of the primary and secondary mediators. The resultant polymorphonuclear leukocyte infiltration, which appears over a period of hours, is necessary for the subsequent, more delayed mononuclear cell inflammatory response.

CONCLUSIONS

Allergic reactions are now recognized to consist of an immediate reaction (the classic allergic reaction) followed by the LPR (Fig. 4). The appreciation of the LPR with its several stages of cellular infiltrations may explain certain enigmas which have confused clinicians. For instance, urticarial reactions, which are associated with cold, heat, light, and pressure, are clearly associated with histamine release, indicating mast cell degranulation. Chronic idiopathic urticaria, which clinically resembles the physical urticarias, is characterized by a perivascular inflammatory response. It seems possible that the inflammation seen in chronic urticaria is the late component of antecedent mast cell degranulation.

It has been appreciated for many years that seasonal exposure to pollen leads to a decreased threshold for the elicitation of nasal allergic responses (28). This effect, known as "priming," is possibly due to the inflammatory response produced by LPR, which would lead to hyperirritability of the nasal mucosa. In a similar manner, it is possible that hyperreactive airways disease (asthma) is also influenced by LPR (see Chapter 16, this volume). Thus, we are at a stage where we recognize that LPR is a direct consequence of mast cell degranulation and that it possibly plays an important role in the pathogenesis and treatment of allergic diseases; but we also recognize that we are not yet perfectly certain of all of the nuances of its generation or control.

REFERENCES

1. Dunnill, M. S. The pathology of asthma, with special reference to changes in the bronchial mucosa. *J. Clin. Pathol.* **13**:27–33, 1960.
2. Kaliner, M. A., Blennerhassett, J., and Austen, K. F. Bronchial asthma. *In* "Textbook of Immunopathology" (P. A. Meischer and H. J. Müller-Eberhard, eds.), pp. 387–401. Grune & Stratton, New York, 1976.

3. Kaliner, M. Mast cell derived mediators and bronchial asthma. *In* "Airway Reactivity" (F. E. Hargreave, ed.), pp. 175–188. Astra Scientific Publications, Ontario, Canada, 1980.

4. Metcalfe, D. D., Donlon, M., and Kaliner, M. The mast cell. *CRC Crit. Rev. Immunol.* **3**:23–74, 1981.

5. Bach, M. K. Mediators of anaphylaxis and inflammation. *Annu. Rev. Microbiol.* **36**:371–413, 1982.

6. Nagy, L., Lee, T. H., and Kay, A. B. Neutrophil chemotactic activity in antigen-induced late asthmatic reactions. *N. Engl. J. Med.* **306**:497–501, 1982.

7. Atkins, P., Zweiman, B., Dyer, J., Bedard, P. M., and Kaliner, M. Antigen inhalation induces systemic increases in histamine and chemotactic activity levels in subjects with rhinitis or asthma. *J. Allergy Clin. Immunol.* **71**(Suppl.):151, 1983.

8. Lee, T. H., Nagy, L., Nagakura, T., Walport, M. J., and Kay, A. B. Identification and partial characterization of an exercise-induced neutrophil chemotactic factor in bronchial asthma. *J. Clin. Invest.* **69**:889–899, 1982.

9. Tannenbaum, S., Oertel, H., Henderson, W., and Kaliner, M. The biologic activity of mast cell granules. I. Elicitation of inflammatory responses in rat skin. *J. Immunol.* **125**:325–335, 1980.

10. Gleich, G. J. The late phase of the immunoglobulin ε-mediated reaction: A link between anaphylaxis and common allergic disease? *J. Allergy Clin. Immunol.* **70**:160–169, 1982.

11. Lemanske, R. F., and Kaliner, M. Mast cell-dependent late phase reactions. *Clin. Immunol. Rev.* **1**:547–580, 1982.

12. Oertel, H., and Kaliner, M. The biologic activity of mast cell granules. III. Purification of inflammatory factors of anaphylaxis (IF-A) responsible for causing late-phase reactions. *J. Immunol.* **127**:1398–1402, 1981.

13. Solley, G., Gleich, G., Jordon, R., and Schroeter, A. The late phase of the immediate wheal and flare skin reaction. Its dependence on IgE antibodies. *J. Clin. Invest.* **58**:408–420, 1976.

14. Lemanske, R. F., Joiner, K., and Kaliner, M. The biologic activity of mast cell granules. IV. The effect of complement depletion on rat cutaneous late phase reactions. *J. Immunol.* **130**:1881–1884, 1983.

15. Lemanske, R. F., and Kaliner, M. The experimental production of increased eosinophils in rat late phase reactions. *Immunology* **45**:561–568, 1982.

16. Lemanske, R. F., Guthman, D. A., Oertel, H., Barr, L., and Kaliner, M. The biologic activity of mast cell granules. VI. The effect of vinblastine-induced neutropenia on rat cutaneous late phase reactions. *J. Immunol.* **130**:2837–2845, 1983.

17. Lemanske, R. F., Guthman, D. A., and Kaliner, M. The biologic activity of mast cell granules. VII. The effect of anti-neutrophil antibody induced neutropenia on rat cutaneous late phase reactions. *J. Immunol.* **131**:929–936, 1983.

18. DeShazo, R. D., Levinson, A. I., Dvorak, H. F., and Davis, R. W. The late phase skin reaction: Evidence for activation of the coagulation system in an IgE dependent reaction in man. *J. Immunol.* **122**:692–698, 1979.

19. Goetzl, E. J., and Austen, K. F. Purification and synthesis of eosinophilotactic tetrapeptides of human lung tissue: Identification as eosinophil chemotactic factor of anaphylaxis. *Proc. Natl. Acad. Sci. U.S.A.* **72**:4123–4127, 1975.

20. Atkins, P. C., Norman, M., Weiner, H., and Zweiman, B. Release of neutrophil chemotactic activity during immediate hypersensitivity reactions in humans. *Ann. Intern. Med.* **86**:415–418, 1977.

21. Atkins, P. C., Norman, M., Zweiman, B., and Rosenblum, F. Further characterization

and biologic activity of ragweed antigen-induced neutrophil chemotactic activity in man. *J. Allergy Clin. Immunol.* **64:**251–258, 1979.

22. Wasserman, S. I., Soter, N. A., Center, D. M., and Austen, K. F. Cold urticaria. Recognition and characterization of a neutrophil chemotactic factor which appears in serum during experimental cold challenge. *J. Clin. Invest.* **60:**189–196, 1977.

23. O'Driscoll, B. R., Lee, T. H., Cromwell, O., and Kay, A. B. Release of high molecular weight neutrophil chemotactic activity from immunologically challenged human lung fragments. *J. Allergy Clin. Immunol.* **71**(Suppl.):146, 1983.

24. Goetzl, E. J. Mediators of immediate hypersensitivity derived from arachidonic acid. *N. Engl. J. Med.* **303:**822–825, 1980.

25. Goetzl, E. J., Goldman, D. W., and Valone, F. H. Lipid mediators of leukocyte function in immediate-type hypersensitivity reactions. *In* "Biochemistry of the Acute Allergic Reactions" (E. L. Becker, A. S. Simon, and K. F. Austen, eds.), pp. 169–182. Alan R. Liss, Inc., New York, 1981.

26. Newball, H. H., Berninger, R. W., Talamo, R. C., and Lichtenstein, L. M. Anaphylactic release of a basophil kallikrein-like activity. I. Purification and characterization. *J. Clin. Invest.* **64:**457–465, 1979.

27. Newball, H. H., Talamo, R. C., and Lichtenstein, L. M. Anaphylactic release of a basophil kallikrein-like activity. II. A mediator of immediate hypersensitivity reactions. *J. Clin. Invest.* **64:**466–475, 1979.

28. Connell, J. T. Quantitative pollen challenges. III. The priming effect in allergic rhinitis. *J. Allergy* **43:**33–44, 1969.

DISCUSSION

Kay: Does human lung release IF-A?

Kaliner: Supernatants from antigen-challenged human lung tissue, when injected into rat skin, cause inflammations precisely like those seen in response to mast cell granules. While this response is only seen in appropriately challenged human lung, we have not purified this activity yet.

Gleich: In the study of the late-phase reaction by Solley *et al.* (G. O. Solley, G. J. Gleich, R. E. Jordan, and A. L. Schroeter, *J. Clin. Invest.* **58:**408, 1976), the reaction was transferred passively into patients who were not atopic, and yet the biopsies showed appreciable eosinophilia. Thus, the occurrence of peripheral blood eosinophilia is not essential for the development of tissue eosinophilia in the late-phase reaction.

Lewis: When you degranulated the rat cutaneous mast cell in situ, the egressing granules stained heterogeneously pink and blue. Is there another basis on which this could be considered to relate to granule heterogeneity?

Kaliner: It appeared that granules released from the skin mast cells might be staining differently. I believe that this observation reflects the depth of the cut and other technical variations and is not a reflection of mast cell granule heterogeneity.

Clark: In your model, did you ever get a late reaction without an early reaction? Did the extent of the late reaction depend on the severity of the early response?

Kaliner: In this animal model, each positive skin test is accompanied by an LPR at 6 to 8 and 24 hrs. There is a direct correlation between the intensity of the early (immediate) allergic reaction and the consequent LPR.

Schwartz: On a weight basis, how much IF-A resides in rat serosal mast cells? Does the quantity vary in resting and activated cells? Does the quantity vary in resting and activated cells? Could this peptide be generated by the actions of chymase and/or carboxypeptidase A that reside in rat serosal mast cells?

What is the basis of the insolubility of IF-A? Is this a highly charged molecule that is ionically bound, either to negatively charged heparin proteoglycan or to the positively charged neutral proteases?

Kaliner: We have not done this type of quantification of IF-A. However, it is so potent that you do not need much to elicit LPR and so the quantity per cell may be very low.

Lichtenstein: In our skin blister studies we found that while most patients developed late reactions (5–8 hr), some did not. The amount of histamine and PGD was significantly greater in the former than the latter.

Kaplan: I have been puzzled for some time by the absence of delayed phase reactions in patients with cold urticaria. Here is a situation in which one can induce a large hive with an ice cube, a circumstance thought to favor late responses. There is also release of histamine and NCA, and in some cases, it is clearly IgE dependent. If products of the mast cell lead to the delayed phase infiltrate, it seems curious that in no case (more than 50 studied) have I seen a delayed reaction. I wonder whether something else is required for the late reaction to be manifest.

Wasserman: Late-phase responses do not occur after single challenges of patients with cold urticaria, even in patients with long-lasting angioedema. Biopsies at intervals up to 48 hr after challenge reveal no infiltrating leucocytes. We feel that this finding reflects deactivation of circulating leucocytes by high concentrations of released chemotactic factors. However, Greaves and Eady (R. A. J. Eady and M. W. Greaves, *Lancet* **1:**336, 1978) have described several patients with cold urticaria who developed leukocytoplastic vasculitis after repeated local cold challenge.

Johansson: Can you initiate a late-phase reaction in your rat model by anti-IgG? Also, in humans, it is possible to get a late-onset asthmatic reaction by repeated bronchial challenges using low doses of allergen which by themselves do not give an immediate response. Have you tried that approach with your anti-IgE?

Kaliner: We have not injected anti-IgG. If we retest human or rat skin we produce an intense LPR. Thus, in myself, repeated skin testing with very dilute extracts of ragweed antigen at the site of a minimal response 1 hr later elicits an impressive LPR.

Askenase: The blueing experiment is very important. Don't you think that a pulse of dye, to separate groups of animals, is required every 15 min?

Kaliner: We did not inject blue dye every 15 min during the course of LPR but did examine if Evans blue dye injected iv at 30 min and at 2, 4, 6, 8, and 24 hr after skin tests in rats were positive. Blueing was only seen at 30 min. Thus we have no evidence for vascular permeability accompanying rat LPR.

Lichtenstein: Perhaps it would be useful to define a late reaction, for readers of the book. Does the reaction have to fade and reappear?

Kaliner: We chose to define late-phase reactions as inflammatory responses appearing hours after an immediate reaction. In the animal models (rat or monkey), this inflammatory response is due initially to polymorphonuclear leucocytes and subsequently to macrophages.

Gleich: In the typical (cutaneous) late-phase reaction the initial pruritus is followed by a period of time, about 2 hr, during which pruritus is largely absent. Then at 2–3 hr, the area again becomes symptomatic with pruritus. Presumably your rats would tell us the same story.

Hargreave: The induction of a dual cutaneous response after injection of two doses over 1 hr, which did not occur after injection of one dose, is probably a result of a more severe allergic reaction, which is one important determinant of the late response.

Wasserman: In experiments in which late-phase reactions occurred in the absence of signs of vasopermeability, was the permeability response assessed by Evans' blue dye or by ^{125}I albumin? The pale center of skin test responses to leukotrienes despite histological evidence of oedema suggests that dye extrusion may differ, in some instances, from ^{125}I-labeled albumin extravasation.

Kaliner: Evans' blue dye binds to albumin and therefore the blueing test is actually a test of vascular permeability to albumin.

Lewis: Intradermal administration of LTC_4 in guinea pigs, followed by intravenous administration of Coomassie blue dye, leads to a region of central pallor surrounded by a blue rim.

CHAPTER 15

An Animal Model of the Late Asthmatic Response to Antigen Challenge

GARY L. LARSEN, MARK P. SHAMPAIN, WILLIAM R. MARSH,
and B. LYN BEHRENS

Department of Pediatrics
National Jewish Hospital and Research Center
National Asthma Center
and University of Colorado School of Medicine
Denver, Colorado, U.S.A.

INTRODUCTION

The observation that allergic patients exposed to allergens can develop both early and late reactions in the respiratory tract dates back more than a century. Despite this knowledge of these late pulmonary responses, the clinical importance of the late asthmatic response (LAR) has only recently been emphasized. An important initial observation was made by Herxheimer in 1952 (1) when he noted patients with LARs had more severe asthma than patients without these reactions. More recent observations have also noted the similarity of LARs and chronic, severe bronchial asthma, in that both require steroids to decrease or abolish symptoms and abnormalities in pulmonary physiology (2,3). In addition, Warner (4) has observed a significant correlation between frequent attacks of asthma and the presence of LARs in children challenged with house dust mite. Recent studies from McMaster University have linked LARs to a basic feature of asthma: airway hyperreactivity to aerosol challenge with histamine or methacholine. Thus, Cockcroft and associates (5) have reported that allergen-induced LARs are associated with an increase in bronchial responsiveness to these drugs while subjects with only an immediate asthmatic response (IAR) do not exhibit this height-

ASTHMA: Physiology,
Immunopharmacology,
and Treatment
THIRD INTERNATIONAL SYMPOSIUM

245

ened reactivity. More recently, these observations have been extended by Cartier and associates (6), who showed that this increased bronchial responsiveness to histamine after the LAR is not due to a reduction in baseline airway caliber alone. These observations suggest that a clearer understanding of the pathophysiology of LARs might help in the approach to patients with severe and/or frequent asthma and could lead to a better understanding of bronchial hyperreactivity.

The pathogenesis of the pulmonary reactions has been unclear (2–4) with both IgE-mediated (7) as well as non-IgE-mediated mechanisms (8) proposed to explain these reactions. Attempts to define the pathogenesis have been limited in the past because of an absence of an acceptable animal model of this reaction., We have recently developed an animal model of LARs to antigen challenge employing rabbits as the test animal (9). This report describes the animal model, summarizes observations made to date, and discusses potential uses of the model in evaluating the pathophysiology of the LAR.

BACKGROUND: THE ANIMAL MODEL

The development of an animal model of LARs began in our laboratory in 1978. At that time, the work of Dolovich and co-workers (10) and Solley and associates (11) had pointed out that the late cutaneous response (LCR) to antigen challenge could be IgE mediated. Several observations in man suggested that LARs, like LCRs, are not all Arthus reactions. First, pollen antigens such as ragweed, which may not cause production of large quantities of IgG antibody, can provoke LARs (7). Second, inhalation of disodium cromoglycate prior to antigen inhalation prevents both IARs and LARs, implying a role for mast cells in the pathogenesis of the late reaction (3). Third, the effect of steroids on LARs parallels that seen with LCRs in that the immediate reaction is not altered while the late response is abolished (2), suggesting the skin and lung may have more in common in terms of mechanisms than just the temporal development of the reaction. These observations raised the possibility that the LAR could also be primarily dependent on an IgE-initiated event for its expression. Work from separate laboratories had shown that rabbits produce a homocytotropic antibody analogous to human IgE (12,13). Based on the studies of Pinckard and co-workers (14), we knew that a proportion of rabbits immunized with antigen within the first 24 hr of life will produce exclusively antigen-specific IgE (homocytotropic antibody), whereas rabbits immunized first at 7 days of age will produce several antibody isotypes to the antigen. Thus, immunizing rabbits to produce only antigen-specific IgE was employed to test the hypothesis that the LAR could occur in the presence of IgE antibody alone.

IMMUNIZATION/IMMUNOLOGIC CHARACTERIZATION

Immunization of New Zealand white rabbits (Dutchland, Denver, Pennsylvania) to preferentially produce homocytotropic antibody to the antigen is started at less than 24 hr of age. In our initial study (9), we used lyophilized *Alternaria tenuis* extract (Lot No. LM1-116, Greer Laboratories, Lenoir, North Carolina), 1 : 20 dilution weight to volume, reconstituted in normal saline. Subsequent studies have also employed ragweed antigen (mixed ragweed, Lot No. LP1-58, Greer Laboratories, or short ragweed, Lot No. 87103FD, Center Laboratories, Port Washington, New York) as the sensitizing antigen. The concentrations of antigen used as well as the timing of the injections is the same for all antigens, and is shown in Table I.

Immunologic characterization is carried out when the rabbits are 3 months old. Antigen-specific homocytotropic antibody (designated IgE) is measured by homologous passive cutaneous anaphylaxis (PCA) by intracutaneous injection of 0.2 ml serum dilutions from the immunized rabbits into the back of naive 3-month-old New Zealand white rabbits. Serums from nonimmunized rabbits and rabbits immunized with other antigens

TABLE I

Immunization Schedule for the Preferential Production of Homocytotropic Antibody (IgE) in New Zealand White Rabbits

Age (days)	Immunization mixture[a]	Route[b]
0	Antigen extract (0.25 ml) + aluminum hydroxide (0.25 ml)	ip
7, 14, 21, 35, 49, 63	Antigen extract (0.25 ml) + normal saline (0.25 ml)	ip
77	Antigen extract (1.0 ml) + aluminum hydroxide (1.0 ml)	sc

[a] Antigen extract, *Alternaria tenuis* or ragweed diluted 1 : 20 weight to volume; aluminum hydroxide, 10 mg/ml suspended in normal saline.

[b] ip, intraperitoneally; sc, subcutaneously.

are used as controls. After a latent period of 3 days, the recipient rabbits
are injected with 5 ml of a 1 : 10 dilution of antigen (weight to volume) and
5 ml of 2.5% Evans blue dye. To assess skin test responsiveness, histamine phosphate and normal saline are injected intracutaneously 10 min
before the extract–dye mixture is given. Bluing of the sites is measured 1
hr after dye administration with a positive response measuring 5 mm or
greater in diameter. Previous experiments have shown that heating positive serum for 2–4 hr at 56°C results in loss of the long-term sensitivity.
No evidence of short-term sensitizing antibody is present when animals
are challenged 4 hr after intracutaneous injections.

Rabbit antigen-specific IgG is measured by heterologous PCA in
Hartley strain guinea pigs and by precipitation assay (15). For these
PCAs, serum dilutions (0.1 ml) are injected intracutaneously into the
backs of the guinea pigs. After a 4-hr latent period, 2.5 ml of antigen (1 : 10
weight to volume) and 1.0 ml of Evans blue dye are given intravenously to
each animal. Controls (histamine, saline, serum) are as described above.
Blueing of lesions is measured at 30 min with a positive response being 5
mm or greater in diameter.

CHALLENGE AND ASSESSMENT OF LUNG FUNCTION

Rabbits are anesthetized with a short-acting barbiturate for placement
of a cuffed endotracheal tube. While they are anesthetized, an esophageal
balloon is placed, and a silastic mouth guard that conforms to the contour
of the animal's mouth is placed to the back of the oropharynx to protect
the esophageal catheter and endotracheal tube from damage by the rabbit's posterior teeth. The guard is secured with adhesive. The animals are
allowed to awaken over 2 hr. For assessment of lung function, the difference between esophageal balloon and proximal endotracheal tube pressure is recorded as transpulmonary pressure (P_{TP}). The endotracheal tube
is connected to a size 00 pneumotachograph (Hewlett-Packard Model
21069B) which is attached to a Hewlett-Packard Model 47203A flow trans-
ducer. The pressure and flow signals are sent to an analog computer
(Hewlett-Packard Respiratory Analyzer Model 8816A), which integrates
flow to tidal volume and computes dynamic compliance (C_{dyn}) by the
technique of von Neergard and Wirz (16) and total pulmonary resistance
(R_L) by the method of electrical subtraction of Mead and Whittenberger
(17). In addition, functional residual capacity (*FRC*) is determined by a
gas dilution technique employing helium. Thus, R_L can also be expressed
in relation to lung volume as specific conductance of the lung ($SG_L = 1/R_L/FRC$).

After baseline lung functions are measured, the animals are challenged with appropriate aerosols. For the challenge, the endotracheal tube is attached to a Vaponephrine nebulizer (Fisons Corp., Bedford, Massachusetts). One milliliter of material (1 : 20 weight/volume of antigen diluted in normal saline, saline alone, or medications such as disodium cromoglycate) is nebulized over 5 min directly into the endotracheal tube of the spontaneously breathing animal. The mass median diameter of the aerosol is approximately 5.6 μm $\pm$ 1.8 (SD) (18). At the end of the challenge, the endotracheal tube is reconnected to the pneumotachograph, and assessment of lung function is repeated at specified intervals over a 6-hr period. Passage of a catheter with suctioning as needed ensures patency of the endotracheal tube. Adequate hydration of the animals is ensured by humidification of respired air as well as by administration of intravenous fluids.

PHYSIOLOGIC RESPONSE TO ANTIGEN CHALLENGE

Actively Immunized Rabbits

The physiologic response to antigen challenge in actively immunized rabbits has been found to depend on the antibody status of the animals studied. As outlined in the initial description of the model (9), when rabbits were immunologically assessed at 3 months of age, 19 rabbits were found to have only IgE to *Alternaria tenuis* (titers of homologous PCA from 1 : 8 to 1 : 128), while 7 animals immunized first at 7 days of age had not only IgE titers similar to those above but had guinea pig PCA titers of 1 : 16 to 1 : 64 as well as precipitin titers of 1 : 8 to 1 : 32. The latter group of rabbits were classed as multiple antibody (E/G) responders. The rabbits with only IgE exhibited biphasic changes in their pulmonary functions as displayed in Fig. 1. An early phase increase in R_L and decrease in C_{dyn} began within 15 min of the challenge and lasted through approximately 30 min. The R_L and C_{dyn} either approached baseline or reached a plateau after 30 min, and a second phase of increased R_L and decreased C_{dyn} began ~1.5–2.0 hr after challenge. The maximum changes in these lung functions were usually reached by 3.5–4.0 hr after challenge with mean values stable during the last 2 hr of the study. Control rabbits, that is, nonimmunized rabbits or rabbits immunized with bovine serum albumin and challenged with *A. tenuis,* remained at or near baseline throughout the 6-hr study period (Fig. 1).

Rabbits with E/G isotypes also exhibited early and late alterations in pulmonary function. As noted in the study (9), the response in this group

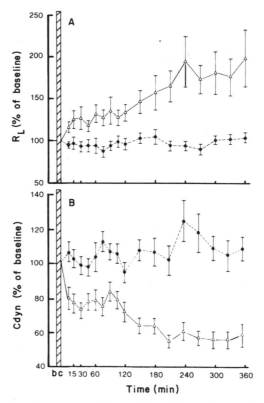

Fig. 1. Changes in pulmonary resistance (A) and dynamic compliance (B) (mean ± SEM), expressed as a percentage of baseline (b) values after aerosol challenge (c) with *Alternaria tenuis* in 19 rabbits producing only the IgE antibody isotype to the antigen (△). The responses to *Alternaria* in 10 rabbits who were either nonimmunized or immunized with another antigen (●) are also shown. Reprinted with permission from Shampain *et al.* (9).

appeared to be blunted compared to the response in the IgE group. To address this in more detail, the following studies were performed. First, results of challenges from rabbits of the same litter with IgE titers of 1 : 8 were compared directly with E/G rabbits with higher IgE titers. Despite the higher IgE titers in the E/G group, the changes in pulmonary function were still reduced when compared with those in rabbits with only IgE, again implying blunting of the response when antibody other than the homocytotropic antibody was present. The second method of addressing this problem was by studying the effects of transfusion of heat-treated serum containing only IgG against *A. tenuis* into rabbits with IgE. The rabbits had their pulmonary response to *A. tenuis* challenge assessed both before and after the transfusion of IgG serum. Both early and late altera-

TABLE II
Mean SG_L 4–6 Hr after Challenge with
Ragweed Antigen E in Three Actively
Immunized Rabbits

Antigen–specific IgE/IgG titers	SG_L (% baseline)[a]
16/0	39.4 ± 9.0
64/512	50.1 ± 3.3
128/2048	86.4 ± 9.1

[a] Mean ± SEM.

tions in R_L and C_{dyn} were significantly reduced by transfusion of serum containing IgG against *A. tenuis*. In contrast, rabbits with only IgE who received transfusions of normal serum exhibited no significant blunting of the response from one study to another.

Recent observations in rabbits immunized with a different antigen (ragweed) also support the observations made above regarding the importance of antigen-specific IgE and IgG in determining the magnitude of the late asthmatic response. As shown in Table II, the mean specific conductance of the lung (SG_L) over the time period from 4 to 6 hr after challenge with ragweed antigen E is related to the titers of antibody present. The largest response was noted in the rabbit with only IgE to ragweed present on immunologic study. In the E/G ragweed-sensitized animals, despite increasing concentrations of IgE, the presence of antigen-specific IgG was associated with less alteration in SG_L during the period of the LAR. Thus, the importance of antibody type (IgE and IgG) in determining the pulmonary response in actively immunized rabbits appears to apply to at least two antigens in this model: *A. tenuis* and ragweed.

Passively Immunized Rabbits

The results outlined in the previous section demonstrate that the LAR can occur in the presence of antigen-specific IgE alone. Because the studies were done in rabbits immunized from birth, however, the possible dependence of the LAR on cellular immune mechanisms resulting from the immunization procedure could not be assessed. To address this, experiments were conducted in which nonimmunized 3-month-old rabbits were transfused with plasma or serum containing IgE antibodies to *Alternaria tenuis,* and then challenged with the antigen to determine if the pulmonary response could be produced in the absence of cellular immune

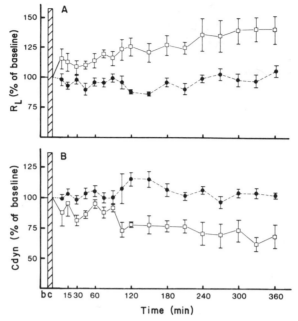

Fig. 2. Changes in pulmonary resistance (A) and dynamic compliance (B) (mean ± SEM) after aerosol challenge (c) with *Alternaria tenuis* in 3 rabbits transfused with plasma containing IgE to this antigen (□) compared with control rabbits transfused with normal rabbit plasma (●). Reprinted with permission from Shampain *et al.* (9).

reactions associated with immunization. As displayed in Fig. 2, these rabbits transfused with IgE alone showed biphasic early and late changes in R_L and C_{dyn} similar to actively immunized rabbits, whereas age-matched control rabbits transfused with nonimmune plasma showed no significant alterations in these lung functions. In the passively sensitized IgE rabbits, the pulmonary response was abolished on restudy 4 weeks after the transfusion, consistent with the expected catabolism of the passively transfused antibody.

As in the studies described above in rabbits immunized from birth, the passively sensitized rabbits also exhibited blunting of the response to antigen challenge in the presence of antigen-specific IgG. As previously described (9), rabbits transfused with plasma or serum containing IgE alone developed larger changes in R_L and C_{dyn} than rabbits transfused with antigen-specific E/G, despite higher IgE titers in the latter group. This observation has been expanded in a recent preliminary report from our laboratory (19). Based on the anti-*Alternaria* titers of the transfused serum, the pulmonary response to antigen challenge was examined in five

TABLE III
Changes in R_L in Passively Immunized
Rabbits 5 Hr after Challenge with
Alternaria tenuis

Antibody status	R_L mean (Range)[a]
E only	232 (160–298)
E/low G (1 : 256)	155 (133–189)
E/high G (1 : 2048)	110 (95–129)
G only	94 (75–109)

[a] Results are expressed as the percent of baseline value with the baseline value equal to 100%. The number of animals in the groups is 3–6.

groups of animals: E only, E/low G, E/high G, G only, and normal serum (control). During the immediate asthmatic reaction, only the first two groups exhibited significant alterations in R_L, SG_L, and C_{dyn}. As shown in Table III, during the LAR, the alteration in R_L was influenced by the relative amount of anti-*Alternaria* IgG present in that as the amount relative to IgE increased, abnormalities in pulmonary function decreased. Similar findings were noted for SG_L and C_{dyn}. Thus, the data to date reviewed in this section demonstrate that the late asthmatic response can be passively transferred, the response is dependent on the presence of antigen-specific IgE, and the response is blocked in a dose-dependent manner by the presence of antigen-specific IgG.

EFFECTS OF DRUGS ON LATE ASTHMATIC RESPONSE

Various classes of medications have been employed in clinical studies of the LAR to ablate or modify this reaction. Human late responses are often poorly reversed by adrenergic agents (2,4). On the other hand, both the immediate and late asthmatic response have been blocked by inhalation of disodium cromoglycate prior to antigen challenge (3,20). In addition, pretreatment of human subjects with steroids has been shown to have no significant effect on the immediate response while abolishing or greatly diminishing the LAR (3,20). To further characterize this animal model of LARs, studies have also been conducted with these three classes of drugs (adrenergic agents, disodium cromoglycate, steroids) to determine if they exert similar actions in the rabbit model.

The initial study employing adrenergic drugs utilized isoproterenol, 0.5

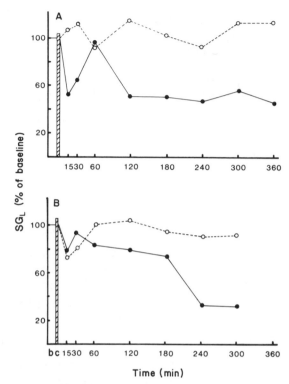

Fig. 3. Alterations in the response to antigen challenge produced by pretreatment with either disodium cromoglycate or methylprednisolone. (A) Changes in SG_L, compared to baseline (b), after challenge (c) with ragweed antigen E in a rabbit immunized from birth with ragweed. For the first study, the animal was pretreated with inhalation of disodium cromoglycate (Cromolyn, ○) and had neither an IAR or LAR. One week later, pretreatment with placebo (saline, ●) did not prevent the development of either response. (B) Changes in SG_L, compared to baseline (b), after challenge (c) with *Alternaria tenuis* in a rabbit immunized with that antigen. Intravenous administration of saline (●) before challenge did not prevent an immediate and late decrease in this lung function while pretreatment with intravenous methylprednisolone (steroids, ○) prevented the late response.

μg/kg/min, given to nine rabbits for 5 min at the end of the 6-hr studies. As previously reported (9), this did not reverse the alterations if R_L and C_{dyn} described above and displayed in Fig. 1. Subsequent studies employing isoetharine HCl (1%) or epinephrine given during the LAR have not reversed this reaction once it has developed (B. L. Behrens, unpublished observations). Whether this represents a failure to reduce airways obstruction primarily caused by mucosal edema and cellular infiltration rather than smooth muscle contraction remains to be determined.

Studies have also been conducted where animals immunized from birth with either *Alternaria tenuis* or ragweed antigen have been studied repetitively to assess if cromolyn inhalation prior to antigen challenge will block the IAR and LAR. An example of two studies in an animal sensitized by immunization with ragweed antigen is shown in Fig. 3A. For the first study, the animal was pretreated by inhalation of 10 mg of disodium cromoglycate 30 min before inhalation of ragweed antigen E, and then observed for 6 hr after exposure to antigen for alterations in lung function. As can be seen, neither an IAR or LAR developed after the challenge. One week later, however, pretreatment with placebo (saline) before the antigen challenge did not block the subsequent development of the asthmatic responses. Similar results have been obtained in experiments where the rabbits have been sensitized to *A. tenuis*. In addition, reversing the order of the experiments (placebo pretreatment the first week followed by cromolyn pretreatment the second week) has not changed the results.

Experiments have also been conducted to delineate the effects of steroid pretreatment on the response to antigen challenge in animals immunized from birth with *A. tenuis* (Fig. 3B). Methylprednisolone, 1.5 mg/kg/dose, has been given intravenously the day before as well as 30 min before antigen challenge. With this pretreatment, the LAR has been abolished or greatly diminished when compared to the response in the same animal when saline pretreatment was given in an identical protocol. As above, the sequence of studies (saline or steroid the first week followed by the alternate pretreatment the following week) has not altered the results. Thus, in this model, the response to these three classes of drugs is similar to responses described in humans.

LATE ASTHMATIC RESPONSE AND NEUTROPHILS

Interest in the role of neutrophils in the LAR has been stimulated by several recent reports. Neutrophil chemotactic activity (NCA) has been identified in the serum of patients with asthma after challenge with antigens to which they have IgE-antibody (21–23). The activity first appears 5–15 min after a positive challenge, but it is not present after a negative antigen challenge or a positive response to methacholine (21). This neutrophil chemotactic activity has not been found in serum when the early asthmatic response has been blocked by disodium cromogycate administration (22). Of interest in terms of the LAR, Nagy and co-workers (23) have demonstrated biphasic increases in NCA after antigen challenge in asthmatics with late reactions. These authors hypothesized that the ap-

TABLE IV
Mean Circulating Neutrophil Counts 5–6 Hr
after *Alternaria tenuis* Challenge in
Immunized and Control Rabbits

Immune status	Circulating neutrophils[a]	n
Immunized	34.6 ± 12.2	8
Control	143.2 ± 24.5	6

[a] Expressed as % of baseline value, mean ± SEM.

pearance of NCA was due to its release from mast cells. Indeed, Terral and co-workers (24) have noted biphasic degranulation of rat peritoneal mast cells after a single nonimmunologic stimulus, thus making this hypothesis more attractive. Thus, NCA is present in serum after antigen challenge, is presumably released from mast cells in the lung, and thus could attract neutrophils to that target organ. The contribution of the neutrophil to the LAR therefore becomes an important area of study.

Our investigations into the role of the neutrophil in the LAR have just begun, but several observations suggest this cell may play an important part in this animal model. First, when we have monitored white blood counts and differentials in both immunized and control rabbits undergoing antigen challenge, we have observed that circulating neutrophils in the immunized rabbits are significantly decreased from prechallenge (baseline) values during the LAR, while control rabbits challenged with the same antigen (Alternaria) have had no LAR and showed an increase in circulating neutrophils at a comparable time (Table IV). In addition, we have observed that rabbits who develop fatal LARs after antigen challenge have precipitous drops in circulating neutrophil levels before death (B. L. Behrens, unpublished observations). Preliminary data from lavages of animals who develop LARs demonstrated the intrapulmonary accumulation of many neutrophils, and lung histology showed neutrophil accumulation in and around airways. Control animals challenged with antigen also have neutrophil accumulation noted in the lung as assessed by lavage and histology, but the magnitude of the response appears to be less. Thus, immunized rabbits who develop LARs have a decrease in circulating neutrophils and an increase in pulmonary neutrophils as the response develops. These observations raise questions about the contribution of the neutrophil to the LAR in this model. The mechanisms through which these cells could contribute to the LAR are many. For example, they could mechanically increase airways obstruction by infiltrating smaller airways. In addition, by migrating through interstitial spaces and epithelial surfaces, they could increase the permeability of the airways to mediators released from these or other cells. This model will allow us to address these questions. The importance of the cell to the LAR can be addressed in studies employing neutrophil depletion and repletion of immunized animals before antigen challenges. The mechanisms through which the neutrophil contributes to the LAR can be studied by correlating information from a morphometric evaluation of the pathology of the developing LAR with a detailed physiologic description of the process. In addition, physiologic and pathologic alterations can be correlated with assays for mediators in serum and/or lavage to further define the pathogenesis of the process.

SUMMARY

We have demonstrated that neonatal rabbits immunized with either *Alternaria tenuis* or ragweed extract preferentially produce homocytotropic antibody (IgE) to that allergen. Aerosol challenge of these rabbits with the sensitizing antigen induced both early and late changes in lung function with an increase in R_L and FRC and a decrease in C_{dyn} and SG_L. The magnitude of the changes in actively immunized rabbits was dependent in part on the quantity of antigen-specific IgE present with greater alterations in lung function noted in animals with higher titers. The presence of antigen-specific IgG appeared to blunt rather than enhance the LAR as noted by comparing responses in rabbits with only IgE to the response in E/G rabbits. In addition, a blunting of the pulmonary responses in IgE rabbits transfused with antigen specific IgG antibody was documented. Transfusion of plasma containing anti-*Alternaria* IgE into nonimmunized rabbits also resulted in biphasic changes in lung function upon aerosol challenge with the antigen, demonstrating that the LAR can occur in the absence of cellular immune mechanisms associated with immunization as long as IgE is present. Passive transfer experiments employing transfusion of nonimmunized rabbits with serum or plasma with differing titers of IgE and IgG again confirmed the blunting of the LAR by the latter immunoglobulin. As in human studies, adrenergic agents did not reverse the LAR while disodium cromoglycate prevented both the IAR and LAR and steroids inhibited only the LAR in this animal model. The observation that neutrophils disappear from the circulation of animals developing an

LAR and accumulate in the pulmonary tissues during this response suggests this cell contributes to the reaction by mechanisms yet to be explained. This model should provide an approach where the pathologic events of a developing LAR can be correlated with physiologic changes, and the contribution of various cells (mast cells, neutrophils) and mediator systems can be defined.

ACKNOWLEDGMENTS

The work reported here was supported by grants HL-27063 and HL-21565 from the National Institutes of Health and Biomedical Research Support Grant SO7RR05842. The authors thank Peter Henson for his review of the manuscript; Brenda Mitchell, Mary Willcox, David Basaraba, and Amelia Behrens for technical assistance; and Georgia Wheeler for her preparation of the manuscript.

REFERENCES

1. Herxheimer, H. The late bronchial reaction in induced asthma. *Int. Arch. Allergy Appl. Immunol.* **3:**323–328, 1952.
2. Hargreave, F. E., Dolovich, J., Robertson, D. G., and Kerigan, A. T. The late asthmatic responses. *Can. Med. Assoc. J.* **110:**415–421, 1974.
3. Booij-Noord, H., Orie, N. G. M., and de Vries, K. Immediate and late bronchial obstructive reactions to inhalation of house dust and protective effects of disodium cromoglycate and prednisolone. *J. Allergy Clin. Immunol.* **48:**344–354, 1971.
4. Warner, J. O. Significance of late reactions after bronchial challenge with house dust mite. *Arch. Dis. Child.* **51:**905–911, 1976.
5. Cockcroft, D. W., Ruffin, R. E., Dolovich, J., and Hargreave, F. E. Allergen-induced increase in non-allergic bronchial reactivity. *Clin. Allergy* **7:**503–513, 1977.
6. Cartier, A., Thomson, N. C., Frith, P. A., Roberts, R., and Hargreave, F. E. Allergen-induced increase in bronchial responsiveness to histamine: Relationship to the late asthmatic response and change in airway caliber. *J. Allergy Clin. Immunol.* **70:**170–177, 1982.
7. Robertson, D. G., Kerigan, A. T., Hargreave, F. E., Chalmers, R., and Dolovich, H. Late asthmatic responses induced by ragweed pollen allergen. *J. Allergy Clin. Immunol.* **54:**244–254, 1974.
8. Pepys, J. Immunopathology of allergic lung disease. *Clin. Allergy* **3:**1–22, 1973.
9. Shampain, M. P., Behrens, B. L., Larsen, G. L., and Henson, P. M. An animal model of late pulmonary responses to *Alternaria* challenge. *Am. Rev. Respir. Dis.* **126:**493–498, 1982.
10. Dolovich, J., Hargreave, F. E., Chalmers, R., Shier, K. J., Gauldie, J., and Bienenstock, J. Late cutaneous allergic responses in isolated IgE-dependent reactions. *J. Allergy Clin. Immunol.* **52:**38–46, 1973.

11. Solley, G. O., Gleich, G. J., Jordan, R. E., and Schroeter, A. L. The late phase of the immediate wheal and flare skin reaction. Its dependence upon IgE antibodies. *J. Clin. Invest.* **58**:408–420, 1976.
12. Zvaifler, N. J., and Robinson, J. O. Rabbit homocytotropic antibody. A unique rabbit immunoglobulin analogous to human IgE. *J. Exp. Med.* **130**:907–929, 1969.
13. Ishizaka, K., Ishizaka, T., and Hornbrook, M. M. A unique rabbit immunoglobulin having homocytotropic antibody activity. *Immunochemistry* **7**:515–528, 1970.
14. Pinckard, R. N., Halonen, M., and Meng, A. L. Preferential expression of anti-bovine serum albumin IgE homocytotropic antibody synthesis and anaphylactic sensitivity in the neonatal rabbit. *J. Allergy Clin. Immunol.* **49**:301–310, 1972.
15. Halonen, M., Fisher, H. K., Blair, C., Butler, C., and Pinckard, R. N. IgE-induced respiratory and circulatory changes during systemic anaphylaxis in the rabbit. *Am. Rev. Respir. Dis.* **114**:961–970, 1976.
16. von Neergaard, K., and Wirz, K. Uber eine methode zur messung der lungenel astizitat am lebenden menschen, inbesondere beim emphysim. *Z. Klin. Med.* **105**:35–50, 1927.
17. Mead, J., and Whittenberger, J. L. Physical properties of human lungs measured during spontaneous respiration. *J. Appl. Physiol.* **5**:779–796, 1953.
18. Mercer, T. T., Goddard, R. F., and Flores, R. L. Output characteristics of several commercial nebulizers. *Ann. Allergy* **23**:314–326, 1965.
19. Behrens, B. L., Marsh, W. R., Henson, P. M., and Larsen, G. L. Passive transfer of the late pulmonary response in an animal model: Relationship of immunologic status to pulmonary physiologic changes. *Am. Rev. Respir. Dis.* **127**(2):65 (abstr.), 1983.
20. Pepys, J., and Hutchcroft, B. J. Bronchial provocation tests in etiologic diagnosis and analysis of asthma. *Am. Rev. Respir. Dis.* **112**:829–859, 1975.
21. Atkins, P. C., Norman, M., Weiner, H., and Zweiman, B. Release of neutrophil chemotactic activity during immediate hypersensitivity reactions in humans. *Ann. Intern. Med.* **86**:415–418, 1977.
22. Atkins, P. C., Norman, M. E., and Zweiman, B. Antigen-induced neutrophil chemotactic activity in man. Correlation with bronchospasm and inhibition by disodium cromoglycate. *J. Allergy Clin. Immunol.* **62**:149–155, 1978.
23. Nagy, L., Lee, T. H., and Kay, A. B. Neutrophil chemotactic activity in antigen-induced late asthmatic reactions. *N. Engl. J. Med.* **306**:497–501, 1982.
24. Terral, C., Modat, G., Michel, F. B., and Lalaurie, M. Non-specific intervention of mast cells during the late reaction after bronchial provocation tests. *In* "The Mast Cell: Its Role in Health and Disease" (J. Pepys and A. M. Edwards, eds.), pp. 123–126. Pitman, London, 1979.

DISCUSSION

Johansson: In the light of your studies, could you explain earlier hypotheses on late-phase reactions in allergic bronchopulmonary aspergillosis, which proposed that this was mediated exclusively by IgG antibody and complement activation?

Larsen: The data presented here do not exclude the possibility that pulmonary responses that take hours to develop cannot be Arthus-type reactions. This model only points out that a late asthmatic response with airways obstruction and hyperinflation can be initiated by antigen-specific IgE, in the absence of antigen-specific IgG. The type of pulmonary response that develops after exposure to an agent probably depends on many factors including the nature of the agent, the site in the lung of the challenge, and the immunologic status of the host.

Turner-Warwick: In view of the intense cellular response you have shown in the extremely peripheral airways, have you any information on the extent of penetration of antigen down the bronchial tree?

Larsen: We have not addressed that question in this animal model. We are administering *Alternaria* extract by nebulization, and from published data expect that the mass median diameter of the aerosol is approximately 5–6 μm (T. T. Mercer, R. F. Goddard, and R. L. Flores, *Ann. Allergy* **23**:314, 1965). The histologic changes have been in the airways, and we have not found evidence of an alveolitis on pathology specimens.

Platts-Mills: Dr. Larsen, this is a very nice model. However, I have two questions: First, how much antigen do you think you are using? You nebulize 1 ml of a 1:20 *Alternaria* solution. Assuming that this contains 1 μg/ml of major allergen then you may be using the equivalent of an annual dose in the ragweed system in 2 min. Could you use *Alternaria* spores? Second, do you know the quantitative relationship between your IgG and IgE measurements? I got the impression from your results that the ratio of IgG antibody:IgE antibody might be very high, perhaps more than 1000:1, which is much higher than the ratios found in hay fever even after desensitization. Therefore, I do not think your results on IgG antibody should be taken as a simple model of the mechanisms of desensitization for inhalant allergens.

Larsen: The dose of the antigen delivered in our challenges is indeed high. We have continued to use this dose, however, so that this factor remains constant, since the immunologic make-up of the animals is the variable under study. Now that we have a better understanding of the factors that determine how a rabbit will respond (for instance, the levels of antigen-specific IgE in the blood), we can reduce the dose of antigen used for challenge, especially in rabbits with raised IgE and little or no IgG, which we would predict will have a severe or fatal response. In terms of your statement regarding the difficulty in applying our data to the clinical uses of immunotherapy for asthma, I agree this needs more evaluation before more definitive statements can be made.

Nadel: Did morphologic studies after steroids and cromolyn provide useful information?

Larsen: Morphologic evaluation after pretreatment with steroids or cromolyn have not yet been undertaken with our model. We agree that these are important studies.

Hargreave: With reference to an earlier question, we found that in patients with allergic bronchopulmonary aspergillosis there was no potentiation of the late cutaneous allergic response in patients who had both IgE and IgG antibodies (L. Umemoto, J. Poothullil, J. Dolovich, and F. E. Hargreave, *J. Allergy Clin. Immunol.* **58**:60, 1976).

Flenley: Why don't patients with pneumonia wheeze? They have a large number of polymorphs in their lungs.

Larsen: The lack of wheezing in most patients with pneumonia may relate to the sites in the lung primarily involved in the process. In addition, just having neutrophils in the airways and/or parenchyma of asthmatics may not contribute substantially to acute episodes of wheezing. That is far from clear at this time. The contribution of these cells to a late asthmatic response remains to be determined.

Grant: *Alternaria* may not have been the best fungus to choose for an animal model, since it seldom causes asthma in man. It might have been preferable to use a fungus such as *Aspergillus fumigatus,* which is well known to produce a "dual" reaction in man. Another point is that there was practically no immediate reaction following *Alternaria* provocation, but a very brisk immediate reaction with ragweed—how can that be explained?

Larsen: *Alternaria* has been shown to cause late asthmatic responses in the patients that we care for at our institution, that is, children with steroid-dependent chronic asthma (M. P. Shampain, unpublished observations). In addition, *Alternaria* has been cited in the literature to be a potent inducer of immediate and late skin and asthma responses in allergic patients, as noted and referenced in our initial description of this model (M. P. Shampain, B. L. Behrens, G. L. Larsen, and P. M. Henson, *Am. Rev. Respir. Dis.* **126:**493, 1982).

In response to your second question, if the immediate asthmatic response to *Alternaria* and ragweed is compared in all rabbits studied to date there are probably no significant differences in the magnitude of the response. Each group contained animals who had either a large or small immediate response. This variability is related both to the immunologic status of the animal, which is known at the time of the study, as well as the reactivity of the animals airway which we did not routinely assess.

McFadden: Could you tell us about the rabbits' breathing patterns? Did they change after antigen exposure? The reason that I ask is that your measurements of pulmonary mechanics are flow- and volume-dependent, and if those change, this may influence your results.

Larsen: The rabbits were anesthetized only for a short time for placement of the endotracheal tube, esophageal ballon, and mouth guard. Only when they were fully awake were baseline lung functions assessed. After challenge, during the immediate asthmatic reaction no consistent changes in the rate or pattern of breathing were noted. During the late asthmatic reaction, the more severely affected rabbits would show a decrease in their respiratory rate as their breathing became laboured. I do not know if these rabbits exhibited uniform changes in their depth of respiration. Lung volume measured both plethysmographically or by a gas dilution technique showed an increase from baseline values during the late reaction.

Askenase: Is it the serum IgE that is actually responsible for the transfer? Have you absorbed out with an anti-IgE to make sure? Does 56°C heat treatment of the serum prevent transfer? Is the "blocking" IgG antigen-specific or possibly antiidiotypic?

Larsen: We believe it is antigen-specific IgE in the serum that is responsible for the transfer of the late asthmatic reaction, but we have not removed IgE from serum with an anti-IgE to conclusively demonstrate this point. Heat treatment of serum from immunized rabbits does ablate the homologous passive cutaneous anaphylaxis activity. In addition, when we heated serum that contained antigen-specific IgE in titers that would normally cause a late response, this ablated our ability to transfer the reaction. I agree that it would be helpful to separate IgE from the serum and use that antibody in some passive transfer studies, and these studies are underway. In addition, we have also initiated work to separate antigen-specific IgG from the serum so that we can then address your last question.

Barnes: You showed that the β-agonist did not reverse the late bronchoconstrictor response. Did you investigate whether giving a β-agonist *prior* to challenge prevented the late response?

Larsen: We have only tried to reverse the late asthmatic response with these drugs once the reaction has developed. We agree it is important to study their effect on the late response when they are given before the antigen challenge.

Morley: Did you attempt to modify the IgE response by infusion of nonspecific IgG? I make this comment as it is possible to modify experimental airway obstruction by large doses of IgG.

Larsen: Normal rabbit serum that did not contain antibodies to *Alternaria* was infused into rabbits that had antigen-specific IgE only, and this did not modify the subsequent asthmatic response. We have not infused large quantities of nonspecific IgG into immunized rabbits, however, to answer the precise question you pose.

Platts-Mills: Do you think your results on repeat application suggest a role for antigen persistence in the LAR?

Larsen: We have no data that addresses the fate of the inhaled antigen. This is an interesting possibility which remains to be answered.

Lessof: If you are looking for parallels with human asthma, Tom Platts-Mills has objected that short challenges with high concentrations are rather artificial. Would you consider using your model to study the effects of repeated low-level exposure over a longer period?

Larsen: These are other studies that will be initiated soon. We do not know what the effect of prolonged exposure to lower doses of the antigen will be, but we intend to study the consequences of repeated challenges over a long time period by monitoring lung function, the composition of bronchoalveolar lavage, and lung pathology.

CHAPTER 16

Bronchial Responsiveness and Late Asthmatic Response

FREDERICK E. HARGREAVE

Department of Medicine
St. Joseph's Hospital and McMaster University
Hamilton, Ontario, Canada

JERRY DOLOVICH

Department of Pediatrics
McMaster University Medical Centre
and McMaster University
Hamilton, Ontario, Canada

INTRODUCTION

Inhalation tests have provided many insights into the pathogenesis of asthma. They have permitted identification of a large number of occupational chemical sensitizers such as toluene diisocyanate and plicatic acid (1). Tests with allergens and chemical sensitizers have shown different patterns of response in different people: asthmatic responses designated isolated early, early followed by late (dual), and isolated late have been observed. Tests with chemical mediators (or their analogs), such as histamine and methacholine, have served to quantify bronchial responsiveness to nonallergic (nonspecific, nonsensitizing) stimuli, which correlates closely with the presence and severity of clinical asthma (2). The experimental demonstration of increases in nonallergic responsiveness from inhalation tests with allergens and chemical sensitizers has illustrated the pathogenesis of the induction of asthma. This chapter will focus on recent studies of bronchial responsiveness to histamine or methacholine that

ASTHMA: Physiology,
Immunopharmacology,
and Treatment
THIRD INTERNATIONAL SYMPOSIUM

illustrate relationships among nonallergic responsiveness, clinical features of asthma, and allergen- and chemical-induced responses.

PRECISION IN MEASUREMENT

Precision in measurement is necessary to interpret results accurately in terms of normal or abnormal and the degree of abnormality. It is just as important in clinical practice as in research. Precision is obtained by regulating technical factors that influence the results. For example, in the method of aerosol generation and inhalation that we use (3,4), which was modified from the one introduced by deVries and co-workers (5), aerosol is generated continuously and inhaled through the mouth by tidal breathing. The factors that might influence the response are nebulizer output, particle size, the apparatus between the nebulizer and the mouth, the variability of tidal breathing, and the duration of inhalation. The effect of each of these has been studied (6–9). The factors that *do* influence the response are nebulizer output (6) and duration of inhalation (9), and these are kept constant at 0.13–0.16 ml/min and 2 min, respectively. Normal saline is inhaled first followed by twofold increasing concentrations of histamine acid phosphate or methacholine chloride. The twofold increases allow better quantitation of the response and prevent unnecessarily severe bronchoconstriction. The response is measured by FEV_1 and a dose–response curve is constructed. The results are expressed as the provocation concentration to cause a fall in FEV_1 of 20% (PC_{20}).

The reproducibility of the measurement of PC_{20} is within a twofold concentration difference (4,10–12). Responsiveness to methacholine correlates closely with responsiveness to histamine, usually also within a twofold concentration difference (4,13), and to prostaglandin $F_{2\alpha}$ (14). People with current episodic symptoms of asthma usually have a PC_{20} less than 8 mg/ml (3,4,11,15–17). Bronchial responsiveness has come to be regarded as increased if the PC_{20} is less than 8 mg/ml.

The measurement is influenced by airway caliber. A reduction in airway caliber does favour increased responsiveness insofar as a smaller muscle contraction is needed to effect an equivalent percentage change in flow rates (18,19). In asthma, however, this factor does not seem to be important when responsiveness is only mildly increased. When PC_{20} was related to the baseline FEV_1, expressed as percentage of the best value after inhaled salbutamol (200 μg), the FEV_1 was generally not reduced below values seen in nonasthmatic subjects until the PC_{20} was below ~0.4 mg/ml (15) (Fig. 1). This relationship suggests that bronchial hyperresponsiveness in asthma is an expression of an increase in bronchial smooth

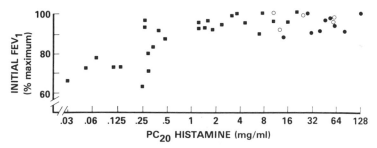

Fig. 1. Relationship between PC_{20} histamine (mg/ml) and initial FEV_1 at the time of the histamine inhalation test. FEV_1 is expressed as a percentage of maximum FEV_1 after inhaled salbutamol (200 μg) measured seven days later. Depicted are 41 subjects; 9 nonasthmatic (●), 5 previous asthmatic (○), and 27 current asthmatic (■). From Ryan *et al.* (15).

muscle responsiveness, and that airway caliber can be an additional factor when responsiveness is moderately to severely increased.

BRONCHIAL RESPONSIVENESS AND ASTHMA

In clinical terms, asthma is still usually defined as a disease characterized by wide variations in resistance, over short periods of time, to flow in the airways of the lungs (20). The wide variations in flow might result from spontaneous bronchoconstriction as with morning dipping, from stimulated bronchoconstriction as with exercise or hyperventilation, or from bronchodilation after treatment with a bronchodilator or corticosteroid. PC_{20} was related to variation in flow rates in this manner: when the PC_{20} was less (the increase in responsiveness was greater), the morning peak flow rate was lower (PFR) (15), the diurnal variation of PFR expressed as the difference between the lowest prebronchodilator and highest postbronchodilator measurement was greater (15) (Fig. 2), the degree of exercise-stimulated bronchoconstriction and lability was greater (21–23), and the response to respiratory heat loss measured by isocapnic hyperventilation of cold dry air also was greater (11,24). The relationships indicated that histamine or methacholine bronchial responsiveness in asthma relates closely to the irritability of bronchial smooth muscle and is an important determinant of morning dipping and exercise-stimulated bronchoconstriction. It is not difficult to appreciate that the effects of endogenous mediators or circulating catecholamines, which probably affect diurnal variations in asthma, may be greater when the bronchial muscle is more responsive.

The level of bronchial responsiveness is also an important determinant of allergen-induced early asthmatic responses (25–27) (Fig. 3). Quantita-

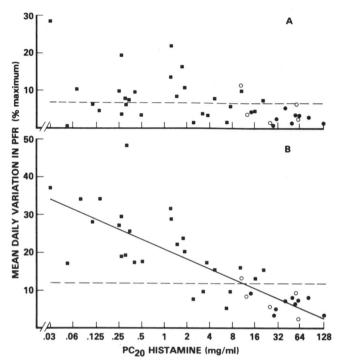

Fig. 2. Relationship between PC_{20} histamine (mg/ml) and variability of PFR during the day. PFR was measured before and after salbutamol (200 μg) at 0600–0800 hr and 1600–1800 hr. Variability was calculated by two methods: (A) the difference between the two PFRs before salbutamol, expressed as a percentage of the higher ($r = -.41$); and (B) the difference between the maximum and minimum of the four PFR results each day, expressed as a percentage of the maximum ($r = -.81$). The horizontal line represents the upper boundary of the 95% confidence interval about the mean of the nonasthmatic subjects; A, 6.7%, and B, 11.8%. Symbols and source as in Fig. 1.

tion of the latter indicates that the PC_{20} and the intensity of the allergic reaction to inhaled allergen are the two main determinants of the early response: the lower the PC_{20}, the less severe the allergic reaction (and presumably the lower the mediator release) required to produce an early asthmatic response of standard severity.

LATE RESPONSES AND INCREASES IN NONALLERGIC BRONCHIAL RESPONSIVENESS

The occurrence of late responses after exposure to sensitizing allergen or chemicals has already been discussed (see Chapter 13, this volume).

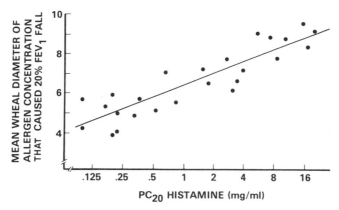

Fig. 3. The relationship between bronchial responsiveness to histamine and the size of the wheal produced by prick tests with the concentration of allergen extract that, when inhaled by tidal breathing for 30 sec, produced a reduction in FEV_1 of 20% or more ($r = -0.91$; $p < .001$). From Hargreave et al. (2).

About 50% of asthmatic people with an early fall in FEV_1 after allergen inhalation also have a late response (28,29). The same dose of the same inhaled allergen in the same person tends to faithfully reproduce the same magnitude of late asthmatic response (28,30,31). Isolated late responses after inhaled allergens are uncommon. In contrast, late asthmatic responses that follow exposure to chemical sensitizers such as plicatic acid frequently occur without a prior early asthmatic response (32).

Late asthmatic responses to allergen and chemical sensitizers are accompanied by increases in nonallergic bronchial responsiveness (32–34) (Fig. 4). Responsiveness might increase from within the normal range into the asthmatic range or might increase further within the asthmatic range. After a single laboratory exposure, the increase in responsiveness might progress over a few days and then persist for days or weeks (34). The magnitude and duration of change in bronchial responsiveness after inhaled allergen relates to the severity of the late response; the more severe the late response, the greater the magnitude and duration of change in PC_{20} (34). When the late response has been particularly severe, it is sometimes followed by recurrent nocturnal asthma (35). This recurrent asthma occurs in association with increases in nonallergic bronchial responsiveness; the recurrent pattern probably results from the fact that the increased responsiveness renders the individual more susceptible to endogenous stimuli with resulting increase in diurnal fluctuation with morning dipping (36).

After experimental laboratory exposure, the responsiveness ultimately returns to baseline. However, in occupational asthma caused by chemical inducers of asthma, cessation of exposure is not always followed by a

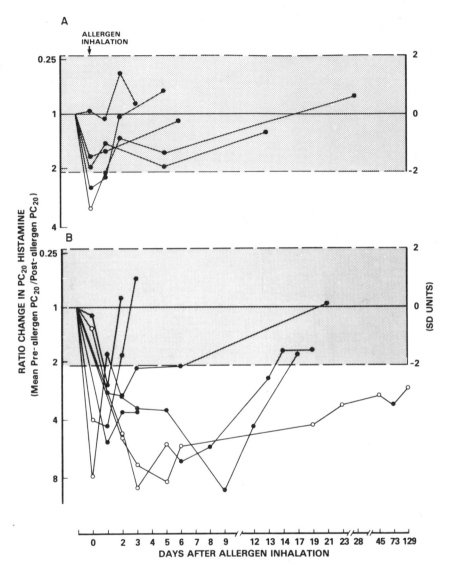

Fig. 4. Changes in PC_{20} histamine after allergen inhalation test (expressed as the mean preallergen PC_{20}/post allergen PC_{20}). (A) Values for subjects with an equivocal allergen-induced late asthmatic response, i.e., a fall in FEV_1 <14% between 3 and 8 hr. (B) Subjects with a definite allergen-induced late asthmatic response, i.e., a fall in FEV_1 >14% between 3 and 8 hr. Shaded areas show the range of variability in $\log_e PC_{20}$ histamine in all subjects before allergen inhalation, expressed with units of the pooled within-subjects standard deviation (1 SD unit = 0.36 on the log scale). Open circles, measurements when FEV_1 was more than 10% below the allergen inhalation baseline value; closed circles, measurements when FEV_1 was within 10% of preallergen inhalation baseline values. From Cartier *et al.* (34).

return to normal in the responsiveness. Moira Chan-Yeung and colleagues followed workers with occupational asthma from western red cedar up to 4 years after they stopped the exposure; one-half of the group persisted with clinical asthma and a low PC_{20} methacholine (37). The persistence of asthma occurred especially in those who had a longer exposure and longer duration of asthma before they left the work. The implication is that the processes involved in late responses are associated with the control of bronchial smooth muscle and that these changes, once induced, may be irreversible.

Late asthmatic responses correlate closely with occupational and seasonal asthma. In occupational asthma, it is uncommon for symptomatic disease to be recognized unless the exposure also elicits late responses (37,38). This may be due to the more common occurrence of late responses, or more likely to the fact that asthma does not progress or become troublesome enough to require attention unless there are late responses and associated increases in nonallergic responsiveness. In keeping with the latter, seasonal asthma caused by ragweed pollen occurred in patients who had greater seasonal changes in responsiveness and experienced dual asthmatic responses in inhalation provocation tests performed out of season (39).

It has been recognized for some time that the severity of the allergic reaction is an important determinant of the late response. In individual subjects, as the dose of antigen and the severity of the early cutaneous or bronchial response increases, the incidence and severity of the late cutaneous (40,41) and late bronchial response, respectively (29,42), increases. However, it has also been recognized that there are differences between subjects in the tendency to develop late responses. For example, one subject may develop a late cutaneous allergic response after only a small early response, while another may require a much larger early wheal (29,42). Similarly, one subject with an early asthmatic response with an FEV_1 fall of 20% may experience no late response while another with the same magnitude of early asthmatic response experiences a severe late asthmatic response (28). Subjects with a greater tendency to develop late cutaneous responses to an antigen also express this tendency in the airways, suggesting a host characteristic common to skin and airways (43) (Fig. 5).

One important characteristic is the level of IgE antibodies. People with higher levels of antibody develop late skin and bronchial responses more readily (28,43,44). Prospective studies now demonstrate that it is generally asthmatics with the highest levels of ragweed-specific IgE antibodies who develop ragweed seasonal asthma (39). Presumably, higher quantities of specific antibodies on mast cells, or perhaps on other cells such as

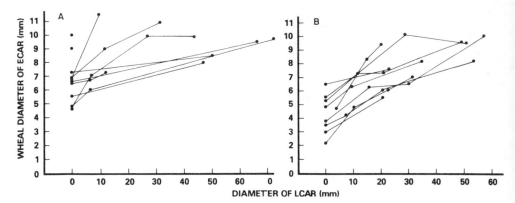

Fig. 5. Results of prick skin tests with allergen extract in persons in whom an allergen inhalation test was followed by an isolated early asthmatic response (A) and dual asthmatic response (B). Wheal diameter of early cutaneous allergic response (ECAR) is plotted against diameter of late cutaneous allergic response (LCAR). The wheal diameters that progressed to late responses were smaller in persons who had dual asthmatic responses. From Clin Allergy, in press.

macrophages, alter the characteristics of kinetics of antigen-stimulated mediator release to create the conditions required for late responses. The level of nonallergic bronchial responsiveness itself is not an important determinant of late asthmatic responses (25,31,45). Late responses to

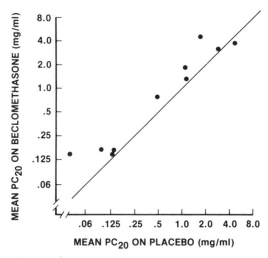

Fig. 6. Mean PC_{20} histamine after 4 weeks treatment with placebo plotted against PC_{20} after 4 weeks of beclomethasone. Unbroken line is the line of identity. A shift to the left indicates a reduction in the level of bronchial hyperresponsiveness. From Ryan et al. (48).

inhaled allergen can occur in asthmatics who have normal bronchial responsiveness as well as those with a severe increase in responsiveness.

The mechanisms that elicit the increase in bronchial responsiveness after late responses are unclear. The measured increases in responsiveness may be partly a function of decreases in airway caliber. However, this is not entirely responsible, since increased responsiveness persists when airflow rates have returned to baseline levels (34,46). Neither does it seem to result from a change in cholinergic function and an increase in reflex bronchoconstriction. Boulet and co-workers measured the effects of a large doses of atropine sulphate on the response to histamine before and after allergen exposure (45). When histamine responsiveness was increased, the effect of atropine on the response to histamine was unchanged; if reflex bronchoconstriction was responsible one would expect the effect of atropine to have been greater.

EPISODIC AND PERSISTING HYPERRESPONSIVENESS

Brief exposure to allergen or chemical inducers of asthma such as toluene diisocyanate or plicatic acid can initiate hyperresponsiveness, which can return to normal when the exposure is discontinued (33,34,37,47). There is asthma at the time of the bronchial injury, but it then subsides.

In contrast, the long-term asthmatic has a persisting increase in bronchial hyperresponsiveness. In some of these, blood eosinophilia, sputum with an excess of eosinophils or lack of complete reversibility of airflow obstruction without treatment with corticosteroids, suggests an ongoing inflammatory reaction. In others, however, there are none of these additional features, but there is an increase in responsiveness with episodic spontaneous or stimulated bronchoconstriction being completely reversed by a bronchodilator. We recently used a group of such subjects in a double-blind cross-over study to compare the effect on bronchial responsiveness of 4 weeks of inhaled beclomethasone dipropianate (400 μg daily) treatment with that of a placebo (48). The subjects had a range of increased responsiveness from mild to severe and a normal or near-normal FEV_1. There was a small but significant improvement in PC_{20} histamine, which was associated with a small nonsignificant improvement in FEV_1 (Fig. 6). The improvement was maximal at the end of the first week and the PC_{20} was then stable. Our interpretation is that there was a component of continuing inflammation that was reversed in the first week, but this failed to explain the continuing hyperresponsiveness. The correction of persisting hyperresponsiveness by any long-term treatment is a key objective as yet unachieved or at least unproved.

CONCLUSION

Current episodic chest tightness, wheezing, or dyspnea in asthma is generally associated with an increase in bronchial responsiveness to chemical mediators. The level of bronchial responsiveness relates closely to the degree of variable airflow obstruction caused by smooth muscle constriction and dilatation. There is evidence that increased responsiveness can be turned on episodically or permanently by inhalation of allergens or chemical inducers of asthma and that this is associated with late asthmatic responses. One determinant of the occurrence of allergen-induced late asthmatic responses seems to be the level of specific IgE antibodies. If these are high, inhaled antigen is likely to elicit a late response and an increase in bronchial responsiveness. The induced increase in responsiveness does not appear to be attributable either to a decrease in airway caliber or an increase in reflex bronchoconstriction. It may be the result of local inflammation. However, established continuing bronchial hyperresponsiveness in asthma cannot as yet be ascribed to continuing inflammation. The mechanisms underlying this chronicity of persisting hyperresponsiveness remain unknown, and pharmacological reversal remains a major therapeutic goal.

REFERENCES

1. Pepys, J., and Hutchcroft, B. J. Bronchial provocation tests in the etiologic diagnosis and analysis of asthma. *Am. Rev. Respir. Dis.* **112:**829–859, 1975.
2. Hargreave, F. E., Ryan, G., Thomson, N. C., O'Byrne, P. M., Latimer, K., Juniper, E. F., and Dolovich, J. Bronchial responsiveness to histamine or methacholine in asthma: Measurement and clinical significance. *J. Allergy Clin. Immunol.* **68:**347–355, 1981.
3. Cockcroft, D. W., Killian, D. N., Mellon, J. J. A., and Hargreave, F. E. Bronchial reactivity to inhaled histamine: A method and clinical survey. *Clin. Allergy* **7:**235–243, 1977.
4. Juniper, E. F., Frith, P. A., Dunnett, C., Cockcroft, D. W., and Hargreave, F. E. Reproducibility and comparison of responses to inhaled histamine and methacholine. *Thorax* **33:**705–710, 1978.
5. deVries, S. K., Goei, J. T., Booy-Noord, H., and Orie, N. G. M. Changes during 24 hours in the lung function and histamine hyperreactivity of the bronchial tree in asthmatic and chronic bronchitis patients. *Int. Arch. Allergy Appl. Immunol.* **20:**93–101, 1962.
6. Ryan, G., Dolovich, M. B., Obminski, G., Cockcroft, D. W., Juniper, E., Hargreave, F. E., and Newhouse, M. T. Standardization of inhalation provocation tests: influence of nebulizer output, particle size and method of inhalation. *J. Allergy Clin. Immunol.* **67:**156–161, 1981.
7. Juniper, E. F., Syty-Golda, M., and Hargreave, F. E. 1984. Histamine inhalation tests: inhalation of aerosol via a facemask on a valve box with mouthpiece. *Thorax* (in press).

8. Heyder, J., Gebbart, J., Rudolf, G., and Strahlhofen, W. Physical factors determining particle deposition in the human respiratory tract. *J. Aerosol Sci.* **11:**505–515, 1980.
9. Cockcroft, D. W., and Berschied, B. A. Standardization of inhalation provocation tests. Dose vs concentration of histamine. *Chest* **82:**572–575, 1982.
10. Ryan, G., Dolovich, M. B., Roberts, R. S., Frith, P. A., Juniper, E. F., Hargreave, F. E., and Newhouse, M. T. Standardization of inhalation provocation tests: Two techniques of aerosol generation and inhalation compared. *Am. Rev. Respir. Dis.* **123:**195–199, 1981.
11. O'Byrne, P. M., Ryan, G., Morris, M., McCormick, D., Jones, N. L., Morse, J. L. C., and Hargreave, F. E. Asthma induced by cold air and its relation to non-specific bronchial responsiveness to methacholine. *Am. Rev. Respir. Dis.* **125:**281–285, 1982.
12. Dehaut, P., Rachiele, A., Martin, R. R., and Malo, J. L. Histamine dose–response curves in asthmatic: Reproducibility and sensitivity of different indices to assess the response. *Thorax* **38:**516–522, 1983.
13. Salome, C. M., Schoeffel, R. E., and Woolcock, A. J. Comparison of bronchial reactivity to histamine and methacholine in asthmatics. *Clin. Allergy* **10:**541–546, 1980.
14. Thomson, N. C., Roberts, R., Bandouvakis, J., Newball, H., and Hargreave, F. E. Comparison of bronchial responses to prostaglandin $F_{2\alpha}$ and methacholine. *J. Allergy Clin. Immunol.* **68:**392–398, 1981.
15. Ryan, G., Latimer, K. M., Dolovich, J., and Hargreave, F. E. Bronchial responsiveness to histamine: Relationship to diurnal variation of peak flow rate, improvement after bronchodilator and airway calibre. *Thorax* **37:**423–4298, 1982.
16. Cockcroft, D. W., Berscheid, B. A., and Murdock, K. Y. Unimodal distribution of bronchial responsiveness to inhaled histamine in a random human population. *Chest* **83:**751–754, 1983.
17. Malo, J. L., Pineau, L., Cartier, A., and Martin, R. R. Reference values of the provocative concentrations of methacholine that cause 6% and 20% changes in forced expired volume in one second in a normal population. *Am. Rev. Respir. Dis.* **128:**8–11, 1983.
18. Benson, M. K. Bronchial hyperreactivity. *Br. J. Dis. Chest* **69:**227–239, 1975.
19. Tattersfield, A. E. Measurement of bronchial reactivity: A question of interpretation. *Thorax* **36:**561–565, 1981.
20. Scadding, G. A. Definition and clinical categorization. *In* "Bronchial Asthma: Mechanisms and Therapeutics" (E. B. Weiss and M. S. Segal, eds.), pp. 19–30. Little, Brown, and Company, Boston, Massachusetts, 1976.
21. Eggleston, P. A. A comparison of the asthmatic responsiveness of methacholine and exercise. *J. Allergy Clin. Immunol.* **63:**104–110, 1979.
22. Anderton, R. C., Cuff, M. T., Frith, P. A., Cockcroft, D. W., Morse, J. L. C., Jones, N. L., and Hargreave, F. E. Bronchial responsiveness to inhaled histamine and exercise. *J. Allergy Clin. Immunol.* **63:**315–320, 1979.
23. Neijens, H. J., Degenhart, J. H., Raatgeep, R., and Kerrebijn, K. F. The correlation between increased reactivity of the bronchi and of mediator releasing cells in asthma. *Clin. Allergy* **10:**535–539, 1980.
24. Weiss, J. W., Rossing, T. H., McFadden, E. R., Jr., and Ingram, R. H., Jr. Relationship between bronchial responsiveness to hyperventilation with cold air and methacholine in asthma. *J. Allergy Clin. Immunol.* **72:**140–144, 1983.
25. Killian, D., Cockcroft, D. W., Hargreave, F. E., and Dolovich, J. Factors in allergen-induced asthma: Relevance of the intensity of the airways allergic reaction and non-specific bronchial reactivity. *Clin. Allergy* **6:**219–225, 1976.
26. Bryant, D. H., and Burns, M. W. Bronchial histamine reactivity: Its relationship to reactivity in the bronchi to inhaled allergens. *Clin. Allergy* **6:**523–532, 1976.

27. Cockcroft, D. W., Ruffin, R. E., Frith, P. A., Cartier, A., Juniper, E. F., Dolovich, J., and Hargreave, F. E. Determinants of allergen-induced asthma; dose of allergen, circulating IgE antibody concentration and bronchial responsiveness to inhaled histamine. *Am. Rev. Respir. Dis.* **120:**1053–1058, 1979.

28. Robertson, D. G., Kerigan, A. T., Hargreave, F. E., Chalmers, R., and Dolovich, J. Late asthmatic responses induced by ragweed pollen allergen. *J. Allergy Clin. Immunol.* **54:**244–254, 1974.

29. Hargreave, F. E., Dolovich, J., Robertson, D. G., and Kerigan, A. T. The late asthmatic responses. *Can. Med. Assoc. J.* **110:**415–424, 1974.

30. Pepys, J., Chan, M., Hargreave, F. E., and McCarthy, D. S. Inhibitory effects of disodium cromoglycate on allergen inhalation tests. *Lancet* **2:**134–137, 1968.

31. Booij-Noord, H., deVries, K., Sluiter, H. J., and Orie, N. G. M. Late bronchial obstructive reaction to experimental inhalation of house dust extract. *Clin. Allergy* **2:**43–61, 1972.

32. Lam, S., Wong, R., and Yeung, M. Nonspecific bronchial reactivity in occupational asthma. *J. Allergy Clin. Immunol.* **63:**28–34, 1979.

33. Cockcroft, D. W., Ruffin, R. E., Dolovich, J., and Hargreave, F. E. Allergen-induced increase in non-allergic bronchial reactivity. *Allergy* **7:**503–513, 1977.

34. Cartier, A., Thomson, N. C., Frith, P. A., Roberts, R., and Hargreave, F. E. Allergen induced increase in bronchial responsiveness to histamine: Relationship to the late asthmatic response and change in airway caliber. *J. Allergy Clin. Immunol.* **70:**170–177, 1982.

35. Newman Taylor, A. J., Davies, R. J., Hendrick, D. J., and Pepys, J. Recurrent nocturnal asthmatic reactions to bronchial provocation tests. *Clin. Allergy* **9:**213–219, 1979.

36. Cockcroft, D. W., Heppner, V. H., and Werner, G. D. Recurrent nocturnal asthma after bronchoprovocation with Western Red Cedar sawdust: Association with acute increase in non-allergic bronchial responsiveness. *Clin. Allergy* **14:**61–68, 1984.

37. Chan-Yeung, M., Lam, S., and Koerner, S. Clinical features and natural history of occupational asthma due to western red cedar (*Thuja plicata*). *Am. J. Med.* **72:**411–415, 1982.

38. Pepys, J., Hargreave, F. E., Longbottom, J. L., and Faux, J. Allergic reaction of the lungs to enzymes of *Bacillus subtilis*. *Lancet* **1:**1181–1184, 1969.

39. Boulet, L. P., Cartier, A., Thomson, N. C., Roberts, R. S., Dolovich, J., and Hargreave, F. E. Asthma and increases in nonallergic bronchial responsiveness from seasonal pollen exposure. *J. Allergy Clin. Immunol.* **71:**399–406, 1983.

40. Dolovich, J., Hargreave, F. E., Chalmers, R., Shier, K. J., Gauldie, J., and Bienenstock, J. Late cutaneous allergic responses in isolated IgE-dependent reactions. *J. Allergy Clin. Immunol.* **52:**38–46, 1973.

41. Gleich, G. J. The late phase of the immunoglobulin E-mediated reaction: A link between anaphylaxis and common allergic disease? *J. Allergy Clin. Immunol.* **70:**160–169, 1982.

42. Joubert, J. R. Factors related to the induction and measurement of the asthmatic response. *In* "Mechanisms of Airways Obstruction in Human Respiratory Disease" (M. A. de Koch, J. A. Nadel, and C. M. Lewis, eds.), pp. 1015–116. AA Balkema, Cape Town, 1979.

43. Boulet, L.-P., Roberts, R. S., Dolovich, J., and Hargreave, F. E. Prediction of late asthmatic responses to inhaled allergen. *Clin. Allergy* (in press).

44. Zetterström, O. Dual skin test reactions and serum antibodies to subtilisin and *Aspergillus fumigatus* extracts. *Clin. Allergy* **8:**77–91, 1978.

45. Boulet, L.-P., Latimer, K. M., Roberts, R. S., Juniper, E. F., Cockcroft, D. W., Thomson, N. C., Daniel, E. E., and Hargreave, F. E. The effect of atropine on allergen-

induced increases in bronchial responsiveness to histamine. *Am. Rev. Respir. Dis.* (in press).

46. Cockcroft, D. W., Cotton, E. J., and Mink, J. T. Nonspecific bronchial hyperreactivity after exposure to western red cedar. *Am. Rev. Dis.* **119:**505–510, 1979.

47. Hargreave, F. E., Dolovich, J., and Boulet, L.-P. Inhalation Provocation Tests. *Semin. Respir. Med.* **4**(3):224–236, 1983.

48. Ryan, G., Latimer, K. M., Roberts, R. S., and Hargreave, F. E. Effect of beclomethasone diproprionate on bronchial responsiveness to histamine in controlled non-steroid dependent asthma. *J. Allergy Clin. Immunol.* (submitted for publication).

DISCUSSION

Flenley: In an individual patient morning dipping often varies in extent from day to day. Can you relate this to variability in responsiveness? Is there any evidence for a diurnal pattern of bronchial hyperresponsiveness?

Hargreave: In the study I described, the correlation was between the PC_{20} measured during the day and the mean PFR measured on waking for 7 days. The PC_{20} is reproducible from day to day, unless altered by some event such as allergen exposure. It is also reproducible at different times of the day, unless altered by a change in airway calibre (A. Rachiele, J. L. Malo, A. Cartier, H. Ghezzo, and R. R. Martin, *Clin. Respir. Physiol.,* **19:**465–469, 1983.

Schwartz: In atopic subjects without clinically apparent asthma, are PC_{20} values altered?

Hargreave: It is usually normal although it is not uncommon for people with no symptoms of asthma to have a mild increase in bronchial responsiveness. However, in these subjects, one can usually demonstrate other objective evidence of abnormally variable airflow obstruction [E. H. Ramsdale, M. Morris, and F. E. Hargreave, *J. Allergy Clin. Immunol.* **71:**143 (abstr.), 1983].

Kerr: Does exposure to occupational allergens such as Western Red Cedar lead to persisting hyperresponsiveness, as measured by the PC_{20}, even after occupational exposure has ceased?

Hargreave: When exposure is discontinued the PC_{20} can improve and return to normal or remain increased. Symptoms of asthma can continue in the latter (M. Chan-Yeung, S. Lam, and S. Koener, *Am. J. Med.* **72:**411, 1982).

Newman Taylor: In support of the view that those with continuing asthma after avoidance of exposure to the inducing agent were those who have suffered the most airway damage, Chan Yeung found that the most important determinant of persistent airway hyperreactivity in those sensitive to western red cedar was continuing exposure after the development of asthma (M. Chan Yeung, S. Lam, and S. Koner, *Am. J. Med.* **72:**411, 1982). An interesting further discriminating factor was the observation that the more severely affected subjects had dual as opposed to isolated late reactions following exposure.

Do you think that increased airway hyperreactivity in some individuals may be a *determinant* as well as a *consequence* of late asthmatic reactions? I have investigated several patients with occupational asthma (especially to diisocyanates) whose initial response to inhalation testing was increased diurnal variation and in whom late asthmatic reactions were subsequently provoked by concentrations of the inhaled agent that were lower than that which had previously failed to provoke such a response. Also, Chan Yeung has reported that following repeated challenges with western red cedar, the late asthmatic reaction become more severe and that the interval between the immediate and late reactions become shorter

(M. Chan-Yeung, G. M. Barton, L. S. MacLean, and S. Grzybowski, *Am. Rev. Respir. Dis.* **108**:1094, 1973).

Hargreave: In group studies increased responsiveness does not seem to be a determinant for developing late reactions (D. Killian, D. W. Cockcroft, F. E. Hargreave, and J. Dolovich, *Clin. Allergy* **6**:219, 1976). However, I agree, in individual subjects bronchial responsiveness does seem to be a determinant; the greater the increase in responsiveness, the greater the magnitude of the fall in FEV_1 in the late response (F. E. Hargreave, E. H. Ramsdale, and S. O. Pugsley, *Am. Rev. Respir. Dis.*, in press).

Warner: The implications of your studies are that the presence of a late asthmatic reaction is more significant in terms of specific allergy diagnosis than the immediate reaction alone. Have you undertaken challenges using different allergens on the same patient to determine whether the late reaction is allergen or patient specific?

Hargreave: I am unaware of any reports of a comparison of the pattern of asthmatic response to different allergens in the same subject.

Oates: Was the correlation of the IgE level with the dual response based on quantification of the specific allergen used in the challenge?

Hargreave: The correlation is with the level of specific antibodies, not total IgE.

Grant: Is it possible that the nature of the antigen (e.g., fungus, chemical, etc.) rather than the antibody level (IgE or IgG) determines whether the asthmatic response is early only, late only, or "dual"?

Hargreave: I don't think so; they occur with different allergens and also following inhalation of anti-IgE (unpublished observations).

Kaliner: Your studies clearly indicate that human pulmonary late-phase reactions are associated with an increase in airway reactivity. Could you speculate as to the role of late-phase reactions in airway hyperreactivity in asthmatics in general?

Hargreave: Retrospective evidence suggests that when late-phase reactions are produced by allergens or by chemical inducers of asthma such as plicatic acid and isocyanates, a permanent increase in responsiveness and asthma can follow (M. Chan-Yeung, S. Lam, and S. Kaener, *Am. J. Med.* **72**:411, 1982). I believe that most, if not all, asthma is acquired as a result of bronchial inflammation and injury.

Gleich: In an open study we administered heparin by nebulization to see whether this would decrease the severity of severe steroid-dependent asthma. While the pulmonary function studies were not improved, the patients did note a marked reduction in cough, suggesting a lessening of irritability. However, the result could equally have been a placebo effect.

Nadel: It is important to know, in patients whose responsiveness does not change after steroids, whether there is evidence of airway inflammation; e.g., neutrophils, eosinophils and epithelial cell desquamation.

Turner-Warwick: I wonder what sort of asthmatics we are discussing considering that bronchial challenge, to demonstrate late reactions, can only be undertaken on relatively mild asthmatics (for ethical reasons). If you take a group of chronic asthmatics with spontaneous and widely varying airflow limitation over short periods of time, as demonstrated on routine records, will formal test of hyperreactivity provide any further information, or will they all be highly reactive?

Hargreave: In people with asthma, if the FEV_1 is reduced and improves by 20% or more after an inhaled β-agonist, the PC_{20} is likely to be lower than about 0.5 mg/ml; i.e., bronchial responsiveness is moderately to severely increased (G. Ryan, K. M. Latimer, J. Dolovich, and F. E. Hargreave, *Thorax* **37**:288, 1982). In clinical practice measurements are most useful when spirometry is normal and when there is doubt about the diagnosis of asthma or the severity of hyperresponsiveness. In this situation measurement of histamine or methacholine responsiveness is more sensitive than are spirometry and measurement of the diurnal variation of peak flow rates.

Warner: We have not found any correlation between the level of IgE antibody on RAST and the presence or absence of late asthmatic reaction (LAR) on challenge with the same allergen (house dust mite). Furthermore, hyposensitisation therapy while abolishing or reducing the LAR in some patients did not produce a change in IgE antibody level. Price *et al.* (J. F. Price, E. N. Hey, and J. F. Soothill, *Clin. Exp. Immunol.* **47:**587, 1982) undertook bronchial challenges with different allergens in the same patient and found the LARs are not necessarily patient specific—in other words, some had LARs to one allergen and an immediate reaction only to a different allergen.

Clark: Do asthmatics patients with no features of allergy display hyperresponsiveness? If so, this draws attention yet again to the importance of bronchial smooth muscle changes as the basic abnormality.

Hargreave: Nonallergic bronchial responsiveness is increased in people with current episodic symptoms of asthma, whether they are atopic or nonatopic.

Platts-Mills: Have you had an opportunity to see whether short-term or prolonged changes in the PC_{20} for histamine occurs after an antigen challenge that has been blocked with DSCG?

Hargreave: There is one controlled study on the effect of regular treatment during the pollen season [S. Rak, E. Millqvist, and O. Löwenhagen, *J. Allergy Clin. Immunol.* **71:**149 (abstr.), 1983]. Sodium cromoglycate appeared to prevent pollen-induced increase in bronchial responsiveness.

Johansson: I agree with you that it is important to use a methodology with high precision, and your PC_{20} method seems to be excellent. However, what is the influence of irritating substances in the inhaled air on the variation in PC_{20}? For instance, does smoking, perhaps even passive smoking, increase the hyperreactivity in a day-to-day fashion?

Hargreave: I don't think that these acute effects have been studied.

CHAPTER 17

Mediators in Exercise-Induced Asthma

T. H. LEE, O. CROMWELL, T. NAGAKURA, and A. B. KAY

Department of Allergy and Clinical Immunology
Cardiothoracic Institute, Brompton Hospital
London, U.K.

INTRODUCTION

Exercise-induced asthma (EIA) is a manifestation of bronchial hyper-reactivity. The typical pattern of response in a subject with EIA is an initial increase in the FEV_1 during the first few minutes of exercise followed by a fall in the FEV_1 that is maximal 5–10 min after the exercise task is discontinued. After this, lung function slowly returns to baseline over the next 30 min, but it may take as long as 1 hr to revert to preexercise values. Although this clinical association has been recognized for many years, the mechanisms involved in its pathogenesis are still incompletely understood.

RESPIRATORY HEAT EXCHANGE THEORY

Evidence for Theory

Deal and his colleagues have suggested that respiratory heat exchange is the initiating stimulus for EIA (1–3). It was shown that cold air potenti-

ASTHMA: Physiology,
Immunopharmacology,
and Treatment
THIRD INTERNATIONAL SYMPOSIUM

ated EIA and that the severity of the airway obstruction was inversely proportional to the ambient temperature and water content of the inspired gas. It was postulated that EIA was directly related to heat exchange that occurred at the bronchial mucosa. This heat exchange is thought to be due to the vaporization of water, which is necessary for the conditioning of the inspired gas by the airways. However, the mechanism whereby respiratory heat exchange causes airflow obstruction in susceptible individuals was not known.

Evidence against Theory

Although recent work has confirmed that the temperature of the airways decreased during exercise or ISH, it usually returns to resting values within 5 min of discontinuing exercise or the ISH procedure (3,4). Airways obstruction, however, progressively increases over the same period of time and does not resolve for 30 to 60 min (5,6). Furthermore, some asthmatics have an exercise-induced late-phase asthmatic reaction (7,8). These observations indicated that other factors must be sustaining the initiating cold air stimulus in the early reaction and in some instances may cause a late asthmatic response. Mast cell mediators may be one of the major factors contributing to these features of bronchial hyperreactivity.

MEDIATOR THEORY

Previous Evidence for Theory

McNeill and his colleagues suggested that chemical mediators such as histamine and slow-reacting substance of anaphylaxis (SRS-A) may be released in EIA and so contribute to bronchoconstriction (9). The demonstration of a refractory period when exercise was repeated within 2 (5) to 4 (10) hr has often been cited as evidence for the depletion of a mediator(s) from certain cells, presumably mast cells, and that time was required for their regeneration. The observation that drugs that inhibit mast cell degranulation *in vitro,* such as disodium cromoglycate (DSCG) (11), β-adrenergic receptor agonists (12), and diethylcarbamazine (13) could prevent EIA has also been cited as evidence in support of the view that mast cell activation plays a role in EIA.

Evidence against Theory

There are a number of DSCG-like drugs, which are orally absorbed and have potent mast cell-stabilizing properties *in vitro* (14) but are ineffective in preventing EIA. Furthermore, recent work has suggested that DSCG may have other properties including inhibition of phosphodiesterase (15), reduction of mucosal hyperreactivity (16), and suppression of neurological reflex mechanisms (17,18). These observations have cast some doubts on the role of mediators in the pathogenesis of EIA. The demonstration that normal subjects will also bronchoconstrict after inhaling cold air, albeit at levels of ventilation in excess of that achievable in any natural environment, has been cited as evidence against the mediator theory since these subjects have no sensitized mast cells (19). Previous studies on circulating mediator concentrations have been unable to resolve whether mast cell degranulation occurs in EIA because of the difficulties in measuring plasma histamine concentrations.

Mediator Measurements

Histamine is rapidly metabolized in the circulation (20,21), and many of the previous assays used for its detection have been insensitive and also nonspecific for the fluorimetric assay. Many of these problems have been overcome using a modification of the double-isotope radioenzymatic method (22), but the technique is expensive and time consuming. Furthermore, histamine measurements have been criticized on the basis that in some situations they might only reflect the degree of basophilia (23). For all these reasons, a search for another marker of mast cell activation would be more rewarding. The mediator chosen to reflect mast cell degranulation does not have to be the only, or indeed the major, mediator released, rather it has to be stable and easily measurable in the circulation or other body fluids. ECF-A tetra- and oligopeptides (24,25), neutral proteases (26), and heparin proteoglycan have potential as markers of mast cell activation, but this approach is yet to be exploited.

Similarly, PGD_2 and the SRS-A leukotrienes might be altered in diseases associated with mast cell degranulation, and radioimmunoassays for the sulphidopeptide leukotrienes (27) and LTB_4 (28) have been described. Nevertheless, much of the recent information on mast cell activation in asthma has been obtained from studies involving heat-stable, neutrophil chemotactic factor (NCF) (29-39). In an attempt to provide information on whether mast cell activation occurs during EIA, we have been studying the circulating levels of NCF and plasma histamine concentration using a double-isotope radioenzymatic assay (22), which has improved the sensitivity of many of the previously available assays.

Recent Evidence

Using these combined techniques, we have demonstrated the appearance of a heat-stable NCF in the sera of 13 atopic asthmatics after treadmill exercise (40). The peak activity was detected at 10 min, and it had returned to prechallenge values by 1 hr. In contrast, no NCF activity was detected in 7 nonasthmatic individuals performing the same exercise task. The NCF provoked by exercise (NCF[EX]) had the same time course of release as NCF produced by antigen bronchial challenge (NCF[AG]) and closely accompanied the development of airflow obstruction. Histamine inhalation challenge that produced a similar magnitude of airways obstruction did not release NCF, suggesting that the elaboration of NCF was the result of the bronchoconstriction alone. NCF release and EIA were inhibited by inhaled DSCG, as previously reported for antigen bronchial challenge. Physicochemical characterization of NCF[EX] and NCF[AG] indicated that they were very similar or identical with a molecular size of approximately 750,000 daltons, elution from DEAE-Sephacel (pH 7.8) at 0.15 M NaCl, an isoelectric point between pH 6.0 and 6.5, and a susceptibility to inactivation by trypsin and chymotrypsin. In a separate study, we were able to demonstrate that plasma histamine concentrations increased in parallel with the elevation in NCF activity after both exercise and antigen challenge, but not following methacholine inhalation challenge (41). The increase in NCF activity was dependent on the duration of the exercise task, and the prior administration of DSCG inhibited not only the rise in NCF but also the increase in plasma histamine concentrations. These observations have confirmed and expanded the results of other workers, who have also detected significant elevations in the concentrations of plasma histamines during EIA (42–46).

Basophils

A basophilia is the normal response to exercise (47) and it has been suggested that exercise-induced elevations in mediator concentrations may be due to a spontaneous release from the postexercise basophilia (23). However, we demonstrated that although there was a similar postexercise basophilia in asthmatics who wheezed (EIA+) and those patients

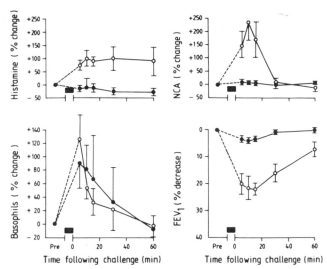

Fig. 1. Percentage changes in plasma histamine, serum NCA, blood basophils, and FEV_1 following treadmill exercise in EIA$^+$ (○) and EIA$^-$ (●) patients. The points represent the mean (±1 SEM) of 13 EIA$^+$ (mean age, 24.7 years; range, 17–35 years) and 7 EIA$^-$ (mean age, 23 years; range, 17–32 years) asthmatics. Following exercise there were significant increases from the baseline preexercise values for histamine and NCA in EIA$^+$ but not EIA$^-$ patients. The degree of significance for the increases in plasma histamine at 5, 10, and 15 min were $p < .025$, $p < .05$ and $p < .05$, respectively. For NCA at 5, 10, and 15 min, these were $p < .05$, $p < .001$, and $p < .005$, respectively. There were also significant rises in blood basophils in EIA$^+$, which at 5 and 10 min were $p < .001$ and $p < .025$, respectively. With EIA$^-$ asthmatics the rise in blood basophil levels was not significant [although with the Wilcoxon rank test, significance was achieved at the 5 min point ($p < .05$)]. When the changes between the EIA$^+$ and EIA$^-$ subjects (in contrast to the change from baseline values in the two groups) were compared, the differences for plasma histamine at 5, 10, and 15 min were $p < .01$, $p < .05$, and $p < .01$, respectively. For NCA at 5 and 10 min, p was <.05 and <.025, respectively. There were no statistically significant differences in basophil counts between the two groups. The mean concentration of histamine before exercise was 0.14 ng/ml (range, 0.05–0.30) in EIA$^+$ and 0.24 ng/ml (range, 0.07–0.41) in EIA$^-$. For NCA, the prechallenge value was 60 neutrophils/10 hpf (range, 15–145) for EIA$^+$ and 73 for EIA$^-$ (range, 24–114). The prechallenge values for basophils were 31 cells/mm^3 for EIA$^+$ (range, 16–50) and 40 cells/mm^3 for EIA$^-$ (range, 10–96). The solid blocks represent the period of exercise and the error bars are the standard error of the mean. The data were analysed using Student's t test.

who did not have EIA (EIA−), mediator release was significantly greater in the EIA+ individuals (Figs. 1 and 2) (48). This finding, taken together with the evidence that DSCG had no effect on mediator release from basophils (49), suggests that these cells are unlikely to be an important source of exercise-induced mediators.

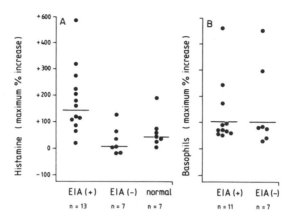

Fig. 2. The maximum percentage increase in plasma histamine levels (A) and basophil (B) counts following treadmill exercise. Blood samples were taken prior to exercise and at 5-, 10-, 15-, 30-, and 60-min intervals after exercise. The maximum increase in plasma histamine in EIA$^+$ patients was significantly different from that in EIA$^-$ asthmatics and normals ($p < .0025$ and $p < .01$, respectively). Changes in basophil counts were not significantly different between the EIA$^+$ and EIA$^-$ groups. Bars represent the geometric means of the groups. Data were analysed using the Mann-Whitney U test.

NONATOPIC ASTHMA

The distinction between atopic and nonatopic asthma has long been emphasized. Mediators of hypersensitivity, which include histamine, leukotrienes, proteases, and chemotactic factors, are believed to play a major role in the development of airways obstruction in atopic subjects. In contrast, it has often been assumed that mast cell mediators do not play an appreciable role in the pathogenesis of nonatopic asthma. However, the difference between these two types of asthma is generally unsatisfactory. Atopic asthmatics may have specific IgE against allergens that bear no clear relationship to the initiation of their symptoms, and there are a number of similar trigger factors, such as exercise, infection, and cold air, which can precipitate an asthmatic attack in both "types" of patients. For these reasons, we have measured circulating mediator concentrations in nonatopic asthmatics during EIA to determine whether there was any evidence of mast cell degranulation in these individuals (50). Our results indicated that nonatopic asthmatics also produced detectable increases in NCF and histamine concentrations during EIA, suggesting that mast cell activation may have occurred in these subjects following exercise and that "sensitized" mast cells are not a prerequisite for mast cell degranulation in EIA.

ASTHMATICS WITHOUT EXERCISE-INDUCED ASTHMA

We had previously shown that there was significant elevation in NCF concentrations in EIA− subjects, although this was substantially less than that in EIA+ individuals (41). At first sight, this would seem to be evidence against the view that mediators play an important role in the pathogenesis of EIA, since mediator release was not accompanied by changes in pulmonary mechanics. However, it must be emphasized that the end organ response is complex and probably depends not only on the concentration of mediators produced, but also on the underlying inflammatory state and the degree of airways reactivity. Hyperreactive airways may respond to a concentration of mediators that has no effect on less reactive bronchi (51–53). It is, therefore, not surprising that some asthmatics, who demonstrate less bronchial reactivity (as evidenced by a lack of EIA), can produce mediators without any detectable airflow limitation.

LATE ASTHMATIC REACTIONS

Since antigen-induced late-phase asthmatic responses are accompanied by elevations in the concentrations of NCF (54) and a rise in NCF also occurred in EIA, we have searched for exercise-induced late reactions. In collaboration with Dr. Yoji Iikura, we have observed exercise-induced late-phase responses in 2 adults and 13 children that were accompanied by elevations in NCF (7). Details of this study are described in Chapter 13 of this volume.

RESPIRATORY HEAT LOSS AND MEDIATOR RELEASE IN EIA

Since RHE is believed to be the initiating stimulus for EIA, we have compared the release of NCF in the same asthmatics, after an identical treadmill exercise task, while inspiring cold/dry (C/D) or warm/humid (W/H) air (55). Mediator release and EIA were only observed after the C/D exercise task and not following exercise whilst breathing fully conditioned air. This suggests that RHE is an important stimulus for bronchoconstriction and the elaboration of mediators. These experiments also indicated that NCF release was not a consequence of the exercise *per se*. Nevertheless, in our patients heat loss from the bronchial mucosa alone was clearly insufficient to produce detectable circulating NCF, as isocap-

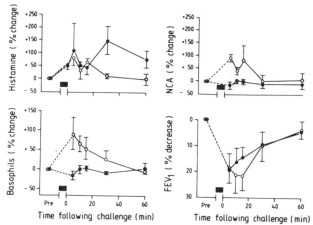

Fig. 3. Percentage changes in plasma histamine, serum NCA, blood basophils, and FEV$_1$ in five patients (mean age, 29 years; range, 19–35 years) who undertook treadmill exercise (○) and isocapnic hyperventilation with cold air (ISH, (●)). Following exercise, there were significant increases from baseline values in histamine at 5 min ($p < .05$), in NCA at 5 min ($p < .05$), and for basophils at 5 and 10 min ($p < .05$ and $p < .05$, respectively). Following ISH, there was a significant elevation in plasma histamine at 30 min ($p < .05$) but not in NCA or basophils. When the changes between exercise and ISH (in contrast to the changes from baseline values in the two groups) were compared, there were significantly greater elevations in plasma histamine at 30 min ($p < .05$) in ISH and significantly higher values for NCA at 5 min ($p < .001$) and basophils at 10 min ($p < .05$) following exercise. The mean concentration of histamine before exercise was 0.11 ng/ml (range, 0.07–0.13) and before ISH, it was 0.10 ng/ml (range, 0.07–0.21). For NCA, the prechallenge mean value was 113 neutrophils/10 hpf (range, 48–153) for exercise and 106 neutrophils/10 hpf (range, 61–170) before ISH. The mean prechallenge values for basophils were 34 cells/mm^3 (range, 22–50) for exercise and 21 cells/mm^3 (range, 15–29) before ISH. The solid blocks represent the periods of exercise or ISH, and the error bars are the standard error of the mean. The data were analysed by Student's t test. The treadmill exercise task and ISH were undertaken as were previously described in detail (48).

nic hyperventilation (ISH) with subfreezing air was not associated with the appearance of this mediator (35,48). Thus, it seems probable that the appearance of NCF in the systemic circulation during EIA was related to the combined stimuli of RHE and exercise. It is possible that ISH released mediators locally in the bronchial mucosa, but that NCF could only be detected in the circulation following exercise. The manner in which exercise facilitates the detection of NCF is unknown, but it may be related to the increased cardiac output of exercise and possible changes in the perfusion of the lungs, which does not occur to the same extent in ISH (56).

This emphasizes that the ability to detect mediators in the systemic circulation depends not only on the concentration of these agents produced locally, but also on the diffusion of these substances into the peri-bronchial circulation and on an adequate blood flow. The suggestion that mediators may be released following ISH would be supported by our preliminary observations that increases in histamine concentrations are detectable after ISH (Fig. 3) and by the observation that antihistamine drugs can cause significant inhibition of ISH-induced asthma (57). Unlike exercise, the elevations in histamine levels in ISH were not accompanied by changes in basophil counts, adding further support to the view that a basophilia is unlikely to be the cause of the changes in histamine concentrations observed during these procedures. A rise in plasma histamine but not NCF after ISH may be related to the fact that histamine is a smaller molecular weight agent than NCF, and may thus gain access into the circulation more easily in this situation, or that the metabolism of histamine and NCF differs after ISH. The mechanism whereby RHE causes mast cell degranulation is unknown. The observation that normal individuals also develop airflow obstruction following ISH (19) suggests that the temperature sensitivity of bronchial mast cells in asthmatics and normals varies only in threshold.

HYPOTHESIS

In an attempt to link clinical features with physiological and experimental findings (55), it is suggested that the hyperventilation associated with exercise leads to RHE and mediator release, and that comparable heat loss with consequent mediator cell activation can also be reproduced by ISH (Fig. 4) (1,2). These mast cell/mediator cell agents may constrict smooth muscle directly or act through reflex mechanisms. The role of mediators in the pathogenesis of EIA may be particularly relevant in those asthmatics in whom the predominant site of airflow obstruction is in the peripheral airways. The EIA in these subjects is inhibited by DSCG but not by anticholinergic agents (58,59), and they tend to have greater bronchial inflammation and higher plasma histamine concentrations (60). The increased bronchial inflammation may interfere with the ability of the mucosa to condition air, thus allowing the cold air stimulus to penetrate further into the intrathoracic airways.

There is another group of asthmatics whose EIA is prevented by the prior administration of either ipratroprium bromide or DSCG (58,59). This suggests that mediators may cause airflow obstruction in these individuals, whose predominant site of airflow obstruction is in the large airways through reflex mechanisms (Fig. 4). Finally there is a small number of

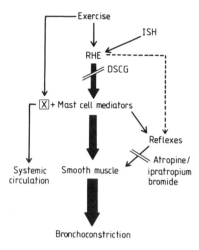

Fig. 4. A hypothesis on the pathogenesis of exercise-induced asthma. DSCG, disodium cromoglycate; //, inhibition by drugs; X, unknown exercise factor. Reproduced by permission of *The Lancet* (55).

asthmatics in which atropine, but not DSCG, inhibited EIA, suggesting that neurological mechanisms may be predominant in the development of bronchoconstriction (61). In this regard, it is important to appreciate that anticholinergic agents may be bronchodilators, thus making it difficult to dissociate the effect of changes in airway geometry from true pharmacological actions. Furthermore, atropine may have other actions, for example, inhibition of mucus secretion (62), an effect on mucociliary transport (63), and even a stabilizing action on the mast cell, which may be important in its efficacy. Therefore, the ability of atropine to block EIA is suggestive but not conclusive evidence of the involvement of a reflex pathway. The presence of such a reflex would be supported by the observation that stimulation of vagal irritant receptors in the upper airways results in bronchoconstriction (64). The mechanism whereby RHE initiates this reflex pathway is not understood, but it may involve changes in bronchial mucosal pH and osmotic gradients (65,66). This hypothesis is supported by the observation that ISH-induced bronchoconstriction, in subjects whose predominant site of airflow obstruction was in the central airways, was inhibited by the prior administration of ipratroprium bromide (67). In contrast, the prior administration of ipratroprium bromide to asthmatics, whose site of obstruction was in the peripheral airways, did not prevent ISH-induced asthma.

REFRACTORY PERIOD

A refractory period after repeated exercise is a characteristic feature of many but not all asthmatics with EIA (5,10). Recent work has shown that there may be two different mechanisms for producing the refractory period (68); 50% of asthmatics made refractory to exercise by repeated running were nonresponsive to a concentration of inhaled allergen, which had previously caused airflow obstruction. This suggests that, although there may be different mechanisms for producing the refractory period, EIA and antigen-induced bronchoconstriction in some patients may share the same final common pathway. This supports the view that, in some subjects, the refractory period may be due to the depletion of mediator stores that need time to replenish. These asthmatics may have the predominant site of airflow obstruction in the peripheral airways, as demonstrated by Wilson et al. (67). Nevertheless, there remains a group of subjects who develop asthma in response to antigen inhalation challenge, despite being made refractory to further EIA. Furthermore, there are asthmatics who can be rendered refractory to further EIA by an initial warm/humid exercise task which causes no RHE. This indicates that there is another mechanism for producing the refractory period apart from mediator depletion, which remains unexplained.

SUMMARY

Elevations in the circulating concentrations of plasma histamine and NCF have been detected during EIA in atopic and nonatopic asthmatics. The changes in mediator concentrations accompanied the development of airflow obstruction and were not observed in normal individuals who undertook an identical exercise task. Although EIA− asthmatics also released mediators after exercise, the increase was significantly less than observed in EIA+ individuals. The elaboration of mediators in susceptible subjects was not due to the treadmill exercise, the postexercise basophilia, or the development of the bronchoconstriction per se; rather it appeared to be caused by respiratory heat exchange resulting from the hyperpnoea of exercise. Since increases in the circulating concentrations of histamine and NCF may reflect mast cell degranulation, these observations suggest that mediators of hypersensitivity are released during EIA and may play a role in its pathogenesis. This view is supported by the observation that the prior administration of DSCG, a mast cell-stabilizing agent, inhibited EIA and mediator release. The demonstration that EIA may have a late-phase response, and the similarity of this to antigen-induced nonimmediate reactions, further implicates the participation of mast cells. Since EIA is a manifestation of bronchial reactivity, these observations may contribute to our understanding of reactive airways disease.

REFERENCES

1. Deal, E. C., Jr., McFadden, E. R., Jr., Ingram, R. H., Jr., and Jaeger, J. J. Hyperpnoea and heat flux: Initial reaction sequence in exercise-induced asthma. *J. Appl. Physiol.* **46:**476–483, 1979.
2. Deal, E. C., Jr., McFadden, E. R., Jr., Ingram, R. H., Jr., Strauss, R. H., and Jaeger, J. J. Role of respiratory heat exchange in production of exercise-induced asthma. *J. Appl. Physiol.* **46:**467–475, 1979.
3. Deal, E. C., Jr., McFadden, E. R., Jr., Ingram, R. H., Jr., and Jaeger, J. J. Esophageal temperature during exercise in asthmatic and non-asthmatic subjects. *J. Appl. Physiol.* **46:**484–490, 1979.
4. McFadden, E. R., Denison, D. M., Waller, J. F., Assoufi, B., Peacock, A., and Sopwith, T. Direct recordings of the temperatures in the tracheobronchial tree in normal man. *J. Clin. Invest.* **69:**700–705, 1982.
5. Haynes, R. L., Ingram, R. H., Jr., and McFadden, E. R., Jr. An assessment of the pulmonary responses to exercise in asthma and an analysis of the factors influencing it. *Am. Rev. Respir. Dis.* **114:**739–752, 1982.
6. Godfrey, S., Silverman, M., and Anderson, S. D. Problems of interpreting exercise-induced asthma. *J. Allergy Clin. Immunol.* **52:**199–209, 1973.
7. Lee, T. H., Nagakura, T., Papageorgiou, N., Iikura, Y., and Kay, A. B. Exercise-induced late asthmatic reactions with neutrophil chemotactic activity. *N. Engl. J. Med.* **308:**1502–1505, 1983.
8. Feldman, C. H., Fox, J., Kraut, E., Feldman, B. R., and Davis, W. J. Exercise-induced asthma (EIA). Treatment for early and late responses. *Am. Rev. Respir. Dis.* **125:**195 (abstr.), 1982.
9. McNeill, R. S., Nairn, J. R., Millar, J. S., and Ingram, C. G. Exercise-induced asthma. *Q. J. Med.* **35:**55–67, 1966.
10. Edmunds, A. T., Tooley, M., and Godfrey, S. The refractory period after exercise-induced asthma: Its duration and relation to the severity of exercise. *Am. Rev. Respir. Dis.* **117:**247–254, 1978.
11. Davies, S. E. Effect of disodium cromoglycate on exercise-induced asthma. *Br. Med. J.* **3:**593–594, 1968.
12. Jones, R. S., Wharton, M. H., and Buston, M. J. The place of physical exercise and bronchodilator drugs in the assessment of the asthmatic child. *Arch. Dis. Child.* **38:**539–545, 1963.
13. Sly, R. M. Effect of diethylcarbamazine pamoate upon exercise-induced bronchospasm. *J. Allergy Clin. Immunol.* **53:**82 (abstr.), 1974.
14. Stokes, T. C., and Morley, J. Prospects for an oral Intal. *Br. J. Dis. Chest* **75:**1–14, 1981.
15. Roy, A. C., and Warren, B. T. Inhibition of cAMP phosphodiesterase by disodium cromoglycate. *Biochem. Pharmacol.* **23:**917–920, 1974.
16. Ryo Ung Yun, K. B., and Townley, R. G. Cromolyn therapy in patients with bronchial asthma. *JAMA, J. Am. Med. Assoc.* **236:**927–931, 1976.
17. Woenne, R., Kottan, M., and Levinson, N. Sodium cromoglycate-induced changes in the dose response curves of inhaled methacholine and histamine in asthmatic children. *Am. Rev. Respir. Dis.* **119:**927–932, 1979.
18. Dixon, M., Jackson, D. M., and Richards, I. M. The action of sodium cromoglycate on 'C' fibre endings in the dog lung. *Br. J. Pharmacol.* **80:**11, 1980.
19. Fanta, C. H., McFadden, E. R., and Ingram, R. H. Effects of cromolyn sodium on the response to respiratory heat loss in normal subjects. *Am. Rev. Respir. Dis.* **123:**161–164, 1981.

20. Beall, G., and Van Arsdell, P. P., Jr. Histamine metabolism in humans. *J. Clin. Invest.* **39:**676–683, 1960.
21. Ind, P. W., Causon, R., and Brown, M. J. A concentration-effect of infused histamine in normal volunteers. *Agents Actions* **12:**12–14, 1982.
22. Brown, M. J., Ind, P. W., Causon, R., and Lee, T. H. A novel double-isotope technique for the enzymatic assay of plasma histamine. Application to estimation of mast cell activation assessed by antigen challenge in asthmatics. *J. Allergy Clin. Immunol.* **69:**20–24, 1982.
23. Howarth, P. H., Pao, G. J.-K., Church, M. K., and Holgate, S. T. The mast cell and basophil in exercise-induced bronchoconstriction. *Thorax* **37:**788 (abstr.), 1982.
24. Kay, A. B., Stechschulte, D., and Austen, K. F. An eosinophil chemotactic factor of anaphylaxis. *J. Exp. Med.* **133:**602–619, 1971.
25. Wasserman, S. I., Austen, K. F., and Soter, N. A. The functional and physicochemical characterisation of three eosinophilotactic activities released into the circulation by cold challenge of patients with cold urticaria. *Clin. Exp. Immunol.* **47:**570–578, 1982.
26. Schwartz, L. B., and Austen, K. F. Acid hydrolases and other enzymes of rat and human mast cell secretory granules. *In* "Biochemistry of the Acute Allergic Reactions" (E. L. Becker, A. S. Simon, and K. F. Austen, eds.), pp. 103–122. Alan R. Liss, Inc., New York, 1981.
27. Levine, L., Magan, R. A., Lewis, R. A., Austen, K. F., Clark, D. A., Marfat, A., and Corey, E. J. Radio-immunoassay of the leukotrienes of SRS-A. *Proc. Natl. Acad. Sci. U.S.A.* **78:**7692–7696, 1981.
28. Lewis, R. A., Mencia-Huerta, J. M., Soberman, R. J., Hoover, D. N., Marfat, A., Corey, E. J., and Austen, K. F. Radioimmunoassay for leukotriene B₄. *Proc. Natl. Acad. Sci. U.S.A.* **79:**7904–7908, 1982.
29. Wasserman, S. I., Soter, N. A., Center, D. M., and Austen, K. F. Cold urticaria. Recognition and characterisation of a neutrophil chemotactic factor, which appears in serum during experimental cold challenge. *J. Clin. Invest.* **60:**180–196, 1977.
30. Atkins, P. C., Norman, M., Weiner, M., and Zweiman, B. Release of neutrophil chemotactic activity during immediate hypersensitivity reactions in humans. *Ann. Intern. Med.* **86:**415–418, 1977.
31. Atkins, P. C., Norman, M., and Zweiman, B. Antigen-induced chemotactic activity in man: Correlation with bronchospasm and inhibition by disodium cromoglycate. *J. Allergy Clin. Immunol.* **62:**149–155, 1978.
32. Atkins, P. C., Zweiman, B., and Rosenblum, F. Further characterisation and biologic activity or ragweed antigen-induced neutrophil chemotactic activity in man. *J. Allergy Clin. Immunol.* **64:**251–258, 1979.
33. Soter, N. A., Wasserman, S. I., Austen, K. F., and McFadden, E. R. Release of mast cell mediators and alterations in lung function in patients with cholinergic urticaria. *N. Engl. J. Med.* **302:**604–608, 1979.
34. Soter, N. A., Wasserman, S. I., Pathak, M. A., Parrish, J. A., and Austen, K. F. Solar urticaria: Release of mass cell mediators into the circulation after experimental challenge. *J. Invest. Dermatol.* **72:**282, 1979.
35. Deal, E. C., Wasserman, S. I., Soter, N. A., Ingram, R. H., and McFadden, E. R. Evaluation of role played by mediators of immediate hypersensitivity in exercise-induced asthma. *J. Clin. Invest.* **65:**659–665, 1980.
36. Martin, G. L., Atkins, P. C., Dunsky, E. H., and Zweiman, B. Effects of theophylline, terbutaline and prednisolone on antigen-induced bronchospasm and mediator release. *J. Allergy Clin. Immunol.* **66:**204–212, 1980.
37. Atkins, P. C., and Zweiman, B. Mediator release in local heat urticaria. *J. Allergy Clin. Immunol.* **68:**286–289, 1981.

38. Nagy, L. Serum neutrophil chemotactic activity and leukocyte count after house dust induced bronchospasm. *Eur. J. Respir. Dis.* **62:**198–203, 1981.

39. Nagy, L. The effect of disodium cromoglycate on serum neutrophil chemotactic activity in antigen-induced bronchospasm. *Allerg. Immunol.* **27:**48–52, 1981.

40. Lee, T. H., Nagy, L., Nagakura, T., Walport, M. J., and Kay, A. B. Identification and partial characterization of an exercise-induced neutrophil chemotactic factor in bronchial asthma. *J. Clin. Invest.* **69:**889–899, 1982.

41. Lee, T. H., Brown, M. J., Nagy, L., Causon, R., Walport, M. J., and Kay, A. B. Exercise-induced release of histamine and neutrophil chemotactic factor in atopic asthmatics. *J. Allergy Clin. Immunol.* **70:**73–81, 1982.

42. Barnes, P. J., and Brown, M. J. Venous plasma histamine in exercise and hyperventilation-induced asthma in man. *Clin. Sci.* **61:**159–162, 1981.

43. Anderson, S. D., Bye, P. T. P., Schoeffel, R. E., Seale, J. P., Taylor, K. M., and Ferris, L. Arterial plasma histamine levels at rest, and during and after exercise in patients with asthma: Effects of Terbutaline aerosol. *Thorax* **36:**259–267, 1981.

44. Ferris, L., Anderson, S. D., and Temple, D. M. Histamine release in exercise-induced asthma. *Br. Med. J.* **1:**1697, 1978.

45. Simon, R. A., Ginsberg, M., Timms, R. M., and Stevenson, D. D. Exercise-induced bronchospasm: A study of plasma mediators. *J. Allergy Clin. Immunol.* **63:**153 (abstr.), 1979.

46. Kerr, R. M., Brach, B. B., Wilson, M. R., Anicetti, V., and Salvaggio, J. E. Change in levels of arterial blood histamine during EIA. *J. Allergy Clin. Immunol.* **63:**153 (abstr.), 1979.

47. Duner, H., and Pernow, B. Histamine and leukocytes in blood during muscular work in man. *Scand. J. Clin. Lab. Invest.* **10:**394–396, 1958.

48. Nagakura, T., Lee, T. H., Assoufi, B. K., Newman-Taylor, A. J., Denison, D. M., and Kay, A. B. Neutrophil chemotactic factor in exercise- and hyperventilation-induced asthma. *Am. Rev. Respir. Dis.* **128:**294–296, 1983.

49. Church, M. K. The role of basophils in asthma. I. Sodium cromoglycate on histamine release and content. *Clin. Allergy* **12:**223–228, 1982.

50. Lee, T. H., Nagakura, T., Cromwell, O., Brown, M. J., Causon, R., and Kay, A. B. Neutrophil chemotactic activity (NCA) and histamine in atopic and nonatopic individuals after exercise-induced asthma. *Am. Rev. Respir. Dis.* **129:**409–412, 1984.

51. Parker, C. D., Bilbo, R. E., and Reed, C. E. Methacholine aerosol as a test for bronchial asthma. *Arch. Intern. Med.* **115:**452–458, 1965.

52. Townley, R. G., Dennis, M., and Itkin, I. H. Comparative action of acetyl-beta methacholine, histamine and pollen antigens in subjects with hay fever and patients with bronchial asthma. *J. Allergy* **36:**121–137, 1965.

53. Juniper, E. F., Frith, P. A., Dunnett, C., Cockcroft, D. W., and Hargreave, F. E. Reproducibility and comparison of responses to inhaled histamine and methacholine. *Thorax* **33:**705–710, 1978.

54. Nagy, L., Lee, T. H., and Kay, A. B. Neutrophil chemotactic activity in antigen-induced late asthmatic reactions. *N. Engl. J. Med.* **306:**497–501, 1982.

55. Lee, T. H., Assoufi, B. K., and Kay, A. B. The link between exercise, respiratory heat exchange, and the mast cell in bronchial asthma. *Lancet* **1:**520–522, 1983.

56. Matalon, S., Dahkoff, N., Nesarajah, M. S., Klocke, F. J., and Fahri, L. E. Effects of hyperventilation on pulmonary blood flow and recirculation time of humans. *J. Appl. Physiol.* **52:**1161–1165, 1982.

57. O'Byrne, P. M., Thomson, N. C., Morris, M., Roberts, R., Daniel, E. E., and Hargreave, F. E. The protective effect of inhaled chlorpheniramine and atropine on bron-

choconstriction stimulated by airway cooling. *Am. Rev. Respir. Dis.* **127**(Suppl.):250, 1983.

58. McFadden, E. R., Ingram, R. H., Haynes, R. L., and Wellman, J. J. Predominant site of flow limitation and mechanisms of post-exertional asthma. *J. Appl. Physiol.* **42**:746–752, 1977.

59. Thomson, N. C., Patel, K. R., and Kerr, J. W. Sodium cromoglycate and ipratropium bromide in exercise-induced asthma. *Thorax* **33**:694–699, 1978.

60. McFadden, E. R., Soter, N. A., and Ingram, R. H. Magnitude and site of airway response to exercise in asthmatics in relation to arterial histamine levels. *J. Allergy Clin. Immunol.* **66**:472, 1980.

61. Godfrey, S., and König, P. Inhibition of exercise-induced asthma by different pharmacological pathways. *Thorax* **31**:137–143, 1976.

62. Richardson, P. S., and Phipps, R. J. The anatomy, physiology, pharmacology and pathology of tracheo-bronchial mucus secretion and the use of expectorant drugs in human disease. *Pharmacol. Ther., Part B* **3**:441–479, 1978.

63. Iravani, J., and Melville, G. N. Mucociliary function in the respiratory tract as influenced by physiochemical factors. *Pharmacol. Ther., Part B* **2**:471–492, 1977.

64. Simmonssen, B. J., Jacobs, F. M., and Nadel, J. A. Role of the autonomic nervous system and the cough reflex in the increased responsiveness of airways in patients with obstructive airways disease. *J. Clin. Invest.* **46**:1812–1818, 1967.

65. Schoeffel, R. E., Anderson, S. D., and Altounyan, R. E. Bronchial hyper-reactivity in response to inhalation of ultrasonically nebulised solutions of distilled water and saline. *Br. Med. J.* **283**:1297–1300, 1981.

66. Anderson, S. D., Schoeffel, R. E., Daviskas, E., and Black, J. L. Exercise-induced asthma (EIA) without airway cooling? *Am. Rev. Respir. Dis.* **127**(Suppl.):228, 1983.

67. Wilson, H. M., Barnes, P. J., Vickers, H., and Silverman, M. Hyperventilation induced asthma—evidence for two mechanisms. *Thorax* **37**:657–662, 1982.

68. Weiller-Ravell, D., and Godfrey, S. Do exercise- and antigen-induced asthma utilise the same pathway? *J. Allergy Clin. Immunol.* **5**:391–397, 1981.

DISCUSSION

Lessof: You suggested that NCF fails to appear in the blood during isocapnic hyperventilation (ISH) because of reduced "washout." How does this tie up with your observation that the very same subjects produced a *greater* rise in blood histamine following ISH than after exercise?

Lee: The difference between the appearance of NCF and histamine in the systemic circulation following ISH is interesting, and it is not easy to explain. Nevertheless, we have speculated that these differences may be related to the much smaller size of histamine, thus facilitating its diffusion into the circulation. Since we do not know the difference, if any, in the metabolism of histamine between ISH and exercise, it is difficult to speculate on other causes for the observed differences.

Oates: Acute changes in the outputs of prostaglandins, which are rapidly metabolized, can best be detected by measuring the levels of proximate metabolites in plasma because of the rapid removal of the prostaglandins themselves. The same is likely to be true of histamine, and changes in histamine clearance may become a function of blood flow to the organ(s) and of clearance, which may change during exercise. Accordingly, measurement of a histamine metabolite might provide a better index of histamine release. This approach also would avoid the problem of *ex vivo* release of histamine from blood basophils.

Flenley: Can you relate the release of NCF to the severity of exercise as assessed by, for instance, minute ventilation, oxygen uptake, and CO_2 output or even cardiac output? More philosophically, do the neutrophils say to the lungs, as it were, "Having got me here, what are you going to do with me?"—in other words, if NCF does contribute to EIA, how does the arrival of neutrophils in the lungs stimulate bronchoconstriction?

Lee: We have not measured minute ventilation, O_2 uptake, and cardiac output. The only dose–response study that we have performed was on asthmatics exercised at 4 mph at a 10–15% incline for 1, 3, and 6 min. We do not want to imply that NCF causes bronchoconstriction. We are using it as a marker for mediator release in these studies.

Wasserman: Changes in plasma histamine noted after various asthma-inducing stimuli may occur both *in vivo* and *ex vivo*, since it may reflect both the number of basophils as well as their intrinsic "releasability." Have you data regarding this latter variable? Have you examined the effect of D_2O upon basophils after such stimuli?

Lee: We have not examined releasability, but Dr. Holgate has done this.

Holgate: We have recently shown a good positive correlation between total blood histamine and plasma histamine levels in normal and asthmatic subjects. We have also demonstrated that basophils in asthmatic subjects have twice the spontaneous release of histamine when measured *in vitro*. This spontaneous releasability is reduced after exercise. (P. H. Howarth, M. K. Church, G. J.-K. Pao, and S. T. Holgate, *J. Allergy Clin. Immunol.*, in press).

Kay: NCA appears to have the potential for causing tissue damage in that it releases enzymes from specific granules of neutrophils and enhances certain neutrophil-mediated cytotoxic reactions. When we have a specific activity, perhaps we can make comparisons with other mediators but until then I think great caution should be exercised in ascribing a cause-and-effect relationship.

Flenley: I respect Professor Kay's proper scientific reticence in equating NCF activity as causally related to EIA but still presume that the major interest of this work to this audience is just that possible relationship. Also, from Dr. Lee's reply I estimate that some of these patients *may* be near their anaerobic threshold, so that *some* (possibly the EIA+) may go over it. Coupled with this is the *possibility* that some (again possibly the EIA+ subjects) may develop modest arterial hypoxaemia on exercise, and this *may* be related to differences in cardiac output or in minute ventilation between EIA+ and EIA–. All of these possibilities could be explored by simple, standard physiological measurements during the exercise.

Lichtenstein: The one thing we do know about histamine is that it is very rapidly cleared. If histamine is infused in amounts which give levels of a few ng/ml and stopped, it is removed from the circulation in less than 2 min. Moreover, experiments with dogs have shown that histamine appears in the blood after antigen challenge very rapidly (<2 min) and is cleared rapidly, that is, it disappears in 10–15 min. Thus it appears to me that you cannot explain the 30–60 min increases in histamine following ISH by clearance problems. There must be continued release. Would you comment?

Lee: Since the rate of catabolism of histamine released locally in the pulmonary tissues is not known, it is still possible that the delay in the appearance of histamine in the circulation is simply due to delayed clearance from the lung into the circulation.

Nadel: In examining the rate of clearance of mediators from tissue to blood, one must consider local blood flow. The release of catecholamines, arachidonic acid, and histamine may modify the appearance of locally released substances into the blood by affecting local blood flow.

Clark: Bronchodilators are effective against EIA but there is debate about their mode of action. One possibility is that they block mediator release, and your study suggests a way of testing this idea. Have you any data on the effects of bronchodilators on histamine and NCA production in EIA?

Lee: This work is being undertaken with Dr. Holgate, and the results are still being analysed.

Dollery: Dr. Philip Ind (in our group) has constructed dose–response curves with intravenous infusions of histamine in man. He was able to show a progressive increase in plasma histamine associated with flushing, a falling diastolic pressure, and this produced a marked systemic response. Thus, increases in plasma histamine associated with a biological response can be measured.

My second point concerns the time course of histamine release. Dr. Hearey in our group has raised wheal and flare responses by injecting antigen into human forearm skin and demonstrated a 10-fold increase (0.1–1.0 ng/μl) in plasma histamine in a draining vein. Histamine release continued (but declined progressively) over an hour. When he and I attempted to match these wheals and flares by injections of histamine, the peak of plasma histamine in the draining vein occurred almost immediately. Thus, the time course of histamine release provoked by antigen was quite different.

Kaplan: An interesting test, given the difference in NCA release with exercise versus ISH, might be to give subcutaneous epinephrine a few minutes before the anticipated increase in mediator release. You could then determine whether a timed increase in cardiac output might allow NCA to appear in the peripheral circulation.

Kaliner: In response to Dr. Dollery's comments, there is quite a difference between measuring histamine in draining venous blood from a local challenge site and measuring it in sustained increases in the system circulation. We infused histamine into humans and recognized that in order to raise plasma histamine systemically, a constant infusion of ~0.1 μg histamine/kg/min is required (M. Kaliner, J. H. Shelhamer, and E. Ottesen, *J. Allergy Clin. Immunol.* **69:**283, 1982). Plasma histamine levels fall to (or below) normal within minutes of stopping histamine infusions. Thus, prolonged increases in plasma histamine indicate an impressive amount of sustained release. By contrast, we have measured plasma histamine after antigen bronchial provocation and found that increases persist only through 30 min and never up to 60 min (P. C. Atkins, P. M. Bedard, B. Zweiman, J. Dyer, and M. Kaliner, *J. Allergy Clin. Immunol.*, **73:**341, 1984). Thus we cannot corroborate your measurements of plasma histamine in humans undergoing ISH.

Morley: Your experimental observations imply that there is an inflammatory response in lung following exercise in some asthmatics. Is there any evidence that exercise in such subjects induces hyperreactivity, and is exercise contraindicated in asthma?

Lee: There is no evidence to suggest that the *early* asthmatic reaction after antigen and exercise is followed by increased reactivity. It would certainly be incorrect to stop asthmatics from exercising until we understand more about mechanisms.

Hargreave: Was the respiratory heat exchange (RHE) the same in your subjects with EIA and those without EIA?

Lee: We did not measure RHE in these subjects.

Gleich: Do patients subjected to exercise demonstrate successive attacks? Or to put the question another way, will the patients become tolerant of exercise? For example, I believe that runners can "run through" an exercise-induced asthmatic episode.

Lee: We have not performed repeated exercise experiments.

Hargreave: The exercise-induced late asthmatic response presented by Dr. Kay seemed to be of a much shorter duration than those recorded after exposure to allergens or chemical sensitizers. They might be produced by a different mechanism in people with a severe increase in bronchial responsiveness, such as diurnal variation.

Lee: We have no data on reactivity in these subjects.

Kay: As Dr. Hargreave said, the exercise-induced late-phase responses were of short duration in the two adults. However, in the children, the time-course pattern was similar to that usually found following allergen challenge.

CHAPTER 18

Airborne Allergen Exposure, Allergen Avoidance, and Bronchial Hyperreactivity

THOMAS A. E. PLATTS-MILLS, E. BRUCE MITCHELL, EUAN R. TOVEY, MARTIN D. CHAPMAN, and SUSAN R. WILKINS

Division of Allergy and Clinical Immunology
Department of Internal Medicine
University of Virginia
Charlottesville, Virginia, U.S.A.
and
Division of Immunology
Clinical Research Centre
Harrow, Middlesex, U.K.

INTRODUCTION

Many patients with asthma will show positive immediate skin tests to inhalant allergens, and in the world, the most common allergen that has been associated with asthma is the dust mite, *Dermatophagoides pteronyssinus* (1,2). Not only do these patients show immediate skin reactions, but when they inhale nebulized dust mite extract in the laboratory, they will develop acute bronchospasm (3,4). This association has been taken by some authors as a direct demonstration that mite allergens are a cause of asthma. On the other hand, there are reasons for doubting the importance of house dust allergens in asthma, even in patients with positive skin tests. The patients are generally not aware that house dust precipitates their attacks of bronchospasm, and they attribute most of their attacks to nonspecific trigger factors, such as exercise, cold air, smoke, and diurnal variations (5,6). This nonspecific bronchial hyperreactivity is clearly a very important feature of asthma, and has been regarded as a constant property of the "asthmatic lung" unrelated to allergens. In addition, it has been pointed out that bronchial provocation often requires a larger quantity of allergen than appears to be present during natural exposure (7).

ASTHMA: Physiology,
Immunopharmacology,
and Treatment
THIRD INTERNATIONAL SYMPOSIUM

297

Because of these doubts, there are many asthma clinics that regard allergens as a relatively minor trigger factor in asthma, and some that do not even carry out skin testing. On the other hand, there are others who find the association between dust mite sensitivity and asthma in school children so striking that they believe that house dust allergens are a major *cause* of asthma (8). In keeping with that belief, some doctors consider that desensitization with house dust and/or housecleaning are major aspects of the treatment for these patients.

We became interested in *Dermatophagoides pteronyssinus* in London simply because a large proportion of the patients in our clinic with asthma, rhinitis, and atopic dermatitis showed strong reactions to this extract. In order to assess the role of dust mites in asthma, we have carried out experiments of two types; the first, to study the allergen and the form in which it becomes airborne in houses (9–11); and the second, to study the effects of prolonged avoidance of dust mites (12). Our results support the view that the striking association between positive skin tests and asthma is not seen because allergens act as a "trigger factor" in asthma but rather because inhaled allergens can make a major contribution to bronchial reactivity.

MITE ALLERGENS

The main problem in purifying allergens from house dust was the extreme complexity of the raw material. As soon as Spieksma and Voorhoorst demonstrated the importance of dust mites, it was only a matter of time before techniques for large-scale culture of *Dermatophagoides farinae* and *D. pteronyssinus* were developed. Initially, cultures were grown on horse dander or human shavings. These extracts contained either horse proteins or human proteins (13). However, by the mid-1970s two approaches had been developed for obtaining mite extracts largely free of culture medium-derived proteins. Some laboratories developed techniques for isolating the mites from culture medium or mite debris. Other laboratories developed techniques for growing mites on modified nonallergenic media. In 1976, we started purifying using whole culture of *D. pteronyssinus* that had been grown on heat-denatured, nonectodermal culture medium of mammalian origin (kindly provided by Bencard, Ltd.).

Using standard techniques to separate proteins and monitoring purification by skin tests, direct RAST, and immunodiffusion, we obtained a partially purified allergen. Although this allergen appeared to be homoge-

TABLE I

**Comparison of the Reported Properties of the Major Allergen from
Dermatophagoides pteronyssinus Purified in Three Different Laboratories[a]**

	Antigen P_1[b]	Dp-42[c]	Dpt 12[d]
SDS–PAGE MW	24,000	25,000–30,000[e]	27,000
Gel filtration MW	<20,000	18,000	—
pI	4.7–7.1	4.6–6.9	5.8–7.0
Assessment of	Skin testing	CRIE[f]	CRIE
major allergen	Antigen-binding RIA	RAST inhibition	RAST
	RAST absorption	Direct RAST	
Source in	Feces and mite	Excrement	Excretory/
mite culture	bodies	fraction	secretion product

[a] Antigen P_1 has been compared directly with both Dp-42 and Dpt 12 by immunodiffusion and shows complete identity.

[b] Chapman and Platts-Mills (9).

[c] Lind *et al.* (16).

[d] Stewart (17).

[e] Different values obtained on separate experiments.

[f] Crossed radioimmunoelectrophoresis.

neous in molecular weight, it showed multiple bands on isoelectric focusing. Subsequent preparative isoelectric focusing demonstrated that a common allergen was present over a very wide pI range of 4.2 to 7.3. This glycoprotein was called *Dermatophagoides* antigen P_1, or antigen P_1. The allergen is very freely soluble, has a molecular weight of 24,000 on SDS, and is present as a major component of the protein in crude aqueous extracts. Indeed, it appeared that antigen P_1 was the single most important protein constituent of *D. pteronyssinus* extract both on SDS and on immunodiffusion (9). These properties are very similar to the physical properties reported for many other inhalant allergens, particularly those from rye grass pollen and ragweed pollen (14,15). By contrast, the amino acid composition of antigen P_1 shows no similarities with those of other allergens (9,14). Since 1980, two other groups have purified the major allergen in *D. pteronyssinus,* and both comparison of properties and direct exchange of reagents confirms that these purifications have all yielded the same protein (Table I). This is of more interest since antigen 42 was purified from a culture grown in Denmark on human dander, while Dpt 12 was separated from mite culture grown on another different medium in Australia. These results left very little doubt that antigen P_1 was, indeed, produced by the mites.

SOURCE OF DUST MITE ALLERGEN

Purified antigen P_1 can be radiolabeled to very high specific activity using the Chloramine T technique. Using the radiolabeled allergen, it was possible to measure anti-mite antibodies using an antigen-binding technique (9,18) and also to develop a sensitive radioimmunoassay (RIA) to measure antigen P_1. This RIA has been used to measure both the allergen content of house dust and also the quantity of allergen in various components of mite culture. Mite cultures contain a variety of mite-derived particles, including live mites, eggs, cuticle, and fecal pellets (Fig. 1). Of these particles, only live mites and fecal pellets contain significant allergen; the mites contain 1.2–3.0 ng antigen P_1 each, and fecal pellets contain 0.1–0.3 ng antigen P_1 each. Examining mite cultures, it was obvious that they contained very large numbers of fecal pellets, and we used two approaches to estimating numbers. First, counting or estimating the number of fecal pellets produced per mite per day, and second, calculating all

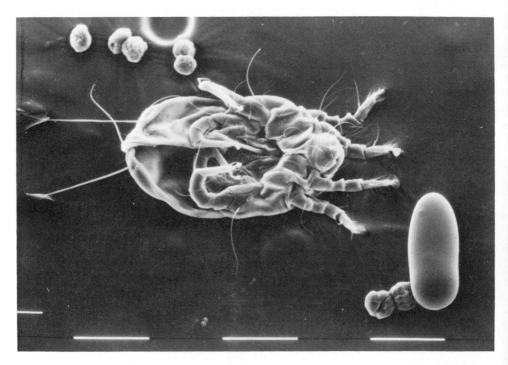

Fig. 1.   Adult *Dermatophagoides pteronyssinus* laid on its back (ventral view) with five fecal particles at the top left and an egg and two fecal particles at bottom right. Bars are 100 μm.

the allergen present in other particles and subtracting. The first technique suggested that >95% of the antigen P_1 accumulated in a culture was in the form of fecal pellets (10). The second calculation suggested that the real figure was lower, but even this lower figure suggested that ~85% of the allergen was in the form of fecal pellets.

Mite feces are well-defined objects. They have a peritrophic membrane, probably made of chitin, which gives them considerable strength. During elution studies, fecal pellets that were kept in saline for 16 hr did not change in shape or size. These elution studies showed that the antigen P_1 in fecal pellets was very rapidly soluble (i.e., 90% eluted in 2 min (10). The average size of fecal pellets is ~20 μm in diameter. It seemed possible that small mites produced particles <10 μm in diameter. When live mites are fixed on their backs, the pellets produced by each animal can be identified and measured. These results showed that even the smallest mites produced particles ~10 μm in diameter (Fig. 2). We concluded that the major form in which mite allergen accumulated in cultures was as spheres of 10–35 μm diameter, which contain ~0.2 ng antigen P_1 in a rapidly soluble form. Interestingly, this quantity of allergen in a sphere of 20 μm diameter represents 10 mg antigen P_1/ml. It should be remembered that the concentrations of this allergen that will give positive intradermal skin tests in allergic patients is ~10^{-4}–10^{-6} μg/ml, while bronchial provocation is often carried out with an extract containing 1 μg antigen P_1/ml.

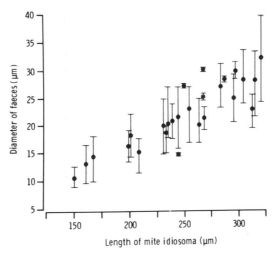

Fig. 2. Correlation between the diameter of fecal particles produced by individual mites (bar indicates the range of values for each mite) and the length of the mite idiosoma ($r = .91$, $p < .001$).

DISTRIBUTION OF DUST MITE ALLERGEN IN HOUSES

Collecting dust samples from different parts of patients' houses showed that antigen P_1 is widely distributed in bedding, mattresses, carpets, furniture, and clothing and demonstrated that the quantities of allergen correlated well with the numbers of *Dermatophagoides pteronyssinus* bodies (11). In English houses, *D. pteronyssinus* is the most important mite; *Euroglyphus maynei* is dominant in a few houses, and *D. farinae* is rare. Air samples from patients' rooms were collected by using a fiberglass filter and a vacuum pump (sampling at 17 liters/min; 1 hr at 17 liters/min = ~1 m^3). In undisturbed bedrooms, airborne allergen was not detected even when sampling for up to 8 hr and even when the filter became dark brown from airborne dust. During vigorous domestic disturbance, such as making beds, vacuum cleaning, etc., as much as 30 ng of antigen P_1 was detected in 30 min (i.e., ~60 ng/m^3). Using a cascade impactor, it was found that >90% of the allergen that became airborne during disturbance was associated with particles that impacted on the first disc (i.e., >10 μm diameter) (Table II) (11). When antiserum to mites was placed in the agar on the discs, it was found that the particles that gave rise to micromancini rings (i.e., contained mite allergen) were mite fecal pellets as judged both from their size and their appearance under electron microscopy (11). The absence of mite allergen in the air of undisturbed rooms, despite the presence of large quantities in bedding, carpets, etc., suggests that the

TABLE II
Airborne Antigen P_1 Collected on a Cascade Impactor in Patients' Houses for Comparison with Nebulized Allergen Extract[a]

Impactor stage	Approximate particle diameter (μm)	Undisturbed bedroom (ng)	Disturbed bedroom (ng)	Mean (%)[b]	Nebulizer (ng)	Mean (%)[c]
1	20–6	<0.3	3.9	<u>88</u>	1	<2
2	15–2	<0.3	0.48	6.7	3.6	10.4
3	5–1	<0.3	<0.3	<2	3.9	11.5
4	2.5–0.3	<0.3	<0.3	<2	17	<u>73.5</u>
Final Filter		<0.3	<0.3	—	<1	<6

[a] Antigen P_1 collected in a layer of 2% agarose on the stages of a cascade impactor was eluted and measured by inhibition radioimmunoassay (11).

[b] Mean value for results during 45 min disturbance in five houses of patients with asthma.

[c] Mean value for two experiments using mite extract nebulized with an acorn nebulizer. Sampled over 10 min and assayed as were the house samples.

allergen-containing particles must be >10 μm in diameter, since particles <5 μm diameter will remain airborne for long periods. After artificial disturbance of dust in the laboratory, the allergen fell very rapidly (Fig. 3). The absence of mite allergen in the air of undisturbed rooms, the particle distribution on the cascade impactor, direct observation of airborne allergen-containing particles, and the rate of fall of allergen after artificial disturbance all lead to the conclusion that antigen P_1 becomes airborne in the form of large particles. These experiments also allow some assessment of a related question, which is, what is the maximum quantity of mite allergen on small particles that could enter the lungs in a house? The highest quantity we have ever observed on the third disc of a cascade impactor was 1.0 ng in 20 min, which contrasts with an estimated ~20–200 ng in similar particles inhaled during 2 min of bronchial provocation. We believe that 1.0 ng in small particles is an overestimate caused by the behavior of the cascade impactor, and that the estimate of <0.3 ng/m^3 from undisturbed rooms may be nearer the truth.

DO CLINICAL SYMPTOMS REFLECT THE PARTICLE SIZE OF INHALED ALLERGENS?

Many asthmatic patients are allergic to cats and cannot enter a house with a cat in it without developing bronchospasm within 20 min. Similarly, people who become allergic to rats often report that they develop bronchospasm within minutes of entering an animal house. In each case, the response of the patients is similar to the response to acute bronchial provocation with nebulized allergen. By contrast, patients who are selectively allergic to dust mites often do not recognize house dust as the major cause of their asthma, and it is most unusual for them to report rapid development of bronchospasm on visiting a particular house. They may associate acute attacks with domestic work, or they may report gradual deterioration after moving the household or visiting a relative. Similarly, asthma occurring in patients with hay fever does not correlate well with pollen counts, and the patients are usually not aware of a direct relationship between pollen exposure and their asthma. As we have shown, mite allergen is not present in the air in small particles, and the bulk of pollen allergen must become airborne as pollen grains. Although some ragweed allergen is present as fragments of pollen grains, this is unlikely to be sufficient to cause bronchospasm (19).

By contrast, significant rat urinary allergen does become and remain airborne in the form of particles <5 μm in diameter (20). It seems likely

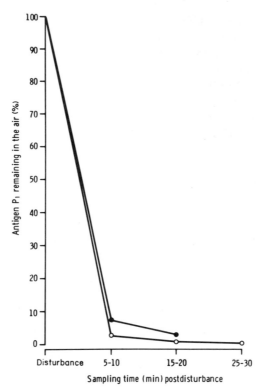

Fig. 3. Falling studies on antigen P_1 in artificially disturbed house dust. Samples were collected using either a filter or a cascade impactor at 17 liters/min. House dust was disturbed in a laboratory room and sampled at various times after disturbance. It is clear from the cascade data that the allergen that was collected on the first disc during disturbance fell very rapidly, since <1% of these particles remained airbourne at 15 min postdisturbance.

Stage	Approximate particle diameter (μm)	Antigen P_1 on stages of cascade impactor (ng)	
		20 min disturbance	15–35 min postdisturbance
1	>20–6	171.0	1.4
2	15–2	13.2	2.0
3	5–1	5.2	0.6
4	2.5–0.3	5.0	0.7
Final filter	<0.5	3.9	1.0

that patients will recognize a direct relationship between allergen exposure and the onset of bronchospasm only if sufficient allergen is airborne in the form of small particles. Many authors in the past have taken the fact that patients are not aware of a direct relationship between mite or pollen exposure and bronchospasm as evidence against a role for these allergens. The alternative explanation is that large particles carrying concentrated allergen contribute to asthma in a way that is not immediately apparent to the patient. There are many well-established occupational causes of asthma in which the patients may not report acute bronchospasm during working hours (21), but nonetheless cessation of exposure leads to improvement and, in some cases, a gradual reduction in bronchial hyperreactivity.

ALLERGEN AVOIDANCE AND BRONCHIAL REACTIVITY

There is a long history of allergen avoidance in asthma. In the early part of this century, it was well known that asthmatic children improved when they went to Switzerland. Storm Van Leeuven developed an allergen-free chamber which was designed to achieve the same results at sea level. In 1929, he reported that 75% of the 400 patients who stayed in the room improved (22), and he concluded that the advantages of Switzerland were largely due to avoidance of airborne particles. The discovery of mites led to increased interest in dust avoidance. Sarsfield *et al.* reported good results by vigorous treatment of bedrooms (i.e., removing carpets, washing all bedding regularly, and covering mattresses) (23). By contrast, most authors found that the advice often given to patients to clean their bedrooms more carefully had little or no effect on symptoms, mite numbers, or allergen levels (24,25). Interestingly, the study of Burr *et al.* used vacuum cleaning of the downstairs room as a placebo treatment (24); the implication being either that mites were only present in the bedroom or that mite exposure was only relevant in the bedroom. Mites and mite allergens can be present throughout a house, and there is no evidence that allergen exposure in the bedroom has any special significance. The bedroom often contains the highest levels of mite allergen, but it is most unlikely that nocturnal asthma is directly caused by exposure at night since it is a common feature of all forms of asthma and often continues after admission to a "mite-free" hospital.

A simple test for bronchial hyperreactivity was first described by Sampter in 1933 (26), and there followed many studies using histamine and methacholine to demonstrate that the lungs of asthmatic patients were nonspecifically sensitive. The first reports suggesting a relationship between bronchial hyperreactivity and allergen exposure come from Tiffeneau in 1955. In 1970, Altounyan reported that patients with "grass pollen asthma" in England, who were hyperreactive to histamine during the pollen season, often lost their hyperreactivity during the following winter (27). An even more striking study was reported the same year on house dust-allergic asthmatic children at a sanatorium in Switzerland. The children showed dramatic falls in bronchial reactivity to histamine when they were tested repeatedly over 1 year (28). However, these authors did not consider the possibility that the improvement was related to avoiding house dust allergens. Several studies have documented falls in bronchial reactivity during weeks or months, after stopping exposure to an industrial allergen (29). In addition, Hargreave and his colleagues have confirmed seasonal changes and demonstrated prolonged increases in nonspecific reactivity following bronchial provocation with allergens (30,31). A recent study has also suggested that vigorous cleaning of the bedrooms of dust-allergic asthmatic children can lead to reduced bronchial reactivity (32).

PROLONGED AVOIDANCE OF HOUSE DUST IN LONDON

Many asthmatic patients in London are strongly skin test-positive to *Dermatophagoides pteronyssinus* and antigen P_1 (18). In order to investigate the effects of prolonged allergen avoidance, we admitted nine of these patients to modified hospital rooms. These rooms were very simple, having no carpets, filtered air, and bedding that was changed every day. The patients were allowed to go out to work or to public places but were instructed to avoid completely houses and domestic animals. In addition, if the patients had positive skin tests to pollens, the studies were carried out over the winter, so that during the study these patients were "avoiding" the inhalant allergens that could be recognized by skin testing. After admission, all the patients improved as judged by peak flow recordings and treatment requirements. Within 1 month, seven of nine had normal or near-normal FEV_1 values and were well enough to undergo repeated histamine provocation. Histamine provocation was carried out at approximately weekly intervals; five of the patients showed a progressive increase of eightfold or greater in the quantity of histamine necessary to cause a 30% fall in FEV_1 (Fig. 4). For the group of seven patients, this increase was highly significant ($p < .005$) (12). In each case this change took many weeks. We would emphasize, first, that all of these patients were on regular treatment prior to admission and that five of seven were

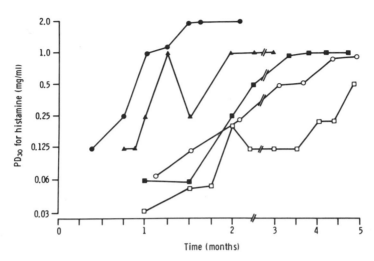

Fig. 4. Time course of changes in bronchial reactivity in patients showing eightfold or greater increase in PD_{30} during prolonged allergen avoidance. Time is given in months after admission. Normal range for PD_{30} histamine in our laboratory is 2.0->8.0 mg/ml. Reprinted from Platts-Mills *et al.* (12), by permission from *The Lancet.*

unfit for bronchial provocation, so that the documented increase in PD_{30} is only the improvement that occurred after their lung function was nearly normal. This is made clear by measurements of FEV_1 taken prior to histamine challenges, which showed no significant change over the period (Fig. 5). Second, these patients were on progressively less treatment so that it is very unlikely that their treatment was responsible for the changes observed. Although we were not able to measure the "total allergen avoidance" achieved by moving patients into hospital rooms, we were able to measure the antigen P_1 concentrations in dust from their houses and in dust from the hospital rooms. The mean level in the houses was 13,600 ng/g (2,552–60,298 SD range) and in the hospital the level was 240 ng/g (100–457 SD range, $p < .001$). This suggests that their exposure to antigen P_1 was <2% of that occurring at home, ignoring the fact that the hospital rooms contained smaller quantities of dust than houses.

IS THERE A RELATIONSHIP BETWEEN PARTICLE SIZE AND BRONCHIAL REACTIVITY?

Both pollen and dust mite allergens are present in the environment in the form of particles that are larger than those which have been tradition-

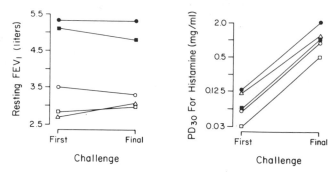

Fig. 5. Relationship between changes in PD_{30} for histamine (B) and prechallenge FEV_1 (A). Data are shown for first and final challenges on the five patients (represented by five symbols) who showed an eightfold or greater increase in PD_{30}.

ally associated with lung diseases. We believe that this finding suggests an alternative explanation of how allergens contribute to asthma. A small proportion of large allergen particles would be expected to enter the lungs, perhaps 5–10% of those inhaled through the mouth (see ref. 2). However, the effect of these particles at one point in the lung could be very marked, because the quantity of allergen in a mite fecal particle or a pollen grain is ~1–10 million times greater than that present in one of the droplets used for bronchial provocation. The patient would probably not be aware of a single event of this kind, although several such particles impacting at the same time might well give rise to bronchospasm. The local inflammation ensuing at the site of impaction would be expected to persist (30) and might well involve a delayed cellular infiltration (33,34,35). Assuming that an inflammatory focus in the lung produced a persistent effect, then repeated episodes (e.g., 5–10 fecal particles or pollen grains per day) could easily produce an accumulating effect on the lung. Thus, an event repeated each day of which the patient was not aware could give rise to bronchial hyperreactivity. The very low quantity of allergen present in each nebulized droplet may explain why it is safe to provoke patients experimentally with such large quantities rapidly. At present, we do not understand the detailed changes involved in bronchial reactivity. We know that these mite-sensitive patients have T cells that proliferate in response to antigen P_1 *in vitro* (36). The range of mediators released from mast cells, T cells, and macrophages, together with increasing awareness of the relationship between immediate hypersensitivity and cutaneous basophil hypersensitivity (33,35), allows considerable speculation about the ways in which a particle carrying very concentrated allergen could contribute to chronic lung changes.

CONCLUSIONS

Our studies support the view that the major contribution of allergens to asthma is their ability to cumulatively increase bronchial reactivity. We also suggest that allergen particles >10 μm in diameter may be peculiarly able to cause the inflammatory foci in the lung that give rise to these persistent changes. If this model is correct, we feel there are three important conclusions: (1) The immunological mechanisms by which allergens contribute to asthma are not restricted to the immediate release of mediators from mast cells or macrophages. (2) The rapid response to bronchial provocation using nebulized allergen extract is not a model of the important contribution of allergens in asthma (30). (3) It should be possible to achieve significant improvement in nonspecific reactivity in many allergic asthmatics by allergen avoidance alone. However, this policy would have to be both vigorous and prolonged.

ADDENDUM

While many of these studies were carried out in England, we have recently assessed a group of house dust-allergic patients in Virginia. Many of these patients were allergic to dust mites as judged by skin tests and serum IgE antibodies. Looking at dust from the houses of 17 dust mite-allergic asthmatics, mites were present in large numbers (~800/g), both *Dermatophagoides farinae* and *D. pteronyssinus*. Using a radioimmunoassay modified to measure allergen derived from both mites, we found allergen levels >10,000 ng antigen P_1/g of fine dust in 16 of the houses. These and similar results obtained in collaboration with Dr. Thomas Smith of Emory University, Atlanta, Georgia, suggest that there are many asthmatic patients in the southeastern United States who are allergic to mites and are exposed to levels of mite allergen similar to those associated with asthma in Europe (11,12,25,37,38).

REFERENCES

1. Voorhorst, R., Spieksma, F. T. M., Varekamp, H., Leupen, M. J., and Lyklema, A. W. The house dust mite (*Dermatophagoides pteronyssinus*) and the allergens it produces. *J. Allergy* **39:**325–339, 1967.

2. Platts-Mills, T. A. E. Type I or immediate hypersensitivity. *In* "Clinical Aspects of Immunology" (P. J. Lachmann and D. K. Peters, eds.), 4th ed., pp. 579–686. Blackwell, Oxford, 1982.
3. Aas, K. Bronchial provocation tests in asthma. *Arch. Dis. Child.* **45:**221–228, 1970.
4. Pepys, J., and Hutchcroft, B. J. Bronchial provocation tests in etiologic diagnosis and analysis asthma. *Am. Rev. Respir. Dis.* **112:**829–859, 1975.
5. Stevenson, D. D., Mathison, D. A., Tan, E. M., and Vaughan, J. H. Provoking factors in bronchial asthma. *Arch. Intern. Med.* **135:**777–783, 1975.
6. Hendrick, D. J., Davies, R. J., D'Souza, M. F., and Pepys, J. An analysis of skin prick test reactions in 656 asthmatic patients. *Thorax* **30:**2–8, 1975.
7. Bruce, C. A., Bias, W. B., Norman, P. S., Lichtenstein, L. M., and Marsh, D. G. Studies of HLA antigen frequencies, IgE levels and specific allergic sensitivities in patients having ragweed hay fever, with or without asthma. *Clin. Exp. Immunol.* **25:**67, 1976.
8. Smith, M. J., Disney, M. E., Williams, J. D., and Goels, Z. A. Clinical significance of skin reactions to mite extracts in children with asthma. *Br. Med. J.* **2:**723–726, 1969.
9. Chapman, M. D., and Platts-Mills, T. A. E. Purification and characterization of the major allergen from *Dermatophagoides pteronyssinus* antigen P_1. *J. Immunol.* **125:**587–592, 1980.
10. Tovey, E. R., Chapman, M. D., and Platts-Mills, T. A. E. Mite faeces are a major source of house dust allergens. *Nature (London)* **289:**592–593, 1981.
11. Tovey, E. R., Chapman, M. D., and Platts-Mills, T. A. E. The distribution of dust mite allergen in the houses of patients with asthma. *Am. Rev. Respir. Dis.* **124:**630–635, 1981.
12. Platts-Mills, T. A. E., Tovey, E. R., Mitchell, E. B., Mozarro, H., Nock, P., and Wilkins, S. R. Reversal of bronchial hyperreactivity during prolonged allergen avoidance. *Lancet* **2:**675–678, 1982.
13. Kawai, T., Marsh, D. G., Lichtenstein, L. H., and Norman, P. S. The allergens responsible for house dust allergy. *J. Allergy Clin. Immunol.* **50:**117–127, 1972.
14. Marsh, D. G. Allergens and the genetics of allergy. *In* "The Antigens" (M. Sela, ed.), Vol. 3, pp. 271–350, Academic Press, New York, 1975.
15. King, T. P. Immunochemical properties of some atopic allergens. *J. Allergy Clin. Immunol.* **64:**159–163, 1979.
16. Lind, P., Korsgaard, J., and Lowenstein, H. Detection and quantitation of Dermatophagoides antigens in house dust by immunochemical techniques. *Allergy* **34:**319–326, 1979.
17. Stewart, G. A. The isolation and characterization of the allergen D.pt 12 from *Dermatophagoides pteronyssinus* by chromatofocussing. *Int. Arch. Allergy Appl. Immunol.* **69:**224–230, 1982.
18. Chapman, M. D., Di Prisco de Fuenmajor, M. C., Pope, F. M., and Platts-Mills, T. A. E. Quantitative assessments of IgG and IgE antibodies to inhalant allergens in patients with atopic dermatitis. *J. Allergy Clin. Immunol.* **73:**27–33, 1983.
19. Busse, W. W., Reed, C. E., and Hoehne, J. H. Demonstration of ragweed antigen in airborne particles smaller than pollen. *J. Allergy Clin. Immunol.* **50:**289–293, 1972.
20. Platts-Mills, T. A. E., Longbottom, J. L., and Wilkins, S. R. Airborne allergens associated with asthma; comparison of dust mite and rat urinary allergens. *J. Allergy Clin. Immunol.* **71:**157, 1983.
21. Karr, R. M., Davies, R. J., Butcher, B. T., Lehrer, S. B., Wilson, M. R., Dharmarajan, V., and Salvaggio, J. E. Occupational asthma. *J. Allergy Clin. Immunol.* **61:**54–65, 1978.
22. Storm Van Leeuwen, W. Asthma and tuberculosis in relation to 'climate allergens.' *Br. Med. J.* **2:**344–347, 1927.

23. Sarsfield, J. K., Gowland, G., Toy, R., and Norman, A. L. Mite sensitive asthma of childhood; trial of avoidance measures. *Arch. Dis. Child.* **49:**716–721, 1974.
24. Burr, M. L., Dean, B. V., Merrett, T. G., Neale, E., St. Leger, A. S., and Verrier-Jones, J. Effects of anti-mite measures on children with mite-sensitive asthma: A controlled trial. *Thorax* **35:**506–512, 1980.
25. Korsgaard, J. Preventive measures in house-dust allergy. *Am. Rev. Respir. Dis.* **125:**80–84, 1982.
26. Sampter, M. Bronchial asthma and histamine sensitivity. *Z. Exp. Med.* **89:**24–35, 1933.
27. Altounyan, R. E. C. Changes in histamine and atropine responsiveness as a guide to diagnosis and evaluation of therapy in obstructive airways disease. *In* "Disodium Chromoglycate in Allergic Airways Disease" (J. Pepys and A. W. Frankland, eds.), pp. 47–53. Butterworth, London, 1970.
28. Kerrebijn, K. F. Endogenous factors in childhood CNSLD. Methodological aspects in population studies. *In* "Bronchitis III" (N. G. M. Orie and R. van der Lende, eds.), pp. 38–48. Royal Vangorcum, Assen, The Netherlands, 1970.
29. Chan-Yeung, M. Fate of occupational asthma. A follow up study of patients with occupational asthma due to western red cedar (Thija Plicata). *Am. Rev. Respir. Dis.* **116:**1023–1029, 1977.
30. Cartier, A., Thomson, N. C., Frith, P. A., Roberts, M., and Hargreave, F. E. Allergen-induced increase in bronchial responsiveness to histamine: relationship to the late asthmatic response and change in airway caliber. *J. Allergy Clin. Immunol.* **70:**170–177, 1982.
31. Boulet, L.-P., Cartier, A., Thomson, N. C., Roberts, R. S., Dolovich, J., and Hargreave, F. E. Asthma and increases in nonallergic bronchial responsiveness from seasonal pollen exposure. *J. Allergy Clin. Immunol.* **71:**399–406, 1983.
32. Murray, A. B., and Ferguson, A. C. Dust-free bedrooms in the treatment of asthmatic children with house dust or house dust mite allergy: A controlled trial. *Pediatrics* **71:**418–422, 1983.
33. Mitchell, E. B., Crow, J., Chapman, M. D., Jouhal, S. S., Pope, F. M., and Platts-Mills, T. A. E. Basophils in allergen-induced patch test sites in atopic dermatitis. *Lancet* **1:**127–130, 1982.
34. Austen, K. F., and Orange, R. P. Bronchial asthma: The possible role of chemical mediators of immediate hypersensitivity on the pathogenesis of subacute chronic disease. *Am. Rev. Respir. Dis.* **112:**423–436, 1975.
35. Mitchell, E. B., Crow, J., Rowntree, S., Webster, A. D. B., and Platts-Mills, T. A. E. Cutaneous basophil hypersensitivity to inhalant allergens: Local transfer of basophil accumulation with immune serum but not IgE antibody. *J. Invest. Dermatol.* (in press), 1984.
36. Rawle, F. C., Mitchell, E. B., and Platts-Mills, T. A. E. T cell responses to the major allergen from the house dust mite *Dermatophagoides pteronyssinus*, Antigen P_1: Comparison of patients with asthma, atopic dermatitis and perennial rhinitis. *J. Immunol.* (in press), 1984.
37. Platts-Mills, T. A. E., Chapman, M. D., Heymann, P. W., Hayden, M. L., and Wilkins, SR. Cross-reacting and noncross-reacting determinants on the major allergen from *D. farinae* and *D. pteronyssinus:* Development of a radioimmunoassay for *Dermatophagoides* derived allergen. (in preparation).
38. Johnson, L. E., Wilkins, S. R., Rawle, F. C., Altman, L. C., Doyle, T., Heymann, P. W., and Platts-Mills, T. A. E. Dust mite allergy; mites and mite allergens in dust from the houses of patients with rhinitis or asthma in Seattle and Charlottesville. *J. Allergy Clin. Immunol.* **73:**119, 1984.

DISCUSSION

Lessof: Your study was a complex one, because you encouraged the patients to take exercise and you took them away from their homes. In occupational asthma, where you have industrial exposure to allergens, you can analyze the effect of changes in work exposure more simply. That lets you look at the cumulative effects on bronchial hyperreactivity that occur with exposure and to look at what happens when the environmental exposure stops. If you abolish exposure for a long period—for example to red cedar, as we heard earlier—you often fail to get a reduction in bronchial reactivity.

Platts-Mills: Our object was to see whether bronchial hyperreactivity in chronic house dust-allergic asthmatics was a reversible phenomenon. Clearly hospital admission involves many different changes, but is none the less the simplest approach to achieving complete or near-complete avoidance of house dust allergens.

McFadden: What therapy were the patients taking during this study? Also, do you have data on the pattern of your patients' airways reactivity? Did it change over time before you used your allergen-free room?

Platts-Mills: On admission all the patients were on continuous treatment with inhaled salbutamol, inhaled cromolyn, and/or beclomethasone dipropionate, as well as long-acting theophylline in two cases. During admission treatment was reduced progressively as the patients improved, so that by the end of the study they were taking the occasional "puffs" of Ventolin or no treatment.

Kay: What was your control group and how did you exclude the effect of regular clinical attendance and possibly better treatment as the cause of improvement in the study group? Also, did any of the patients have allergic conjunctivorhinitis? If so, you could have assessed changes in mucosal sensitivity using the appropriate challenge.

Platts-Mills: To a large degree the patients acted as their own controls, since they were chronically ill and on continuous treatment prior to the study. Furthermore, there is extensive evidence that allergic asthmatic patients who remain at home do not show greater than twofold changes in reactivity to inhaled histamine. I would be surprised if regular clinical attendance would reduce bronchial reactivity, and since all the patients had progressively less pharmacological treatment during the study, I do not think our results could be attributed to "better treatment." We did not carry out any studies on conjunctivorhinitis, as none of the patients continued to have rhinitis while they were in the study.

Gleich: Your presentation could be interpreted as a challenge to the concept of "intrinsic asthma" as used by Rackemann. Would you comment?

Platts-Mills: I do not think our studies are a challenge to the concept of "intrinsic asthma." I would agree with you entirely that there are many patients who have entirely negative skin tests and low serum IgE. My comments are restricted to those patients who have strongly positive skin tests to dust mite extract.

Gleich: I should also point out the studies by Agarwal *et al.* (M. K. Agarwal, J. W. Yunginger, M. C. Swanson, and C. E. Reed, *J. Allergy Clin. Immunol.* **68:**194, 1981) who have shown that amorphous allergens, such as mouse urine-derived allergens, can be measured by collecting the allergens on filters, eluting them from the filters, and finally measuring them by specific radioimmunoassay.

Platts-Mills: I was aware of Dr. Agarwal's studies, and we have similar data on the rat urinary allergen (T. A. E. Platts-Mills, J. L. Longbottom, and S. R. Wilkins, *J. Allergy Clin. Immunol.* **71:**157, 1983).

Flenley: Most of particles of 20-μm diameter will presumably deposit in the nose, in natural breathing. Could this obstruct the nose, by a presumed allergic inflammatory response with mucosal swelling, and thereby lead to a greater chance of deposition of 20-μm particles in the airways? Could this occur, or does deposition in the nose trigger a bronchial constriction, and if so how?

Platts-Mills: Yes, I agree that all particles of this size inhaled into the nose will impact in the nose. I also like the concept that nasal blockage leads to mouth breathing and thus to more particles entering the lung. However, some dust mite-allergic asthmatics do not have blocked noses. Most of the evidence is against any direct reflexes from the nose to the lungs.

Tattersfield: Could you give some more information about the progress of these patients when they left hospital, since this provides a natural experiment of repeat exposure to house dust mite? What happens to children who visit Switzerland when they return home? How long does it take for their asthma to return to its previous level?

Platts-Mills: The subsequent events were very variable, because the patients were "educated" during the admission and changed their rooms. However, none of them had acute trouble on returning home, and several remained relatively unreactive to histamine for several months.

Morley: Might I suggest that your estimate of natural exposure to allergen may be an underestimate, because humans are surrounded by an envelope of warm air that rises by convection so that there is transportation to the mouth and nose from material disturbed by walking or other activities. A realistic estimate requires sampling close to the face of ambulant subjects.

Platts-Mills: Yes, it would be very helpful to do studies with individual monitors for dust allergen exposure.

Warner: I have difficulty persuading my patients to stay in hospital for long periods to do this sort of study, but like many others I have looked at histamine challenge in and out of the pollen season in pure seasonal asthmatics. As expected, there were increases in bronchial reactivity during the season, but surprisingly these changes were less marked than those that occurred after a single grass pollen bronchial challenge in the winter. The significant increases in reactivity in the pollen season occurred predominantly in patients who had had a dual reaction (immediate and late-phase reactions) following bronchial challenge.

Platts-Mills: I would expect to find considerable variation in the relationship between immediate responses to allergen provocation and subsequent prolonged effects. However, I think the general experience is that bronchial provocation can be carried out without risk of severe delayed effects, and I would be surprised if bronchial challenge with threshold dosage of allergen would cause as much effect as a pollen season.

Johansson: Like you, I am fascinated by the extremely low figures for allergen exposure that one can calculate from, for example, the pollen counts. But are these figures really valid for anyone but birds in flight? Could not humans, each time they get close to a grass field or a dusty room, get exposed to doses of allergens 10,000–1,000,000 higher than that calculated from the pollen counts? And if so, is not this short-time/high-dose exposure quite similar to the provocation inhalation test?

Platts-Mills: Yes. I think it possible to be exposed to large numbers of pollen grains or dust particles; inhaling 1000 pollen grains, one would expect more than 100 particles to enter the lung. Under these conditions the number of particles entering the lung is still much lower than bronchial provocation. However, the quantity of allergen, that is, approximately 10 ng, might be close to that used for bronchial provocation and it is not surprising that these patients can sometimes develop acute bronchospasm.

Kay: Was the absence of mites the only difference between your dust-free room and the patient's bedroom? What about temperature, humidity, nocturnal activities, etc.?

Platts-Mills: It would not be simple to control for all the variables that occur during a prolonged admission, but our rooms were designed to allow the patients to lead a "normal" existence during their admission. The temperature would not be different from an average house, while humidity was probably lower.

Hargreave: Natural exposure to large particles like pollen can trigger asthma and increase bronchial responsiveness quickly (L.-P. Boulet, A. Cartier, N. C. Thomson, R. S. Roberts, J. Dolovich, and F. E. Hargreave, *J. Allergy Clin. Immunol.* **71**:399, 1983). The rapidity of onset of asthma will depend on the degree of exposure and the degree of hypersensitivity.

Platts-Mills: Certainly some patients who are exposed to large numbers of pollen grains or large quantities of house dust may report rapid onset of asthma. However, many of these allergic patients are not aware of a direct relationship between their symptoms and allergen exposure.

Clark: The change in reactivity you and others have observed takes many months. Do you have any ideas as to the mechanism to explain this slow recovery?

Platts-Mills: I do not think we have a real answer, but I do not think that immunological mediator release or cellular infiltration could take months to reverse. I think one has to postulate some indirect effect of lymphokines, eosinophil major basic proteins, or mediators on nerves or nerve endings to explain the slow time course of recovery.

CHAPTER 19

Respiratory Heat Exchange and the Asthmatic Response*

E. R. McFADDEN, JR., B. M. PICHURKO, N. A. SOTER,
and E. W. RINGEL

Shipley Institute of Medicine
and Respiratory Diseases Division
Brigham and Women's Hospital
Harvard Medical School
Boston, Massachusetts, U.S.A.

and

I. N. MEFFORD

Department of Chemistry
Boston College
Chestnut Hill, Massachusetts, U.S.A.

INTRODUCTION

Since the Second International Symposium on asthma in 1979, a great deal of progress has been made in our understanding of many aspects of the immunobiology and pathogenesis of this disease. One particular facet of the asthmatic diathesis that has received much attention during this period has been exercise-induced asthma (EIA). Through the efforts of a number of laboratories, it is now appreciated that the development of airway obstruction in this condition results in part from the thermal exchanges that take place within the intrathoracic airways during the heating and humidification of inspired air (1–5). The purpose of the present work is to briefly review what has been learned about this phenomenon and to explore the possible mechanisms by which a fall in airway temperature can induce bronchoconstriction.

* Supported in part by Grants HL 17382 and HL 17873 from the National Heart, Lung and Blood Institute.

ASTHMA: Physiology,
Immunopharmacology,
and Treatment
THIRD INTERNATIONAL SYMPOSIUM

HEAT TRANSFER IN THE RESPIRATORY TRACT

During inspiration, it is generally accepted that the incoming gas is heated and humidified in a coupled fashion so that it is fully saturated with water vapor at body temperature by the time it reaches the alveoli. To accomplish this task, heat and water move from the mucosa to the incoming air as a direct function of the temperature and vapor pressure gradients that exist and as an inverse function of the linear velocity of the gas and the geometry of the exchanging surface. As the temperature of the air rises, its capacity to hold water increases, and it is humidified by evaporation from the airway lining. The process of humidification accounts for the vast majority of the total heat transferred, but it does not warm the air because the thermal energy utilized in generating water vapor remains in latent form until it is released by condensation. The net effect of these thermal exchanges is to cool the mucosa on inspiration so that recovery of heat and water can occur during expiration.

In the expiratory phase of respiration, the air is now warmer than the mucosa, and so as the air leaves the alveoli it gradually undergoes a decrease in temperature and water content as it moves toward the mouth. In normal people during quiet breathing in a typical room, the average temperature of the expired gas exiting the nose or mouth is 32–33°C. Raising the level of ventilation and/or decreasing the temperature of the inspired air causes a marked reduction in expired temperatures, and during exercise in a frigid environment, values in the mid-20s are not unusual (3). This drop in expired temperatures is an important mechanism for the conservation of water, for as the temperature of the gas decreases so does its ability to hold moisture, allowing water condensation back onto the mucosa.

Until recently, it was taught that the heating and humidification of inspired air was a process that did not involve the intrathoracic airways. However, recent data demonstrate that this is not the case. Thermal maps of the airways of normal man have now been constructed for a variety of inspired air conditions during both quiet breathing and periods of hyperventilation (6), and the data from these studies demonstrate that the conditioning of inspired air is a continuous process that begins with the entrance of the air into the body and involves as much of the tracheobronchial tree as necessary to complete the task. During quiet breathing, most of the heating and humidification occurs in the upper airways. However, as the heat-exchanging capacity of the nose and mouth is taxed by lowering the temperature of the air and/or elevating minute ventilation, the point at which the air reaches body conditions progressively moves deeper into the periphery of the lung. During this process, substantial decreases in the temperature of the tracheobronchial tree occur, and when large amounts of frigid air are inhaled, temperatures as low as 19–20°C have been recorded in the trachea; values in the mid-20s are not unusual in the right lower lobe (6,7). Thus, substantial cooling can occur in normal subjects. As yet, there are no data on individuals with asthma.

It is important to emphasize that the ability of the respiratory tract to recover heat and water, thus helping to maintain the body's thermal homeostasis, is based on the degree to which air is cooled during expiration; and this, in turn, is a direct function of how much the temperature of the mucosa decreases during inspiration. Low inspired air temperatures produce greater convective cooling of the mucosa, whereas low humidity causes greater evaporative cooling. With both conditions, increasing ventilation facilitates the mucosal losses. It is easy to appreciate that the most severe degree of airway cooling will occur when frigid, therefore dry, air is inhaled at high-minute ventilation. Thus, it is the temperature and humidity of the climate and the physical activity of the individual that ultimately determine the degree and extent to which the tracheobronchial tree cools. The association between these events and the development of airway obstruction is detailed below.

AIRWAY COOLING AND EIA

The first observation that EIA could be influenced by climatic conditions was published in 1864 by H. H. Salter (8). Salter noted that the obstructive response of asthmatics could be accentuated if they exercised in a cold environment, and he postulated that the "rapid passage of fresh cold air over the bronchial mucous membrane" either stimulated the airways directly or did so indirectly by producing "irritability of the nervous system." The importance of these thoughts went unrecognized for more than a hundred years until Strauss and associates (1) began their studies on the effects of inspired air conditions on the exercise response in asthmatics. Working first with cold air, Strauss *et al.* were able to provide objective confirmation of the qualitative observations of Salter that the combination of a frigid inspirate and exercise increased the obstruction. Subsequently, using a variety of inspired air conditions, a number of investigators (2–5) showed that the severity of the bronchoconstriction that follows exercise could be altered at will be changing the thermal environment in which the challenge was performed. For a fixed minute ventilation, humidification of the inspirate reduces the severity of the response (2,5) while drying and cooling the air increases it (1,3). Consequently, for a given set of inspired air conditions, high levels of ventilation result in greater responses than do low levels (9). Inhaling air preconditioned to body temperature and humidity during exercise prevents the obstruction from developing (2,3,9). Further investigations demonstrated that exercise per se was not an essential ingredient and voluntary hyperventilation was found to produce the exact same mechanical response as exercise when ventilation and inspired air conditions were matched (9,10).

Taken as a group, these studies suggested that the development of airway obstruction could be related to the conditioning of inspired air, and thus, to the local thermal environment within the intrathoracic airways. Analysis of the data in the above investigations from the standpoint of respiratory heat exchange demonstrated that this was indeed the case and that there was a direct relationship between the degree of airway cooling that developed in asthmatics during exercise or hyperventilation and the magnitude of the subsequent bronchoconstriction (3,11). Hence, the phenomenon of EIA can be directly linked to the physiology of heat exchange. The link, however, is a complex one and multiple factors appear to be involved. As soon as exercise or hyperventilation ceases, the airways immediately begin to rewarm and reach their resting temperatures within a few seconds (6); however, the obstruction progressively worsens from the end of exercise until it reaches a peak 5–10 min later, and then slowly abates over the next 30–60 min (12,13). Therefore, airway cooling is only the initiating event; clearly, something else must be happening to sustain the airway response. The nature of the second reaction sequence and the factors influencing it are presently unknown.

STUDIES ON THE PATHOGENESIS OF THE SECOND REACTION SEQUENCE

The mechanism by which airway cooling produces an increase in the resistive work of breathing is currently a matter of intense investigation. The most popular postulate presently is that mediators of immediate hypersensitivity are somehow involved in the process, and three lines of evidence have evolved to support this view. The first is that cromoglycate, a mast cell-stabilizing drug, inhibits EIA, and so mast cells must somehow be involved. The second is that mast cell-associated mediators have been detected in the peripheral circulation in parallel with alterations in pulmonary mechanics in some patients; and the third is the observation that repetitive exercise challenges diminish the intensity of the subsequent obstruction, thus suggesting the consumption of an essential mediator. Taken at face value, the reasoning used to support mast cell involvement appears quite strong. However, close examination of the available data base reveals unexplained difficulties and inconsistencies that limit the uniform acceptance of this theory.

Cromolyn sodium has actions independent of mast cell stabilization, and this factor must be taken into account in interpreting studies using this drug. Cromolyn has been found, to block vagal afferent discharges in the lungs of animals (14) and to blunt sulfur dioxide-induced airway obstruction in both normal and asthmatic people (15,16), yet there is no evidence to suggest that mast cells are involved in either process. Similarly, cromolyn also has been shown to attenuate the changes in mechanics that develop in response to airway cooling in normal subjects who do not have sensitized mast cells in their airways (17). In this latter situation, direct measurements of airway temperature have shown that cromolyn limits the amount of cooling that occurs, perhaps through an effect on the bronchial vasculature (18).

A number of investigators have searched for mediators of immediate hypersensitivity in the peripheral circulation during thermal challenges, with conflicting results. In some studies, the development of EIA has been shown to be associated with elevations of plasma histamine (19—21) and serum neutrophil chemotactic factor (NCF) (21,22); others have failed to confirm these findings (23,24). In several of the investigations showing positive results (19,21,22), the changes observed were quite small, and it has not yet been shown that the mediators present were derived from pulmonary mast cells or that they were causally related to the development of the obstruction. In fact, in one of the positive studies, significant mediator release was observed in asthmatic subjects who did not develop any change in pulmonary mechanics with exercise (21).

In the investigations reported prior to this meeting, none has recorded mediator release with voluntary hyperventilation (19,24,25). Since there are data from one group that indicate that only airway cooling, and not exercise, is essential for the release of NCF (24), the negative findings alluded to above are somewhat puzzling. To explain them, it has been postulated that exercise and isocapnic hyperventilation are different stimuli that have different effects on airway mast cells. However, the hyperpnea of both exercise and voluntary hyperventilation (1) produce the same degree of obstruction when inspired air conditions and ventilations are matched (9,10,21); (2) are modified similarly by various drugs (13,26–30); and (3) produce identical thermal effects throughout the intrathoracic airways (31), thus this thesis does not appear to be very likely. In this context, the paper of Holgate and associates (32) in this symposium is of great importance. In a carefully controlled series of studies, these investigators found variable patterns of mediator release in response to a number of challenges. For example, unlike other investigators, they found a kinetic release of NCF with both exercise and hyperventilation; however, they could not detect histamine with either. Thus, it is probable that there are some as yet undefined factors at work in controlling the appearance, or lack thereof, of mediators in the peripheral circulation during bronchoprovocations, and until they can be identified and controlled, the situation is likely to remain confused.

With respect to the third line of evidence used to support mediator involvement in EIA, it has been recognized for over 20 years that when repetitive bouts of exercise are performed by asthmatics over short periods of time, the severity of the obstructive response diminishes (33–35). This phenomenon is the so-called refractory period, and it has given rise to the notion that a stored mediator that is critical to the reaction is being depleted and needs time for resynthesis (35,36). While this was an attractive explanation when originally formulated, many investigators now believe it to be unsatisfactory for a variety of reasons. For example, there is no evidence that mast cells become depleted of their mediator content with repetitive challenges, and no one has identified a mast cell-associated spasmogen that is critical to the development of the obstructive response. Further, the mediator-depletion hypothesis does not take into account the profound neurohumoral compensations occurring with exercise that are designed to improve pulmonary performance. Since the refractory period has been shown to depend upon the amount of physical exertion a subject performs rather than the degree of bronchoconstriction that develops (36), this could very well be an important omission.

Despite the difficulties in interpretation, the available information about the refractory period suggests that one might be able to make use of this phenomenon to gain some insights into how airway cooling produces obstruction. If the mechanism underlying the loss of response to an exercise stimulus could be uncovered, it might be possible to begin to isolate the factors that influence the development of the airway constriction and so sort out their relative contributions. It might also be possible to clarify the role played by mast cell mediators.

In an effort to achieve these aims, we had a number of asthmatic subjects undergo repetitive challenges on a cycle ergometer under controlled inspired air conditions. Prior to, and at 2-min intervals during and after the first challenge, peak expiratory flow rates (PEFR) were measured and venous blood was drawn. The latter was analyzed for catecholamines, histamine, and NCF activity. Six minutes after completion of the work load, while the subjects were experiencing acute bronchospasm, they were reexercised and the above measurements were repeated. With this protocol, we wished to observe the pattern of change that would develop in pulmonary mechanics and plasma catecholamine levels with repetitive exercise. Equally, we wished to determine if the catecholamine release associated with strenuous physical exertion would act as a form of auto-treatment. If this were the case, then the second exercise challenge should reverse the bronchospasm induced by the first and catecholamines should rise concomitantly. In addition, we hoped to record the kinetics of any mediator of immediate sensitivity that might be released and to determine how repetitive challenges influenced blood levels.

During the performance of the initial challenge, the subjects developed bronchodilatation, which was followed by bronchoconstriction when exercise ceased. Peak flow increased 16% during exercise and then fell 22%, as compared with control values 6 min after the subjects stopped pedaling. During the second challenge, bronchodilatation once again developed, but this time it was of sufficient magnitude to totally resolve the subjects' airway obstruction. Now PEFR rose an average of 43% and reached levels comparable to the values that were present prior to the commencement of the first challenge. When the subjects ceased work the second time, the bronchoconstriction once again recurred.

Preliminary results indicate that the plasma levels of catecholamines paralleled the changes in mechanics. During the first exercise task, norepinephrine rose approximately 40%, and then fell with the cessation of exercise and the onset of bronchoconstriction. When exercise was resumed, the same pattern recurred, but in this circumstance the levels both during and after exercise were substantially higher than in the first challenge. No consistent changes were found with either NCF or histamine.

These results demonstrate that the predominant airway effect of exercise in asthmatics is bronchodilatation, which develops in concert with increases in circulating catecholamine levels. Repeating the exercise challenge causes the plasma levels of norepinephrine to rise even more, thus further enhancing the degree of relaxation. Hence, in a sense repetitive exercise can be thought of as a form of auto-treatment. In addition to their effects on airway smooth muscle, the circulating adrenergic agonists also influence the bronchial vasculature and so could also alter airway cooling and heat exchange. It is not yet known how long the elevated plasma levels persist, but since the pharmacologic action of these agents is known to last for at least 30 min following a single administration, it is likely that they contribute significantly to the development of the refractory period.

The failure to find mediators in the peripheral circulation is disappointing, and so the role that mast cells play in the pathogenesis of the refractory period specifically, and of EIA in general, remains unsettled. While it is possible that mediators were released and we failed to detect them for technical reasons, we believe this to be unlikely because we have found them in other circumstances (25,37). Irrespective of whether mediators are involved or not, it is clear that the postexercise obstructive response in asthmatics derives from an interplay of competing stimuli, and that the application of repetitive challenges may provide a useful model to explore these interactions.

REFERENCES

1. Strauss, R. H., McFadden, E. R., Jr., Ingram, R. H., Jr., and Jaeger, J. J. Enhancement of exercise-induced asthma by cold air breathing. *N. Engl. J. Med.* **297:**743–747, 1977.
2. Strauss, R. H., McFadden, E. R., Jr., Ingram, R. H., Jr., Deal, E. C., Jr., and Jaeger, J. J. Influence of heat and humidity on the airway obstruction induced by exercise in asthma. *J. Clin. Invest.* **61:**433–440, 1978.
3. Deal, E. C., Jr., McFadden, E. R., Jr., Ingram, R. H., Jr., Strauss, R. H., and Jaeger, J. J. The role of respiratory heat exchange in the production of exercise-induced asthma. *J. Appl. Physiol.: Respir., Environ. Exercise Physiol.* **46:**467–475, 1979.
4. Chen, W. Y., and Horton, D. J. Heat and water loss from the airways and exercise-induced asthma. *Respiration* **34:**305–313, 1977.
5. Bar-Or, O., Neuman, I., and Dotan, R. Effects of dry and human climates on exercise-induced asthma in children and pre-adolescents. *J. Allergy Clin. Immunol.* **60:**163–168, 1977.
6. McFadden, E. R., Jr., Pichurko, B. M., Bowman, K. F., Solway, J., Burns, S., Dowling, N., and Ingram, R. H., Jr. Thermal mapping of the airways in man. *Fed. Proc., Fed. Am. Soc. Exp. Biol.* **41:**1357 (abstr.), 1983.
7. McFadden, E. R., Jr., Denison, D. M., Waller, J. F., Assourfi, B., Peacock, A., and Sopwith, T. Direct recordings of the temperatures in the tracheobronchial tree in normal man. *J. Clin. Invest.* **69:**700–705, 1982.
8. Salter, H. H. "On Asthma: Its Pathology and Treatment." Blanchard & Lea, Philadelphia, Pennsylvania, 1864.
9. Deal, E. C., Jr., McFadden, E. R., Jr., Ingram, R. H., Jr., and Jaeger, J. J. Hyperpnea and heat flux. The initial reaction sequence in exercise-induced asthma. *J. Appl. Physiol.: Respir., Environ. Exercise Physiol.* **46:**476–482, 1979.
10. Bungaard, A., Ingemann-Hansen, T., Schmidt, A., Halkjaer-Kristensen, J., and Bloch, I. Influence of temperature and relative humidity of inhaled gas on exercise-induced asthma. *Eur. J. Respir. Dis.* **63:**239–244, 1982.
11. Deal, E. C., Jr., McFadden, E. R., Jr., Ingram, R. H., Jr., and Jaeger, J. J. Observa-

tions on esophageal temperature during exercise in asthmatic and non-asthmatic subjects. *J. Appl. Physiol.: Respir., Environ. Exercise Physiol.* **46**:484–490, 1979.

12. Godfrey, S. Exercise-induced asthma. *J. Allergy* **33**:229–237, 1978.
13. Haynes, R. L., Ingram, R. H., Jr., and McFadden, E. R., Jr. An assessment of the pulmonary response to exercise in asthma and an analysis of the factors influencing it. *Am. Rev. Respir. Dis.* **114**:739–752, 1976.
14. Dixon, M., Jackson, D. M., and Richard, I. M. The action of sodium cromoglycate on "C" fibre endings in the dog lung. *Br. J. Pharmacol.* **70**:11–13, 1980.
15. Snashall, P. D., and Baldwin, C. Mechanisms of action of sulphur dioxide induced bronchoconstriction in normal and asthmatic man. *Thorax* **37**:118–123, 1982.
16. Sheppard, D., Nadel, J. A., and Boushey, H. A. Inhibition of sulfur dioxide-induced bronchoconstriction by disodium cromoglycate in asthmatic subjects. *Am. Rev. Respir. Dis.* **124**:257–259, 1981.
17. Fanta, C. H., McFadden, E. R., Jr., and Ingram, R. H., Jr. Effects of cromolyn sodium on the response to respiratory heat loss in normal subjects. *Am. Rev. Respir. Dis.* **123**:161–164, 1981.
18. Pichurko, B. M., McFadden, E. R., Jr., Bowman, K. F., Burnes, S., Dowling, N., and Ingram, R. H., Jr. The influence of cromolyn sodium on airway temperature. *Clin. Res.* **31**:513 (abstr.), 1983.
19. Barnes, P. J., and Brown, M. J. Venous plasma histamine in exercise- and hyperventilation-induced asthma in man. *Clin. Sci.* **61**:159–162, 1981.
20. Anderson, S. D., Bye, P. T. P., Schoeffel, R. E., Seale, J. P., Taylor, K. M., and Ferris, L. Arterial plasma histamine levels at rest, and during and after exercise in patients with asthma: Effects of terbutaline aerosol. *Thorax* **36**:259–267, 1981.
21. Lee, T. H., Brown, M. J., Nagy, L., Causon, R., Walport, M. J., and Kay, A. B. Exercise-induced release of histamine and neutrophil chemotactic factor in atopic asthmatics. *J. Allergy Clin. Immunol.* **70**:73–81, 1982.
22. Lee, T. H., Nagy, L., Nagakura, T., Walport, M. J., and Kay, A. B. Identification and partial characterization of an exercise-induced neutrophil chemotactic factor in bronchial asthma. *J. Clin. Invest.* **69**:889–899, 1982.
23. Morgan, D. J. R., Phillips, M. J., Moodley, I., Elliot, E. V., and Davies, R. J. Histamine, neutrophil chemotactic factor and circulating basophil levels following exercise in asthmatic and control subjects. *Clin. Allergy* **12**(Suppl.):29–37, 1982.
24. Lee, T. H., Assoufi, B. K., and Kay, A. B. The link between exercise, respiratory heat exchange and the mast cell in bronchial asthma. *Lancet* **1**:520–522, 1983.
25. Deal, E. C., Jr., Wasserman, S. I., Soter, N. A., Ingram, R. H., Jr., and McFadden, E. R., Jr. Evaluation of the role played by mediators of immediate hypersensitivity in exercise-induced asthma. *J. Clin. Invest.* **65**:659–665, 1980.
26. Resnick, A. D., Deal, E. C., Jr., Ingram, R. H., Jr., and McFadden, E. R., Jr. A critical assessment of the mechanism by which hyperoxia attenuates exercise-induced asthma. *J. Clin. Invest.* **64**:541–549, 1979.
27. Breslin, F. J., McFadden, E. R., Jr., and Ingram, R. H., Jr. The effect of cromolyn sodium on the airway response to hyperpnea and cold air in asthma. *Am. Rev. Respir. Dis.* **122**:11–16, 1980.
28. Deal, E. C., Jr., McFadden, E. R., Jr., and Ingram, R. H., Jr. Effects of atropine on potentiation of exercise-induced bronchospasm by cold air. *J. Appl. Physiol.: Respir., Environ. Exercise Physiol.* **45**:238–243, 1978.
29. Griffin, M. P., Fung, K. F., Ingram, R. H., Jr., and McFadden, E. R., Jr. Dose-response effects of atropine on thermal stimulus–response relationships in asthma. *J. Appl. Physiol.: Respir., Environ. Exercise Physiol.* **53**:1576–1582, 1982.

30. Rossing, T. H., Weiss, J. W., Breslin, F. J., Ingram, R. H., Jr., and McFadden, E. R., Jr. Effects of inhaled sympathomimetics on the obstructive response to respiratory heat loss. *J. Appl. Physiol.: Respir., Environ. Exercise Physiol.* **52:**1119–1123, 1982.
31. Pichurko, B. M., McFadden, E. R., Jr., and Sullivan, B. P. Comparison of the intrathoracic thermal events produced by exercise and voluntary hyperventilation in man. (In preparation.)
32. Holgate, S. T., Church, M. K., Cushley, M. J., Robinson, C., Mann, J. S., and Howarth, P. H. Pharmacological modulation of airway calibre and mediator release in human models of bronchial asthma. Chapter 24, this volume.
33. McNeill, R. S., Nairn, J. R., Millar, J. S., and Ingram, C. G. Exercise-induced asthma. *Q. J. Med.* **35:**55–67, 1966.
34. James, L., Faciane, J., and Sly, R. M. Effect of treadmill exercise on asthmatic children. *J. Allergy Clin. Immunol.* **57:**408–416, 1976.
35. Edmunds, A. T., Tooley, M., and Godfrey, S. The refractory period after exercise-induced asthma: Its duration and relation to the severity of exercise. *Am. Rev. Respir. Dis.* **117:**247–254, 1978.
36. Ben-Dov, I., Bar-Yishay, E., and Godfrey, S. Refractory period after exercise-induced asthma unexplained by respiratory heat loss. *Am. Rev. Respir. Dis.* **125:**530–534, 1982.
37. Soter, N. A., Wasserman, S. I., Austen, K. F., and McFadden, E. R., Jr. Release of mast-cell mediators and alterations in lung function in patients with cholinergic urticaria. *N. Engl. J. Med* **302:**604–608, 1980.

DISCUSSION

Kay: We have consistently been able to detect NCA following EIA and yet you apparently have not. Why do you think this is?

McFadden: We are disappointed not to have found mediator release and are certainly willing to consider that the differences between our results and yours could be due to technical difficulties. If such is the case, perhaps we can work out some way of detecting and correcting them if present.

Holgate: With reference to the effect of cromoglycate on airway temperature, it has long been known that intravenous cromoglycate causes vasodilatation. With a variety of cromolyn-like compounds administered orally or by aerosol, a number of patients also complain of a feeling of heat and may flush.

McFadden: I was unaware of these studies, thank you.

Lichtenstein: I don't know who suggested that mediator depletion is responsible for the refractory period, but it is highly unlikely. One can challenge the nose, for example, and get the same histamine release each time. Further, the amount of histamine released from human bronchi challenged *in vitro* is just several percent. *In vivo* it would be much less.

McFadden: I believe that it was originally postulated by McNeill *et al.* in the late 1960s (R. S. McNeill, J. R. Nairn, and J. S. Millar, *Q. J. Med.* **35:**55, 1966) and then again by several investigators relatively recently (L. James, J. Faciane, and R. M. Sly, *J. Allergy Clin. Immunol.* **57:**408, 1976; A. T. Edmunds, M. Tooley, and S. Godfrey, *Am. Rev. Respir. Dis.* **117:**247, 1978).

Dollery: I have two questions: (1) What was the exercise load used in the experiments on exercise-induced asthma? (2) What is the relationship between the temperatures you measure (which I suppose are air temperatures) and the temperature in the bronchial wall?

While I have no difficulty in believing that the wall temperature also falls, I suggest that the changes are much less because of the much greater thermal capacity of the tissues. If this is the case is it not highly speculative to suggest that temperatures may be attained at which calcium transport fails?

McFadden: The level of exercise was moderately severe, resulting in a ventilation of 60–70 liters/min. We know that the bronchial wall cools because we have found the temperature in the retrotracheal oesophagus to fall during exercise (E. C. Deal, Jr., E. R. McFadden, Jr., R. H. Ingram, Jr., and J. J. Jaeger, *J. Appl. Physiol.* **46**:484, 1979). We have not yet measured the transairway temperatures, nor have we completed our studies on the heat capacity of the airways. I meant only to speculate about the magnitude of local thermal effects.

Kaliner: Are you not also avoiding nasal breathing and thereby removing an effective warming device which is ordinarily present under normal circumstances? What is the influence of nasal breathing on air temperature under the condition you describe?

McFadden: Exercising subjects switch from nose to oral breathing at ventilations ranging from 30 to 60 liters/min. Thus at the level of exercise we used, measurements made during mouth breathing seem appropriate.

Hogg: Data from Sandra Anderson's laboratory, presented at the American Thoracic Society meeting this year, showed that the response could be produced without cooling [S. A. Anderson, R. E. Schoeffel, E. Daviskas, and J. L. Black, *Am. Rev. Respir. Dis.* **127**:228(A), 1983]. Others, including Elwood *et al.* from our laboratory, have shown that hyper- or hypoosmolar challenge can produce a similar response [R. K. Elwood, J. C. Hogg, and P. D. Pare, *Am. Rev. Respir. Dis.* **125**:61(A), 1982]. As a change in osmolarity on the airways surface might either change the epithelium or degranulate mast cells, the change you observe might be due to water loss rather than heat loss.

Barnes: I would like to raise a number of points. We agree that adrenaline does not rise during exercise in asthmatics in contrast to normal subjects exercised to the same extent. Do you have data from nonasthmatic control subjects for comparison? Also, the small increase in noradrenaline in exercise will not reflect pulmonary sympathetic nerve activity (which is trivial in comparison with cardiovascular sympathetic nerve activity), and therefore its effects on the airways will be related to its effects as a circulating hormone. These are likely to be unimportant since noradrenaline has almost no effect on β_2-adrenoceptor-mediated responses within the physiological range of concentrations. It is more likely that the bronchodilatation of exercise results from vagal withdrawal (J. B. Warren, *Clin. Sci.* 1983, in press).

McFadden: Thank you for your comments. We do have data on normal controls but at this time we have not yet completed our analysis.

Barnes: We have shown that a refractory period can be demonstrated in some patients after hyperventilation challenge (N. M. Wilson, P. J. Barnes, H. P. Vickers, and M. Silverman, *Thorax* **37**:657, 1982). Presumably hyperventilation is not associated with significant bronchodilatation. Would you predict that calcium channel blockers would be deleterious in exercise induced asthma by causing bronchial vascular dilatation? In fact, they have a protective effect (P. J. Barnes, N. M. Wilson, and M. J. Brown, *Thorax* **36**:726, 1981).

Nadel: Referring to Dr. Dollery's comment, the fluid phrase "heat sink" should be determined to a large extent by blood flow. Thus, this is another example of the possible importance of bronchial blood flow in airway regulation.

Lee: I would agree that mediator depletion is unlikely to be the only cause of the refractory period. However, how do you explain Simon Godfrey's observation that only 50% of asthmatics made refractory to further EIA by repeated exercise were nonresponsive to a concentration of antigen that had previously been shown to cause airflow obstruction (D. Weiler-Ravell and S. Godfrey, *J. Allergy Clin. Immunol.* **68:**391, 1981)? If catecholamines are responsible for the refractory period, one might expect that all asthmatics should be protected from antigen challenge.

McFadden: I am afraid that I cannot comment knowledgeably about the studies that you are citing, because I do not remember all of the technical details.

Tattersfield: In normal subjects the bronchodilatation that occurs during exercise can be blocked completely by β-blocking drugs, so presumably in normal subjects, at least, the bronchodilatation is due to catecholamines not vagal withdrawal.

Kaplan: Could you expound upon your idea that affecting calcium fluxes in either direction will lead to improvement in exercise-induced bronchoconstrictions? From your explanation of initial vessel constriction followed by "paradoxical" vasodilation with bronchoconstriction associated with the latter, one might conclude that a calcium channel blocker would make it worse.

McFadden: In the scheme that I proposed, if the bronchial vasculature plays a role in exercise-induced asthma, then any drug that delays either the initial contraction or the later dilation of this vascular bed would alter local heat transfer and shift the stimulus–response curve to the right for any given thermal load.

CHAPTER 20

The Effect of Mucosal Inflammation on Airways Reactivity*

J. C. HOGG, W. C. HULBERT, C. ARMOUR, and P. D. PARE

Pulmonary Research Laboratory
St. Paul's Hospital
University of British Columbia
Vancouver, British Columbia, Canada

INTRODUCTION

At the Asthma II meeting, we presented data on the physiologic abnormalities that occurred with antigen challenge in *Ascaris*-sensitive monkeys (1). This showed that antigen challenge with a fairly large molecular weight antigen caused a physiological response within seconds, which suggested to us that the antigen must react with mast cells on the airway surface. We speculated that the mediators released by this interaction would change the mucosal permeability and allow antigen to penetrate to a larger number of mast cells in the submucosa. We also suggested that the known relationship between epithelial damage and airways hyperreactivity might be related to a permeability change associated with the onset of the inflammatory reaction. We have subsequently obtained data that bear on several aspects of this hypothesis (2–6), but in this presentation I would like to focus on the nature of change in epithelial permeability that occurs in the airway mucosa when it is acutely inflamed.

* Supported by the Medical Research Council of Canada and the Canadian Tobacco Manufacturers' Council.

AIRWAY MUCOSAL INFLAMMATION

To facilitate the discussion, I would like to spend a few moments discussing the nature of the inflammatory reaction of a mucus membrane. Lord Florey studied this problem extensively in both the gastrointestinal tract and (to a lesser degree) in the respiratory tract of animals and man. He summarized his findings in his book (7) in which he stated that an inflammatory reaction in a mucus membrane had certain features that

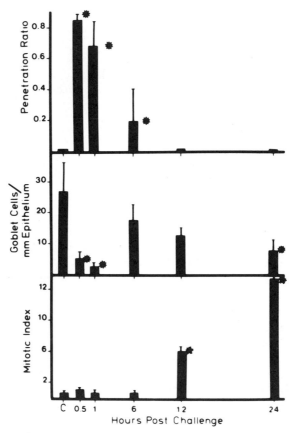

Fig. 1. Penetration of the epithelium by horseradish peroxidase is maximally increased at 0.5 to 1 hr after smoke exposure (100 puffs whole cigarette smoke). This increased permeability is associated with goblet cell discharge. As permeability returns to control values, the epithelium begins to regenerate, as indicated by an increased mitotic index. *, p ≤ .05. [Modified from ref. (2) with permission from authors and publisher.]

were common to all inflamed tissue as well as two features that were specific for mucus membranes. The common features include vascular dilatation, increased permeability of blood vessels with formation of an exudate of plasma proteins, and the emigration of leukocytes from the vascular space into the interstitial space and onto the membrane surface. The additional features are the increase in mucus secretion and the desquamation of epithelial cells. Jennings and Florey (8) showed that the irritation of the surface of the colon could cause the goblet cells to empty and that removal of the irritant caused them to fill again within a few hours. Recent studies from our laboratory (2) have shown similar changes in airways irritated by cigarette smoke in which goblet cells empty and then recover (Fig. 1). Early studies by Florey *et al.* (9) established that stimulation of either the afferent or efferent vagus nerve produced secretion of the bronchial glands. These early observations have been confirmed and elegantly extended by Nadel (10–13) and his colleagues, who have shown that the glands can be reflexly stimulated from sites in the nose, larynx, and airways. This means that local irritation of the airways is capable of increasing mucus secretion by reflex stimulation of the bronchial glands as well as by emptying the goblet cells.

THE RELATIONSHIP BETWEEN MUCOSAL PERMEABILITY AND INFLAMMATION

Using a fixation technique that involves perfusion of fixative through the bronchial circulation (14), it has been possible to show that edema forms in the interstitial space between the basal and superficial epithelial cells during the exudative phase of an inflammatory reaction (Fig. 2). Subsequently, inflammatory cells collect in this space and the surface epithelium is separated leaving the basal cell layer below. These changes are associated with an increased mucosal permeability during the exudative phase of the inflammatory reaction when the epithelial edema forms, and a return to normal permeability when the superficial epithelium is sloughed leaving the basal cell layer (compare Figs. 1 and 2). This return to normal permeability probably relates to the fact that the basal cells cover a greater surface area than the superficial cells and therefore provide a smaller paracellular pathway per unit surface area than does surface epithelium. Clearly the rapid return to normal permeability does not mean that the epithelium has returned to normal. The change in airway permeability produced by acute inflammation is however a transient phenomena that occurs only during the initial exudative phase of the reaction.

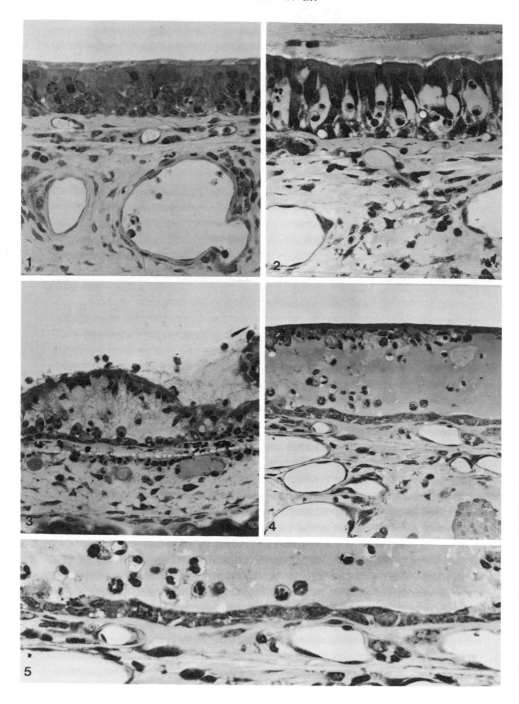

AIRWAY MUCOSAL PERMEABILITY AND REACTIVITY IN ASTHMA

A characteristic feature of asthmatic patients is that as they hyperreact to nonspecific stimuli, a relationship between airways hyperreactivity and permeability would be expected in these patients. Elwood *et al.* (15) have recently examined the airway mucosal permeability of asthmatic patients and compared it to that observed in subjects with normal airways. They found (Table I) that, while the asthmatics had a marked increase in airways reactivity, there was no increase in mucosal permeability. This result would not be expected if there was a simple direct relationship between mucosal permeability and reactivity. However, in the light of a

TABLE I

	N	$PI_{10}{}^{b}$	PI_{25}	PI_{60}	$t_{1/2}{}^{c}$
Normals	9	10.7 ± 4.4	14.0 ± 4.9	19.3 ± 5.3	66 ± 19
Asthmatics	10	7.2 ± 6.2	11.1 ± 9.9	13.9 ± 10	88 ± 39
		NS^{d}	NS	NS	NS
Nonsmokers	8	9.3 ± 5.7	15.0 ± 8.2	23.0 ± 8.9	110 ± 62
Asymptomatic smokers	10	29 ± 14.4	33.4 ± 10.1	34.4 ± 9.3	42 ± 16
		$p < .001$	$p < .001$	$p < .001$	$p < .005$

[a] Data for normals and asthmatics from Elwood *et al.* (15); data for nonsmokers and asymptomatic smokers from Kennedy *et al.* (20).

[b] $$PI = \frac{\text{Counts} \times \text{ml of blood} \times \text{kg body wt}}{\text{Counts for lungs on completion of aerosol delivery}}.$$

[c] $t_{1/2}$ is time for one-half the counts delivered to the lungs to disappear. The difference between normal subjects reported by Elwood *et al.* (45) and Kennedy *et al.* (20) reflect an attempt at central delivery in study of Elwood *et al.*

[d] NS, not significant.

Fig. 2. Histology following smoke exposure when the lungs are fixed by perfusion of the bronchial circulation as described in ref. (14). (1) Normal epithelial mucosa; (2) minor epithelial edema; (3) confluent epithelial edema where superficial cells lift off; (4) severe epithelial edema; (5) higher magnification of (4) showing squamous basal cell layer. We believe that the increased permeability shown in Fig. 1 is caused by the initial disruption of the epithelium during the exudative phase of the reaction and that the return to normal is associated with a squamous basal cell layer. As these cells are larger and have a small paracellular pathway per unit surface area they form an excellent barrier. (See text for further explanation.)

clearer appreciation of the nature of the change in permeability associated with an injured epithelium, we believe that the result may be reasonable. Asthmatics are known to shed large numbers of cells into their sputum and show marked squamous metaplasia with active turnover of the epithelial cells (16). It therefore seems possible that when asthmatics are in a quiescent phase, their airways might be expected to be relatively impermeable because the epithelium is being actively repaired. Why they remain hyperreactive during the repair phase is not clear, but it could be due to some other aspect of the inflammatory reaction or possibly occur because intact irritant nerve endings remained above the squamous epithelial surface. We are presently investigating this problem but have no results to report.

AIRWAYS PERMEABILITY AND REACTIVITY IN CIGARETTE SMOKERS

The relationship between airways reactivity, permeability, and inflammation is also of interest with respect to asymptomatic cigarette smokers. Several laboratories have now shown that these people have an increased airway permeability (17,18), and one study (19) has suggested that they have increased airways reactivity. These observations led Kennedy *et al.* (20) to examine the relationship between reactivity and permeability in asymptomatic smokers. She found (Table I) that the smokers had an increased permeability, but this was not associated with an increased airways reactivity. This observation is also against a simple hypothesis linking permeability to reactivity. In the study of Kennedy *et al.*, however, the smokers had physiological evidence of peripheral airways abnormality (increased $\Delta N_2 L$, CC and decreased V_{50}), which others have shown to be related to inflammation in terminal and respiratory bronchioles. This makes it possible that the site of permeability in smokers' lungs may be in the peripheral airways, whereas the nerve endings of the irritant receptors, which must be exposed to lower airways reactivity, are in the central airways.

AIRWAYS PERMEABILITY AND REACTIVITY IN GUINEA PIGS

In order to test the hypothesis that increased permeability and increased airways reactivity are associated with inflammation of the central

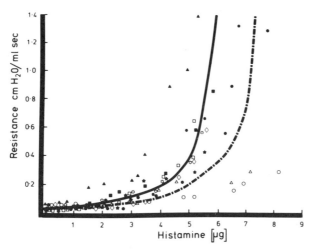

Fig. 3. Histamine dose–response curves (no drug pretreatment) performed on normal (not exposed: solid line on graph) guinea pigs and on guinea pigs 0.5 hr after cigarette smoke exposure (dot-dash line) when their epithelial permeability was maximal. The data show that the smoke-exposed animals are less reactive than the nonexposed animals ($n = 5$ for both).

airways, we have returned to the study of the guinea pig. In particular, we have tried to examine the relationship between permeability and reactivity using a constant stimulus of cigarette smoke, which we know produces tracheobronchial inflammation and increased permeability of the trachea

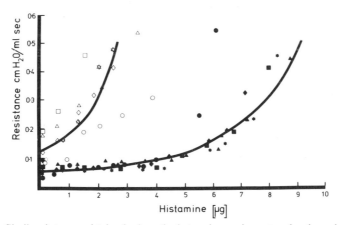

Fig. 4. Similar data are obtained when the beta adrenergic system has been blocked by propranolol (10 mg/kg) and the parasympathetic pathway has been blocked by atropine (5 mg/kg). This points out that the smoke-exposed animals (0.5 hr; open symbols) with increased permeability are much more reactive than the control animals (not exposed; solid symbols) ($n = 5$ for both).

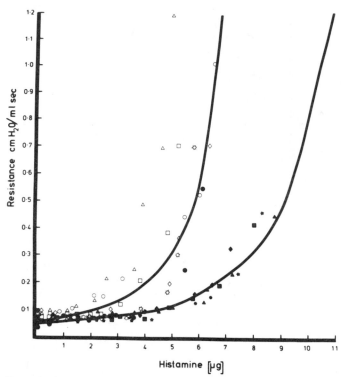

Fig. 5. Data obtained with similar conditions comparing animals exposed to cigarette smoke (open symbols) to control animals (solid symbols) 24 hr after the exposure ($n = 5$, both). These data show that the reactivity of these animals is returning toward the control level at this time.

(Fig. 1) (2). To measure airways reactivity in the guinea pig, we have developed a simple technique for performing a histamine dose–response curve. We found (21) that the inflammatory reaction caused by cigarette smoke does not produce an increase in airways reactivity without drug intervention (Fig. 3). However, when the experiment was repeated with both beta sympathetic and parasympathetic blockade, there was a marked increased airways reactivity at the time of the greatest increase in permeability (Fig. 4) that returned towards the control values after 24 hr (Fig. 5). This is consistent with an increased reactivity of the muscle at the time the histamine dose response was performed but it does not prove that it is due to increased permeability. However, as examination of isolated muscle preparations from these animals (Fig. 6) showed no difference between airways from smoke-exposed reactive animals and the control ani-

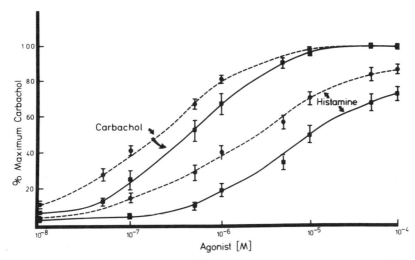

Fig. 6.   Data from isolated muscle studied in an organ bath. These data show that the smooth muscle from smoke-exposed animals (solid line) with hyperreactive airways are not more responsive than that of the controls (dashed line) ($n = 5$, both).

mals, we attributed the increased reactivity to the fact that more agonist could reach the muscle through the permeable airways.

SUMMARY

These data show that there is no simple relationship between permeability and reactivity. Indeed, this relationship can only be obtained in experimental animals with autonomic blockade. It therefore seems much more likely that an increased reactivity relates primarily to factors that control smooth muscle activity. The fact that the inflammatory reaction is associated with mediator release, which can affect epithelial permeability and smooth muscle function, makes it seem likely that changes in reactivity and permeability during an inflammatory reaction occur as part of the inflammatory reaction but are not directly related to each other.

REFERENCES

1. Hogg, J. C., Pare, P. D., Boucher, R. C., Michoud, M. C., Guerzon, G., and Moroz, L. Pathologic abnormalities in asthma. *In* "Asthma: Physiology, Immunopharmacology,

and Treatment" (L. M. Lichtenstein, K. F. Austen, and A. S. Simon, eds.), Vol. 2, pp. 1–9. Academic Press, New York, 1977.

2. Hulbert, W., Walker, D. C., Jackson, A., and Hogg, J. C. Airway permeability to horseradish peroxidase in guinea pigs: The repair phase after injury by cigarette smoke. *Am. Rev. Respir. Dis.* **123:**320–326, 1981.

3. Hogg, J. C. Bronchial mucosal permeability and its relationship to airways hyperreactivity. *J. Allergy Clin. Immunol.* **67:**421–425, 1981.

4. Michoud, M. C., Pare, P. D., Boucher, R. C., and Hogg, J. C. Airway responses to histamine and methacholine in *Ascaris suum*–allergic rhesus monkeys. *J. Appl. Physiol.* **45:**846–851, 1978.

5. Guerzon, G. M., Pare, P. D., Michoud, M. C., and Hogg, J. C. The number and distribution of mast cells in monkey lungs. *Am. Rev. Respir. Dis.* **119:**59–66, 1979.

6. Boucher, R. C., Pare, P. D., and Hogg, J. C. The relationship between airway hyperreactivity and hyperpermeability in the *Ascaris suum*–sensitive rhesus monkey. *J. Allergy Clin. Immunol.* **64:**197–201, 1979.

7. Florey, Sir H. Secretion of mucus in the inflammation of mucus membranes. *In* "General Pathology" (Sir H. Florey, ed.), 3rd ed., Chapter 6. Lloyd Luke Medical Books Ltd., London, 1962.

8. Jennings, M. A., and Florey, H. W. Autoradiographic observations on mucus cell of stomach and intestine. *Q. J. Exp. Physiol. Cogn. Med. Sci.* **41:**131, 1956.

9. Florey, H., Carlstone, H. M., and Wells, A. Q. Mucus secretion in the trachea. *Br. J. Exp. Pathol.* **13:**269, 1932.

10. Nadel, J., and Davis, G. Autonomic regulation of mucus secretion and ion transport in airways. *In* "Asthma: Physiology, Immunopharmacology, and Treatment" (L. M. Lichtenstein, K. F. Austen, and A. S. Simon, eds.), p. 197. Academic Press, New York, 1977.

11. Nadel, J. A., Davis, D., and Phipps, R. J. Control of mucus secretion and ion transport in airways. *Annu. Rev. Physiol.* **41:**369, 1979.

12. Nadel, J. A., and Davis, D. Parasympathetic and sympathetic regulation of secretion of submucosal glands in airways. *Fed. Proc., Fed. Am. Soc. Exp. Biol.* **39:**3075, 1980.

13. Nadel, J. A. Autonomic control of airway smooth muscle and airway secretions. *Am. Rev. Respir. Dis.* **115**(Suppl.):117, 1977.

14. Hulbert, W. C., Forster, B., Laird, W., Pihl, C., and Walker, D. C. An improved method for fixation of the respiratory epithelial surface with the mucous and surfactant layers. *Lab. Invest.* **47:**354, 1982.

15. Elwood, R. K., Kennedy, S., Belzberg, A., Hogg, J. C., and Pare, P. D. Respiratory mucosal permeability in asthma. *Am. Rev. Respir. Dis.* **128:**523–527, 1983.

16. Naylor, B. The shedding of the mucosal and the bronchial tree in asthma. *Thorax* **17:**69, 1962.

17. Jones, J. G., Minty, B. D., Lawler, P., Hullands, G., Crawley, J. C. W., and Vealle, N. Increased alveolar epithelial permeability in cigarette smoke. *Lancet* **1:**66–68, 1980.

18. Mason, G. R., Uszler, J. M., Effros, R. M., and Reid, E. Rapidly reversible alterations in pulmonary epithelial permeability induced by smoking. *Chest* **83:**6–11, 1983.

19. Gerrard, J. W., Cockcroft, D. W., Mink, J. T., Cotton, D. J., Poonwalla, R., and Dosman, J. A. Increased non-specific bronchial reactivity in cigarette smokers with normal lung function. *Am. Rev. Respir. Dis.* **122:**577, 1980.

20. Kennedy, S. M., Elwood, R. K., Wiggs, B. J., Pare, P. D., and Hogg, J. C. Increased airway mucosal permeability of smokers: Relationship to airway reactivity. *Am. Rev. Respir. Dis.* **129:**143–148, 1984.

21. Hulbert, W. C., McLean, T., Pare, P. D., and Hogg, J. C. The relationship between cigarette smoke-induced airway inflammation and histamine reactivity in guinea pigs. *Clin. Invest. Med.* **6**:76, 1983.

DISCUSSION

Lessof: Would you care to speculate a little more on what happens to the goblet cells?

Hogg: The goblet-cell discharge occurs at the height of the exudative phase of the inflammatory response, and this is fairly common in inflammatory reactions of mucous membranes. I think it is possible that this is the event that pulls the cells apart at their corners, but this is not proven as yet.

Clark: Your original publication showed horseradish peroxidase (HRP) in goblet cells after allergen challenge with HRP. Can you explain this observation?

Hogg: You refer to the study of Richardson *et al.* (J. B. Richardson, J. C. Hogg, T. Touchard, and D. L. Hall, *J. Allergy Clin. Immunol.* **172**:181, 1973). We believe those changes were the result of cell death so that the cells picked up the HRP. I believe the transport is paracellular in nature and do not think there is any transport through the cells.

Flenley: If the occurrence of squamous metaplasia explains the poor correlation between permeability and reactivity in human asthma, shouldn't this mean that mucociliary clearance is severely impaired, even if only locally, in even moderately severe asthmatics as they have considerably increased bronchial reactivity?

Hogg: The lesions would certainly interfere with mucociliary clearance locally. The question is—how widespread are the lesions? We have not quantitated this. I believe there is evidence that asthmatics have poor mucociliary clearance.

Kay: What is the evidence for believing that single goblet cells recover? Have goblet cells been cultured?

Hogg: Our data show a rapid recovery in the number of goblet cells. This occurs in a time period that we believe is too short to form a new cell and so we interpret the finding as indicating synthesis of new contents by the goblet cell. I believe that the goblet cells have been studied in explant cultures, but I do not know of single-cell culture studies of goblet cells.

Barnes: Do histamine or other inflammatory mediators increase permeability in man [using, for instance, ^{99m}TcDTPA as described by Jones *et al.* (J. G. Jones, D. Royston, and B. D. Minty, *Am. Rev. Respir. Dis.* **127**:S51, 1983)]?

Hogg: Yes, and it has also been shown *in vivo* in animals (R. C. Boucher, V. Rango, P. D. Pare, S. Inveu, L. A. Moroz, and J. C. Hogg, *J. Appl. Physiol.* **45**:939, 1979).

Clark: Studies at Guy's Hospital by Rees and Eiser have shown histamine to increase lung permeability [P. J. Rees, D. Shelton, N. Eiser, T. J. H. Clark, and N. M. Maisey, *Thorax* **38**:713 (abstr.), 1983].

Gleich: A comment and two questions:

Mezey *et al.* (R. J. Mezey, M. A. Cohn, R. J. Fernandez, A. J. Januskiewicz, and A. Wanner, *Am. Rev. Respir. Dis.* **118**:677, 1978), as well as others, have shown decreased mucociliary clearance in asthma (as Dr. Flenley suggested in his earlier question). Then to the questions. First, what do you believe is the mechanism of the epithelial damage in your smoke model in the guinea pig? Second, were the asthmatics you studied actually desquamating their epithelium? For instance, did they have Creola bodies in their sputum?

Hogg: One assumes that something in the tobacco smoke injures the epithelial cell and that this results in an inflammatory reaction, but the precise mechanism is obscure. We did not study the sputum on these patients at the same time as the permeability investigations were undertaken. With respect to the changes that occurred in the animal studies, this would have been interesting to do.

Turner-Warwick: If you used the Gareth Jones technique (J. G. Jones, D. Royston, and B. D. Minty, *Am. Rev. Respir. Dis.* **127:**S51, 1983) in which they alleged that changes in permeability are in the alveoli, then the discordance between permeability and bronchial hyperreactivity would be explained. Do you think this is a possible explanation?

Hogg: I don't know. In the studies on asthmatics the protocol for delivery of the aerosol should have favoured central deposition. However, in the smokers' studies the protocol did not. I would guess that in the smokers the increased permeability relates to a respiratory bronchiolitis, but more studies need to be done.

CHAPTER 21

β-Adrenoceptors in Asthma and Their Response to Agonists

PETER J. BARNES and PHILIP W. IND

Department of Medicine
Royal Postgraduate Medical School
London, U.K.

COLIN T. DOLLERY

Department of Clinical Pharmacology
Royal Postgraduate Medical School
London, U.K.

INTRODUCTION

β-Adrenergic agonists are the most widely used and effective bronchodilators for the treatment of asthma. Because β-agonists restore asthmatic airway function towards normal, it was suggested that there may be a defect in airway β-adrenoceptor function in asthma. This was supported by the observation that β-adrenergic antagonists increase bronchoconstriction in asthmatic subjects. We review the function and regulation of β-receptors in normal and asthmatic airways and discuss the role of β-agonists as bronchodilators. Where possible, we have presented evidence from human rather than animal studies, although information about airway β-receptor function in asthma is limited.

FUNCTION AND LOCALISATION OF AIRWAY β-RECEPTORS

Direct receptor binding studies using radiolabelled β-adrenoceptor antagonists have shown the density of β-receptors in lung from several

ASTHMA: Physiology,
Immunopharmacology,
and Treatment
THIRD INTERNATIONAL SYMPOSIUM

TABLE I
Function of Airway β-Adrenoceptors

Site	Function
Smooth muscle	Relaxation
Mast cell	Inhibit mediator release
Submucosal gland	Increase mucus secretion
Epithelium	Increase fluid transport and mucociliary clearance
Microvasculature	Decrease permeability
Cholinergic nerves and ganglion	Decrease neurotransmission

species, including man, to be higher than in any other tissue (1–3). β-Agonists affect many aspects of pulmonary function, including airway and vascular smooth muscle tone, secretion from airway glands and mast cells, fluid transport across epithelium, and secretion of surfactant; this suggests that β-receptors must be localised to many different cell types within the lung (Table I).

Airway Smooth Muscle

β-Agonists potently relax smooth muscle from human trachea and bronchi (4) and peripheral lung strips (5), suggesting that β-receptors are present in smooth muscle of large and small airways (Fig. 1). Using an autoradiographic technique, the density of β-receptors in mammalian airway smooth muscle can be shown to increase progressively from trachea to terminal bronchioles (6,7). *In vivo,* dose-dependent bronchodilation to inhaled β-agonists has been demonstrated in normal subjects using sensitive tests of large and small airway function (8,9), but the relationship between tests of airflow, which depend on airway radius, and smooth muscle tone is complex and makes detailed study of airway β-receptor function difficult *in vivo*. In human airway smooth muscle, relaxation is mediated by β_2-adrenoceptors (5,10), and direct binding studies of human lung confirm that β_2-adrenoceptors predominate (3,11). In canine tracheal smooth muscle, binding studies show that while β_2-receptors predominate, approximately 20% of β-receptors are of the β_1-subtype. Functional studies of the same muscle indicate that β_2-receptors mediate relaxation to exogenous β-agonists, whereas β_1-receptors mediate relaxation to sympathetic nerve stimulation (12). This supports the proposal that β_1-receptors are regulated by sympathetic nerves, whereas β_2-receptors are influenced by circulating catecholamines (13). In human airway smooth

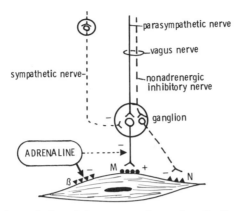

Fig. 1. Autonomic regulation of airway smooth muscle cells. Parasympathetic fibres in the vagus nerve relay in ganglia located in the airway and activate excitatory muscarinic cholinergic receptors (M) on airway smooth muscle cells. Sympathetic nerves relay in ganglia close to the thoracic spinal cord and do not directly innervate airway smooth muscle, but may supply parasympathetic ganglia. The dominant adrenergic influence on airway smooth muscle is circulating adrenaline, which activates β_2-adrenoceptors (β) on smooth muscle cells. A nonadrenergic inhibitory nervous system is also carried in the vagus and activates specific receptors on airway smooth muscle (N). The neurotransmitter of this nervous system may be vasoactive intestinal peptide.

muscle, which has no direct sympathetic innervation, there is no evidence for functional β_1-receptors *in vitro* (10), and the β_1-selective agonist, prenalterol, has no bronchodilator action in asthmatic subjects (14).

Mast Cells

β-Agonists inhibit mast cell mediator release from passively sensitised human lung fragments *in vitro,* suggesting the presence of functional β-receptors on pulmonary mast cells (15,16), which are of the β_2-subtype (17). This has been confirmed in isolated human lung mast cells (18). Direct binding studies revealed a high density of β_2-receptors in a well-differentiated canine mastocytoma cell line in which β-receptors are functional (19). Isoprenaline inhibits canine tracheal mast cell degranulation *in vivo* (20), but it has been difficult to confirm an effect of β-agonists on human airway mast cells *in vivo*. Infusion of adrenaline causes a fall in the elevated plasma histamine concentration of asthmatic subjects (21), but intravenous propranolol, while causing bronchoconstriction in asthmatics, is not associated with a rise in plasma histamine concentration (22). However, interpretation of changes in plasma histamine concentration as an index of mast cell mediator release must be cautious. Mast cell degranulation as assessed by the immediate skin reaction to intradermal antigen in atopic subjects is not influenced by an orally administered β-agonist or antagonist (23), but topical nasal application of β-agonist inhibits allergen-induced rhinitis (24).

Secretions

β-Agonists increase airway mucus secretion in several animal species (25), including man (26). In animals β-agonists also increase active ion transport and fluid secretion across airway epithelium (25). Autoradiography has confirmed the presence of β-receptors in epithelium of airways from trachea to bronchioles and in submucosal glands (6,27). β-Agonists also increase cAMP, as measured immunocytochemically in airway epithelium and glands (28). Several studies have reported increased mucociliary clearance *in vivo* after β-agonists, although this has not been found consistently (see ref. 29).

Microvascular Permeability

Histamine-induced microvascular leakage in lung and airways is reduced by β-agonists (30), and the high density of β-receptors lining the alveolar wall may be localised to capillary endothelial cells (6).

Cholinergic Neurotransmission

β-Agonists modulate cholinergic nerve stimulation of airway smooth muscle (31), and direct recording from tracheal parasympathetic ganglion cells shows a β-adrenergic inhibitory effect (32).

Thus, β-agonists may produce bronchodilation, not only by a direct effect on bronchial smooth muscle, but also by modulating release of mast cell mediators, by reducing excitatory cholinergic neurotransmission, and by reducing mucosal oedema. Although β-receptors are present in high density in lung and airways, their physiological function in normal man is uncertain since β-antagonists have no detectable effect on airway function (33) or on mucociliary clearance (29). Presumably activation of airway β-receptors becomes functionally important only under conditions of stress such as anaphylactic shock.

REGULATION OF AIRWAY β-RECEPTORS

The only endogenous agonists that may influence β-receptors are noradrenaline (β_1-selective), released from sympathetic nerves, and adrenaline (β_2-selective), released from the adrenal medulla, which functions as a circulating hormone (Fig. 1).

Sympathetic Innervation of Airways

Although the airways receive a dense parasympathetic innervation via the vagus nerve, sympathetic innervation is sparse and variable between species (34). Histological studies using fluorescence histochemistry, electron microscopy, and specific immunocytochemistry have shown few, if any, adrenergic axons in human airway smooth muscle (35–37). Functional studies using electrical field stimulation of isolated human airways similarly provided no evidence for inhibitory sympathetic nerves (35,38), and this is supported by the lack of effect of cocaine, an inhibitor of neuronal uptake of noradrenaline, on noradrenaline dose–response curves in isolated human airways and lung strips (10). Infusion of tyramine, which directly releases noradrenaline from sympathetic nerves, does not produce bronchodilation in asthmatic subjects despite a significant cardiovascular effect (39). This suggests that in humans sympathetic innervation is not important in the regulation of airway tone *in vivo*.

Histological studies have demonstrated, however, that adrenergic axons within the airways supply bronchial blood vessels, submucosal, glands and ganglia (34,36,37).

Circulating Catecholamines

β-Agonists are potent bronchodilators and airway smooth muscle has a high density of β-receptors, yet airway smooth muscle is not directly innervated by adrenergic axons, which suggests that circulating catecholamines may play a role in the regulation of bronchial tone. In normal subjects administration of β-antagonists, either systemically or by inhalation, has no effect on either resting airway tone (33) or on bronchial reactivity (40); but in asthmatics, β-blockers cause bronchoconstriction (41). This suggests that in asthmatic subjects catecholamines may be protective against bronchoconstrictor influences. It is only with the recent development of specific and sensitive assays that accurate measurement of normal circulating concentrations of catecholamines in plasma has been possible (42). In asthmatics, plasma concentrations of noradrenaline and adrenaline at rest are no different from those in age-matched normal subjects and are not correlated with the severity of bronchoconstriction (43). Increased bronchoconstriction in asthmatics at night is closely related to the normal circadian fall in circulating adrenaline, suggesting that the normal concentration of plasma adrenaline may be protective in asthmatics (21).

The fall in plasma adrenaline at night correlates with a rise in plasma histamine, indicating that adrenaline may have indirect effects on bronchial tone by modulation of mast cell mediator release. Although the coincidence of these circadian rhythms does not prove a causal relationship, the demonstration that infused adrenaline lowers plasma histamine at night is suggestive. The normal plasma catecholamine rise during exercise is blunted in asthmatics who develop exercise-induced bronchoconstriction, compared with matched controls, although there is no impairment in the much larger catecholamine response to insulin-induced hypoglycaemia (44) or in the catecholamine response to infused histamine (45). Furthermore, when bronchoconstriction is induced by isocapnic hyperventilation at rest, there is no increase in plasma catecholamines during the "stress" of bronchoconstriction (44). These studies indicate that there may be a partial defect in catecholamine response in asthmatics, which would have the effect of exacerbating provoked bronchoconstriction, although the mechanism for this remains unclear.

Nonadrenergic Inhibitory Innervation

A nonadrenergic inhibitory nervous system similar to that described in the gut has also been found in human lung (Fig. 1). Electrical field stimulation of isolated human airways produces relaxation that is not blocked by β-antagonists but is reduced by the nerve-conduction blocker tetrodotoxin (35,38). Thus, the dominant inhibitory nervous control of human airways is nonadrenergic. Whether function of this system is impaired in asthma is difficult to determine, because neither the nervous pathways nor the neurotransmitter are known and no specific antagonists are available. There is convincing evidence that in guinea pig trachea the neurotransmitter involved in nonadrenergic relaxation may be vasoactive intestinal peptide (VIP) (46). Exogenous VIP causes relaxation of human airway smooth muscle *in vitro* (38) and also stimulates submucosal gland secretion and airway epithelial ion transport in other species (47,48). Furthermore, peptidergic nerves, particularly those showing VIP-like immunoreactivity, have been found to supply airway smooth muscle, glands, and ganglia in human lung (49).

β-RECEPTOR DYSFUNCTION IN ASTHMA

As a result of animal experiments, Szentivanyi (50) proposed that a generalised impairment in β-receptor function may be the underlying abnormality in atopy and asthma. This proposition is unlikely to be correct, because treatment of normal subjects with β-antagonists does not make them asthmatic nor does it increase bronchial reactivity (40). However, it is possible that asthma may lead to a secondary impairment in β-receptor function. This may affect not only airway smooth muscle (tipping the balance in favour of cholinergic and possibly α-adrenergic constrictor influences), but may also increase secretion of mast cell mediators, increase bronchial vascular permeability, and increase cholinergic neurotransmission, all of which would contribute to airway narrowing.

This hypothesis was supported by early studies showing impaired metabolic, cardiovascular, and leucocyte cAMP responses to β-agonists (51,52) and a reduction in lymphocyte β-receptor density in asthmatics compared to normal subjects (53). However, the same reduction in β-receptor function and density are also produced in both normal and asthmatic subjects as a result of treatment with β-agonists (54–56). Moreover, the reduced β-receptor density on circulating leucocytes persists for up to 2 weeks after stopping β-agonists (56). This strongly suggests that at least some of the impairment in β-receptor function in asthma results from tachyphylaxis resulting from previous bronchodilator therapy. There are conflicting reports of whether untreated asthmatics have an abnormality in β-receptor function. Some authors have found no differences in β-adrenergic metabolic responses (57) or in leucocyte β-receptor density (56,58) between normal and untreated asthmatic subjects. Others have reported an impairment in cardiovascular and metabolic responses to β-agonists in untreated asthmatics (59), although the magnitude of these changes is very small.

Similarly, reduced β-receptor density has been found in lymphocytes of untreated asthmatics, the magnitude of which increases with severity of bronchoconstriction (60). After antigen challenge, asthmatics but not normal subjects show a reduction in leucocyte β-receptor density and cAMP response to isoprenaline (61). Taken together, these studies suggested that an intrinsic generalized defect in β-receptors is unlikely in asthma but that some relatively small impairment may be secondary to the disease, although the magnitude of the impairment is less than that resulting from β-adrenergic therapy. The mechanism by which asthma might produce these changes in β-receptor function is unclear. Autoantibodies to the β_2-receptor have been demonstrated in the serum of some asthmatics (62), although their presence in only a small proportion of asthmatic and also in nonatopic normal individuals makes their significance questionable.

The most important question is whether there is a defect in airway β-receptor function in asthma, but this has been difficult to answer because differing baseline measurements and previous β-agonist therapy confused interpretation. In asthmatics who develop spontaneous nocturnal wheezing, no impairment in airway responses to inhaled or infused β-agonist is found when bronchoconstriction is maximal, providing no evidence that impaired β-receptor function contributes to increased bronchoconstriction in these individuals (63). No significant differences were found in dose–response curves to an inhaled β-agonist between normal and very mild asthmatic subjects (64). When dose–response curves in more severe asthmatics and normal subjects are compared, however, a significantly higher dose of β-agonist is required to produce 50% maximal bronchodilatation, and this is significantly correlated with severity of bronchoconstriction (65). However, interpretation is difficult because a larger dose of β-agonist may be required in asthmatics to overcome the greater initial bronchoconstriction, and the distribution of inhaled drugs is abnormal in asthmatic airways. Comparison of airway β-receptor function between normal and asthmatic subjects *in vivo* is therefore misleading. A more promising approach may be to study airway smooth muscle *in vitro*. It is very difficult to obtain such tissue from asthmatic subjects, however, and even when it is available β-adrenergic function may have been compromised by previous therapy or by hypoxia. In a preliminary report, airway smooth muscle from three asthmatics (one of whom was untreated) showed markedly reduced responses to isoprenaline in comparison to nonasthmatic controls (66), but airways from another patient, who died during an asthmatic attack, responded normally to β-agonists (67).

Because pulmonary β-receptor function is difficult to study in human asthma, animal models have been developed, although none of these closely mimics human disease. In *Ascaris*-sensitive dogs, airway smooth muscle cAMP content is reduced compared with nonallergic control animals, although the cyclic AMP response to isoprenaline is unchanged (68). In a guinea pig model of allergic asthma, there is a 20% reduction in total pulmonary β-receptor density but isoprenaline-induced adenylate cyclase activation is unchanged, indicating no overall functional impairment of β-receptors (69). Similarly, there is no difference in pulmonary β-receptor density *in vitro* between patients with normal and obstructed airway function (3). However, autoradiographic studies have indicated that alveolar β-receptors account for >90% of all β-receptors in lung (6), so any change in airway β-receptors is likely to be obscured when whole lung homogenates are examined.

Thus, the critical question of whether airway β-receptor function is impaired in asthma is unresolved; it is likely that any such defect would be minor since asthmatics respond so effectively to inhaled β-agonist therapy. It is possible that airway β-receptor function might be more impaired in acute severe exacerbations of asthma, although this is difficult to evaluate as luminal obstruction by mucus plugs and oedema would cause an apparent reduction in response to β-agonists.

β-AGONISTS AS THERAPY

β-Agonists are the most effective bronchodilator drugs available for the treatment of asthma. The main therapeutic effect probably results from stimulation of smooth muscle β_2-receptors, although effects on stabilisation of pulmonary mast cells, enhancement of mucociliary clearance, and a reduction of inflammation may contribute.

β-Agonist Drugs

Adrenaline was the first β-agonist used in treatment and was later replaced by the more specific β-agonists isoprenaline (isoproterenol) and orciprenaline (metaproterenol). The suspicion, although unproven, that isoprenaline in particular may have been responsible for the "epidemic" of young asthma deaths in the United Kingdom and other countries in the 1960s, led to the introduction of selective β_2-adrenoceptor agonists in the 1970s. These include salbutamol (albuterol), rimiterol, terbutaline, fenoterol, reproterol, and pirbuterol in Europe and isoetharine, terbutaline, and salbutamol in the United States. Differences in β_2 selectivity have been claimed but are generally clinically unimportant. Unwanted effects, which are dose related, include palpitations, tremor, and restlessness. Tachycardia is probably secondary to β_2-receptor-mediated reduction in peripheral vascular resistance although this may also be caused by stimulation of atrial β_2-receptors, and cardiac β_1-receptor stimulation occurs at high doses. Tremor results from stimulation of skeletal muscle β_2-receptors. These side effects tend to disappear with continuation of the drug reflecting the development of tolerance (70). Metabolic effects (increase in plasma free fatty acids, insulin, glucose, and lactate and reduction in plasma potassium) are usually seen only after large systemic doses (71). β-Agonists may increase ventilation–perfusion mismatch by causing pulmonary vasodilatation in vessels previously constricted by hypoxaemia. This may result in a fall in arterial oxygen tension. Although this is usually small (3–5 mm Hg), occasionally in those with severe bronchoconstriction it may be large, although it is prevented by giving additional inspired oxygen (72).

Isoprenaline and rimiterol are conjugated in the gut wall and therefore are relatively inactive when swallowed (but may be absorbed sublingually). Isoprenaline, rimiterol and isotharine are degraded by catechol-O-methyl transferase and therefore have a shorter duration of action than other β_2-agonists.

Route of Administration

The inhalation of β-agonists as particles of 2–4 μm results in their delivery to the conducting airways. This route of administration is logical, rapidly effective, and virtually free from side effects. Pressurised canister inhalers deliver 25–100 μl of a metered dose of β-agonist in fluorocarbon propellant with each "puff," but <10% of each dose actually reaches the airways even with optimal technique (29). Many patients, particularly the elderly, the arthritic, or young children are unable to achieve this efficiency even with careful instruction, and modified pressurised aerosols and a nonpressurised dry powder dispenser have been introduced. It is unclear to what extent inhaled β-agonists act only locally or are absorbed and delivered via the pulmonary circulation to peripheral airways.

Oral administration of β-agonists requires 20–80 times the inhaled dose of the same drug to achieve a similar bronchodilator action. This is slower in onset but longer in duration and is associated with much higher plasma concentrations of drug and therefore greater side effects. Administration of β-agonists by intermittent positive pressure ventilation (IPPV) and wet nebuliser may produce greater bronchodilatation than by metered dose inhaler, although this may be due to the dose administered and distribution of the drug in the airways (72). In acute severe asthma, β-agonists given by nebuliser appear to be more effective than those given either by the intravenous route or by IPPV (73,74).

Acute Severe Asthma

During severe acute exacerbations, asthmatics may appear less responsive to their usual β-agonist inhalers, although they may respond to higher doses given by nebuliser or by IPPV. This may be explained by reduced β-receptor function or by impaired access of inhaled drug because of luminal narrowing by mucosal oedema and inflammatory secretions.

β-ADRENOCEPTOR TOLERANCE

Reports of patients developing tolerance (tachyphylaxis, resistance, subsensitivity) to β-agonists and the suggestion that this might have been a factor in asthma deaths has resulted in more than 30 studies of bronchial β-receptor subsensitivity, and the topic has been reviewed (75).

Airways *in Vitro*

Tachyphylaxis to β-agonists in human bronchial smooth muscle has been demonstrated *in vitro* (4,76), although the concentration of β-agonist necessary is high and the degree of desensitization produced is variable.

Airways *in Vivo*

Tolerance has been found in normal human airways after high-dose inhaled salbutamol (8,57,64) although others have not confirmed this (77,78). In asthmatic subjects, β-agonist tolerance in the airways has been demonstrated in some studies (54,79) but not in others (58,64,70). It is likely that the dose and route of administration of β-agonist, the period of "washout" of prior β-adrenergic therapy, the continuation of drugs such as steroids and theophylline (which may modify development of tolerance), and individual variability may account for the conflicting results. Nevertheless, it is clear that airway β-receptor tolerance can occur, although its magnitude is small and there is no evidence that it is clinically important.

Nonairway β-Receptors

By contrast, tolerance of nonairway β-receptor responses such as tremor (70), increased heart rate (80), metabolic responses (57,81), and white cell cAMP production (54,55) is readily induced in normal and asthmatic subjects. There is also suggestive evidence that β-receptor tolerance may also be more easily produced in pulmonary mast cells than in airway smooth muscle *in vitro* (82) and possibly *in vivo* (58). The relative resistance of airway smooth muscle β-receptors to desensitisation is unlikely to be due to differences in agonist concentration at the receptor site, since after inhaled β-agonist concentrations must be very high in the airways but low in extrapulmonary tissues where tolerance is easily demonstrated (54). It is possible that airways have a relatively high proportion of "spare" receptors that protect against the development of tolerance *in vivo* (76,83).

Mechanism

The underlying mechanism of desensitisation in airway smooth muscle, as in other tissues, is due to a reduction in β-receptor density and also to a fall in the proportion of receptors in the high-affinity state (84). Airway smooth muscle β-receptors are down regulated to the same extent as those in lung parenchyma (84), but may be less susceptible to downregulation than β-receptors in other tissues such as spleen (85).

CORTICOSTEROIDS AND β-RECEPTOR FUNCTION

Corticosteroids modify airway β-receptor function, although whether this is relevant to their effectiveness in asthma is uncertain. *In vitro,* steroids potentiate the effects of β-agonists on bronchial smooth muscle (86), prevent β-receptor tachyphylaxis (87), and increase the rate of recovery of β-adrenergic responsiveness after tachyphylaxis (4). *In vivo,* steroids similarly reverse tolerance to inhaled β-agonist in dogs (88) and in normal man (8). The mechanism by which steroids affect β-receptor function has been studied by radioligand binding. Steroids increased the density of β-receptors (by 70%) in rat lung membranes (89), increased the proportion of β-receptors in the high-affinity binding state in human leucocytes (90), and reversed the fall in leucocyte β-receptor density after β-agonists in normal and asthmatic subjects (91). Increased airway smooth muscle β-receptor density has been shown by autoradiography in fetal rabbit lung after steroids (92). This increase in β-receptor density after steroids may involve an increase in receptor synthesis, since inhibitors of protein synthesis prevent the β-receptor increase in cultured human lung cells (93). Thus steroids may play a beneficial role in asthma by preventing or reversing β-receptor desensitisation, presumably by a direct action on the β-receptor, although this effect is likely to be very minor in relation to their more important antiinflammatory role.

SUMMARY

β-Adrenoceptor agonists remain the most effective bronchodilators currently available. They may have beneficial effects in asthma, not only by direct relaxation of airway smooth muscle but also by inhibition of inflammatory mediator release from pulmonary mast cells, by modulation of cholinergic bronchoconstrictor effects, by reduction of airway microvascular permeability and oedema, and by increase of mucociliary clearance. There is no anatomical or functional evidence for a significant direct sympathetic innervation of human airway smooth muscle, although ganglia, submucosal glands, and vessels receive an adrenergic supply. Airway smooth muscle β-receptors must therefore by physiologically regulated by circulating adrenaline. Although β-adrenoceptor antagonists cause bronchoconstriction in asthmatic subjects but not in normal subjects, there is no evidence that plasma adrenaline concentrations are raised in stable asthma. Moreover, there may be a blunting of catecholamine response to certain bronchoconstrictor stimuli, such as exercise and hyperventilation. The reduction in metabolic and cardiovascular responses to β-agonists, which has been described in asthmatic subjects, may be largely explained by tolerance due to previous β-agonist therapy. However, some impairment in these responses has been described in untreated asthmatics. There is little information about whether airway β-receptor responses are diminished in asthma because of the difficulties in comparing normal and asthmatic subjects. The bronchodilator response to inhaled β-agonists in asthma argues against an important defect in airway β-receptor function, however. While tolerance to the extrapulmonary effects of β-agonists can be readily demonstrated, it has proved difficult to show a reduction in airway response after prolonged β-agonist treatment. The mechanism whereby airway β-receptors are protected in this way remains obscure. Steroids increase airway β-receptor responsiveness, but this is likely to be of only minor importance in comparison with their antiinflammatory role in asthma.

REFERENCES

1. Rugg, E. L., Barnett, D. B., and Nahorski, S. R. Coexistence of beta₁ and beta₂ adrenoceptors in mammalian lung: Evidence from direct binding studies. *Mol. Pharmacol.* **14:**996–1005, 1978.
2. Barnes, P., Karliner, J., Hamilton, C., and Dollery, C. Demonstration of alpha₁-adrenoceptors in guinea pig lung using [³H]prazosin. *Life Sci.* **25:**1207–1214, 1979.

3. Barnes, P. J., Karliner, J. S., and Dollery, C. T. Human lung adrenoceptors studied by radioligand binding. *Clin. Sci.* **58**:457–461, 1980.
4. Davis, C., and Conolly, M. E. Tachyphylaxis to beta adrenoceptor agonists in human bronchial smooth muscle: Studies in vitro. *Br. J. Clin. Pharmacol.* **10**:417–423, 1980.
5. Goldie, R. G., Paterson, J. W., and Wale, J. L. A comparative study of β-adrenoceptors in human and porcine lung parenchyma strip. *Br. J. Pharmacol.* **76**:523–526, 1982.
6. Barnes, P. J., Basbaum, C. B., Nadel, J. A., and Roberts, J. M. Localization of β-adrenoceptors in mammalian lung by light microscopic autoradiography. *Nature (London)* **299**:444–447, 1982.
7. Barnes, P. J., Basbaum, C. B., and Nadel, J. A. Autoradiographic localization of autonomic receptors in airway smooth muscle: Marked differences between large and small airways. *Am. Rev. Respir. Dis.* **127**:758–762, 1983.
8. Holgate, S. T., Baldwin, C. J., and Tattersfield, A. E. Beta-adrenergic agonist resistance in normal human airways. *Lancet* **2**:375–377, 1977.
9. Barnes, P. J., Gribbin, H. R., Osmanliev, D., and Pride, N. B. Partial flow-volume curves to measure bronchodilator dose-response curves in normal man. *J. Appl. Physiol.* **50**:1193–1197, 1981.
10. Zaagsma, J., van der Heijden, P. J. C. M., van der Schaar, M. W. G., and Bank, C. M. C. Comparison of functional β-adrenoceptor heterogeneity in central and peripheral airway smooth muscle of guinea-pig and man. *J. Recept. Res.* **3**:89–106, 1983.
11. Engel, G. Subclasses of beta-adrenoceptors. A quantitative estimation of beta₁- and beta₂-adrenoceptors in guinea-pig and human lung. *Postgrad. Med. J.* **57**(Suppl. 1):77–83, 1981.
12. Barnes, P. J., Nadel, J. A., Skoogh, B.-E., and Roberts, J. M. Characterization of beta-adrenoceptor subtypes in canine airway smooth muscle by radioligand binding and physiological responses. *J. Pharmacol. Exp. Ther.* **225**:456–461, 1983.
13. Ariens, E. J. The classification of beta-adrenoceptors. *Trends Pharmacol. Sci.* **2**:170–173, 1981.
14. Lofdahl, C.-G., and Svedmyr, N. Effects of prenalterol in asthmatic patients. *Eur. J. Clin. Pharmacol.* **23**:297–303, 1982.
15. Assem, E. S. K., and Schild, H. O. Beta-adrenergic receptors concerned with the anaphylactic mechanism. *Int. Arch. Allergy Appl. Immunol.* **45**:62–69, 1969.
16. Orange, R. P., Kaliner, M. A., Laraia, P. J., and Austen, K. F. Immunological release of histamine and slow reacting substance of anaphylaxis from human lung. II. Influence of cellular levels of cyclic AMP. *Fed. Proc., Fed. Am. Soc. Exp. Biol.* **30**:1725–1729, 1971.
17. Peters, S. P., Schulman, E. S., Schleimer, R. P., MacGlashan, D. W., Newball, H. H., and Lichtenstein, L. M. Dispersed human lung mast cells. Pharmacologic aspects and comparison with human lung tissue fragments. *Am. Rev. Respir. Dis.* **126**:1034–1039, 1982.
18. Butchers, P. R., Skidmore, I. F., Vardey, C. J., and Wheeldon, A. Characterisation of the receptor mediating antianaphylactic effects of beta-adrenoceptor agonists in human lung tissues in vitro. *Br. J. Pharmacol.* **71**:663–667, 1980.
19. Phillips, M. J., Barnes, P. J., and Gold, W. M. Characterization of purified drug mastocytoma cells: Autonomic membrane receptors and pharmacologic modulation of histamine release. *J. Immunol.* (in press).
20. Brown, J. K., Leff, A. R., Frey, M. J., Reed, B. R., Lazarus, S. C., Shields, R., and Gold, W. M. Characterization of tracheal mast cell reactions in vivo. Inhibition by a beta-adrenergic agonist. *Am. Rev. Respir. Dis.* **126**:842–848, 1982.

21. Barnes, P. J., FitzGerald, G., Brown, M. J., and Dollery, C. T. Nocturnal asthma and changes in circulating epinephrine, histamine and cortisol. *N. Engl. J. Med.* **303:**263–267, 1980.
22. Ind, P. W., Brown, M. J., Barnes, P. J., and Dollery, C. T. Effect of propranolol on mediator release in asthmatics. *Thorax* **37:**21P (abstr.), 1982.
23. Miyatake, A., Ind, P., and Dollery, C. T. Dose response curves to intradermal histamine, codeine and antigen in man: Effect of pretreatment with salbutamol and propranolol. (Submitted for publication.)
24. Borum, P., and Mygind, N. Inhibition of the immediate allergic reaction in the nose by the beta-2 adrenostimulant fenoterol. *J. Allergy Clin. Immunol.* **66:**25–32, 1980.
25. Nadel, J. A., Davis, B., and Phipps, R. J. Control of mucus secretion and ion transport in airways. *Annu. Rev. Physiol.* **41:**369–381, 1979.
26. Phipps, R. J., Williams, I. P., Richardson, P. S., Pell, J., Pack, R. J., and Wright, N. Sympathetic drugs stimulate the output of secretory glycoprotein from human bronchi in vitro. *Clin. Sci.* **63:**23–28, 1982.
27. Barnes, P. J., and Basbaum, C. B. Mapping of adrenergic receptors in mammalian trachea using an autoradiographic method. *Exp. Lung Res.* **5:**183–194, 1983.
28. Lazarus, S. C., Basbaum, C. B., and Gold, W. M. Cellular localization of cyclic AMP in the trachea of dog, cat and ferret. *Am. Rev. Respir. Dis.* **125:**244 (abstr.), 1982.
29. Pavia, D., Bateman, J. R. M., and Clarke, S. W. Deposition and clearance of inhaled particles. *Bull. Eur. Physiopathol. Respir.* **16:**335–366, 1980.
30. Persson, C. G. A., Ejefalt, I., Grega, G. J., and Svensjo, E. The role of β-receptor agonists in the inhibition of pulmonary edema. *Ann. N.Y. Acad. Sci.* **384:**544–556, 1982.
31. Vermiere, P. A., and Vanhoutte, P. M. Inhibitory effects of catecholamines in isolated canine bronchial smooth muscle. *J. Appl. Physiol.* **46:**787–791, 1979.
32. Baker, D. J., Herbert, D. A., and Mitchell, R. A. Cholinergic neurotransmission in airway ganglia: Inhibition by norepinephrine. *Physiologist* **25:**225 (abstr.), 1982.
33. Tattersfield, A. E., Leaver, D. G., and Pride, N. B. Effects of beta-adrenergic blockade and stimulation of normal human airways. *J. Appl. Physiol.* **34:**613–619, 1973.
34. Richardson, J. B. Nerve supply to the lungs. *Am. Rev. Respir. Dis.* **119:**785–802, 1979.
35. Richardson, J. B., and Beland, J. Nonadrenergic inhibitory nervous system in human airways. *J. Appl. Physiol.* **41:**764–771, 1976.
36. Sheppard, M. N., Kurian, S. S., Henzen Logmans, S. C., Michetti, F., Cocchia, D., Cole, P., Rush, R. A., Marangos, P. J., Bloom, S. R., and Polak, J. M. Neuron-specific enolase and S-100. New markers for delineating the innervation of the respiratory tract in man and other animals. *Thorax* **38:**333–340, 1983.
37. Partanen, M., Laitinen, A., Hervonen, A., and Toivanen, M. Catecholamine- and acetylcholinesterase-containing nerves in human lower respiratory tract. *Histochemistry* **76:**175–188, 1982.
38. Davis, C., Kannan, M. S., Jones, T. R., and Daniel, E. E. Control of human airway smooth muscle: In vitro studies. *J. Appl. Physiol.* **53:**1080–1087, 1982.
39. Ind, P. W., Scriven, A. J. I., and Dollery, C. T. Use of tyramine to probe pulmonary noradrenaline release in asthma. *Clin. Sci.* **64:**9P (abstr.), 1983.
40. Townley, R. G., McGeady, S., and Bewtra, A. The effect of beta-adrenergic blockade on bronchial sensitivity to acetyl-beta-methacholine in normal and allergic rhinitis subjects. *J. Allergy Clin. Immunol.* **57:**358–366, 1976.
41. McNeill, R. S., and Ingram, C. G. Effect of propranolol on ventilatory function. *Am. J. Cardiol.* **18:**473–475, 1966.
42. Barnes, P. J. Endogenous plasma adrenaline in asthma. *Eur. J. Respir. Dis.* **64:**559–563, 1983.

43. Barnes, P. J. Ind, P. W., and Brown, M. J. Plasma histamine and catecholamines in stable asthmatic subjects. *Clin. Sci.* **62**:661–665, 1982.
44. Barnes, P. J., Brown, M. J., Silverman, M., and Dollery, C. T. Circulating catecholamines in exercise and hyperventilation-induced asthma. *Thorax* **36**:435–440, 1981.
45. Ind, P. W., Brown, M. J., and Barnes, P. J. Sympathoadrenal responses in asthma. *Thorax* **38**:702, 1983.
46. Matsuzaki, Y., Hamasaki, Y., and Said, S. I. Vasoactive intestinal peptide: A possible transmitter of nonadrenergic relaxation of guinea-pig airways. *Science* **210**:1252–1253, 1980.
47. Peatfield, A. C., Barnes, P. J., Bratcher, C. Nadel, J. A., and Davis, B. Vasoactive intestinal peptide stimulates cyclic AMP formation in airway submucosal glands and epithelium. *Am. Rev. Respir. Dis.* **128**:89–93, 1983.
48. Nathanson, I., Widdicombe, J. H., and Barnes, P. J. Effect of vasoactive intestinal peptide across dog tracheal epithelium. *J. Appl. Physiol.* **56**:1844–1848, 1983.
49. Dey, R. D., Shannon, W. A., and Said, S. I. Localization of VIP-immunoreactive nerves in airways and pulmonary vessels of dogs, cats and human subjects. *Cell Tissue Res.* **220**:231–238, 1981.
50. Szentivanyi, A. The beta adrenergic theory of the atopic abnormality in bronchial asthma. *J. Allergy* **42**:203–232, 1968.
51. Cookson, D. V., and Reed, C. E. A comparison of the effects of isoproterenol in normal and asthmatic subjects. *Am. Rev. Respir. Dis.* **88**:636–643, 1963.
52. Parker, C. W., and Smith, J. W. Alteration in cyclic adenosine monophosphate metabolism in human bronchial asthma. I. Leucocyte responsiveness to β-adrenergic agents. *J. Clin. Invest.* **52**:48–58, 1973.
53. Kariman, K. β-adrenergic receptor binding in lymphocytes from patients with asthma. *Lung* **158**:41–51, 1980.
54. Nelson, H. S., Raine, D., Doner, H. C., and Posey, W. C. Subsensitivity to the bronchodilator action of albuterol produced by chronic administration. *Am. Rev. Respir. Dis.* **116**:871–878, 1977.
55. Conolly, M. E., and Greenacre, J. K. The lymphocyte β-adrenoceptor in normal subjects and patients with asthma: The effect of different forms of treatment on receptor function. *J. Clin. Invest.* **58**:1307–1316, 1976.
56. Galant, S. P., Durisetti, L., Underwood, S., Allred, S., and Insel, P. A. Beta-adrenergic receptors of polymorphonuclear particulates in bronchial asthma. *J. Clin. Invest.* **65**:577–585, 1980.
57. Holgate, S. T., Stubbs, W. A., Wood, P. J., McCaughey, E. S., Alberti, K. G. M. M., and Tattersfield, A. E. Airway and metabolic resistance to intravenous salbutamol: A study in normal man. *Clin. Sci.* **59**:155–161, 1980.
58. Tashkin, D. P., Conolly, M. E., Deutsch, R. I., Hui, K. K., Littner, M., Scarpace, P., and Abrass, I. Subsensitization of beta-adrenoceptors in airways and lymphocytes of healthy and asthmatic subjects. *Am. Rev. Respir. Dis.* **125**:185–193, 1982.
59. Shelhamer, J. H., Metcalfe, D. D., Smith, L. J., and Kaliner, M. Abnormal adrenergic responsiveness in allergic subjects: Analysis of isoproterenol-induced cardiovascular and plasma cyclic adenosine monophosphate responses. *J. Allergy Clin. Immunol.* **66**:52–61, 1980.
60. Brooks, S. M., McGowan, K., Bernstein, I. L., Altenau, P., and Peagler, J. Relationship between numbers of beta-adrenergic receptors in lymphocytes and disease severity in asthma. *J. Allergy Clin. Immunol.* **63**:401–406, 1979.
61. Meurs, H., Koeter, G. H., deVries, K., Kauffman, H. F. The beta-adrenergic system and allergic bronchial asthma: Changes in lymphocyte beta-adrenergic receptor number

and adenylate cyclase activity after an allergen-induced attack. *J. Allergy Clin. Immunol.* **70:**272–280, 1982.

62. Venter, J. C., Fraser, C. M., and Harrison, L. C. Autoantibodies to β₂-adrenergic receptors: a possible cause of adrenergic hyporesponsiveness in allergic rhinitis and asthma. *Science* **207:**1361–1363, 1980.

63. Barnes, P. J., FitzGerald, G. A., and Dollery, C. T. Circadian variation in adrenergic responses in asthmatic subjects. *Clin. Sci.* **62:**349–354, 1982.

64. Harvey, J. E., and Tattersfield, A. E. Airway response to salbutamol: Effect of regular salbutamol inhalations in normal, atopic and asthmatic subjects. *Thorax* **37:**280–287, 1982.

65. Barnes, P. J., and Pride, N. B. Dose-response curves to inhaled beta-adrenergic agonists in normal and asthmatic subjects. *Br. J. Clin. Pharmacol.* **15:**677–682, 1983.

66. Paterson, J. W., Lulich, K. M., and Goldie, R. G. The role of β-adrenoceptors in bronchial hyperreactivity. *In* "Bronchial Hyperreactivity" (J. Morley, ed.), pp. 19–38, Academic Press, London, 1982.

67. Svedmyr, N. L. V., Larsson, S. A., and Thiringer, G. K. Development of "resistance" in beta-adrenergic receptors of asthmatic patients. *Chest* **69:**479–483, 1976.

68. Rinard, G. A., Rubinfield, A. R., Brunton, L. L., and Mayer, S. A. Depressed cyclic AMP levels in airway smooth muscle from asthmatic dogs. *Proc. Natl. Acad. Sci. U.S.A.* **76:**1472–1476, 1979.

69. Barnes, P. J., Dollery, C. T., and MacDermot, J. Increased pulmonary α-adrenergic and reduced β-adrenergic receptors in experimental asthma. *Nature (London)* **285:**560–571, 1980.

70. Larsson, S., Svedmyr, N., and Thiringer, G. Lack of bronchial beta-adrenoceptor resistance in asthmatics during long-term treatment with terbutaline. *J. Allergy Clin. Immunol.* **59:**93–100, 1977.

71. Taylor, M. W., Gaddie, J., Murchison, E., and Palmer, K. N. V. Metabolic effects of oral salbutamol. *Br. Med. J.* **2:**22–23, 1976.

72. Paterson, J. W., Woolcock, A. J., and Shenfield, G. M. Bronchodilator drugs. *Am. Rev. Respir. Dis.* **120:**1149–1188, 1979.

73. Williams, S., and Seaton, A. Intravenous or inhaled salbutamol in severe acute asthma? *Thorax* **32:**555–558, 1977.

74. Lawford, P., Jones, B. J. M., and Milledge, J. S. Comparison of intravenous and nebulised salbutamol in initial treatment of severe asthma. *Br. Med. J.* **1:**84, 1978.

75. Jenne, J. W. Whither beta-adrenergic tachyphylaxis? *J. Allergy Clin. Immunol.* **70:**413–416, 1982.

76. Avner, B. P., and Jenne, J. W. Desensitization of isolated human bronchial smooth muscle to β-receptor agonists. *J. Allergy Clin. Immunol.* **68:**61–57, 1981.

77. Walters, E. H., Bevan, M., and Davies, B. H. Interactions between response to inhaled prostaglandin E₂ and chronic beta-adrenergic agonist treatment. *Thorax* **37:**430–437, 1982.

78. Higgs, C. M. B., Richardson, R. B., and Laszlo, G. The effect of regular inhaled salbutamol on the airway responsiveness of normal subjects. *Clin. Sci.* **63:**513–517, 1982.

79. Jenne, J. W., Chick, T. W., Strickland, R. D., and Wall, F. J. Subsensitivity to beta responses during therapy with a long acting β-2 preparation. *J. Allergy Clin. Immunol.* **59:**383–390, 1977.

80. Conolly, M. E., Davies, D. S., Dollery, C. T., and George, C. F. Resistance to beta-adrenergic stimulants (a possible explanation for the rise in asthma deaths). *Br. J. Pharmacol.* **43:**389–402, 1971.

81. Harvey, J. E., Baldwin, C. J., Wood, P. J., Alberti, K. G. M. M., and Tattersfield, A. E. Airway and metabolic responsiveness to intravenous salbutamol in asthma: effect of regular inhaled salbutamol. *Clin. Sci.* **60:**579–585, 1981.

82. Van der Heijden, P. J. C. M., and Zaagsma, J. Desensitization of smooth muscle and mast cell adrenoceptors in the airways of guinea pig. *In Receptors and Cold* (J. Zaagsma, G. K. Terpstra, H. Meurs, eds.), pp. 128–134, Excerpta Medica, 1984.

83. Avner, B. P., and Wilson, S. Possible existence of "spare" β-receptors in rat tracheal smooth muscle. *Proc. West. Pharmacol. Soc.* **22:**177 (abstr.), 1979.

84. Brown, J. K., Jones, C. A., Walters, E. H., Barnes, P. J., Nadel, J. A., and Roberts, J. M. Exposure to isoproterenol down regulates beta-adrenergic receptors in airway smooth muscle. *Am. Rev. Respir. Dis.* (in press).

85. Hasegawa, M., and Townley, R. G. Differences between lung and spleen susceptibility of beta-adrenergic receptors to desensitization by terbutaline. *J. Allergy Clin. Immunol.* **71:**230–238, 1983.

86. Townley, R. G., Ree, B. R., FitzGibbons, T., and Adolphson, R. L. The effect of corticosteroids on the beta-adrenergic receptors in bronchial smooth muscle. *J. Allergy* **45:**118 (abstr.), 1970.

87. Mackenzie, C. W. Dexamethasone inhibits isoproterenol desensitization of bovine tracheal strips. *Fed. Proc., Fed. Am. Soc. Exp. Biol.* **42:**1048, 1982.

88. Stephan, W. C., Chick, T. W., Avner, B. P., and Jenne, J. W. Tachyphylaxis to inhaled isoproterenol and the effect of methylprednisolone in dogs. *J. Allergy Clin. Immunol.* **65:**105–109, 1980.

89. Mano, K., Akbarzadeh, A., and Townley, R. G. Effect of hydrocortisone on beta-adrenergic receptors in lung membranes. *Life Sci.* **25:**1925–1930, 1979.

90. Davis, A. O., and Lefkowitz, R. J. In vitro desensitization of beta-adrenergic receptors in human neutrophils. Attenuation by corticosteroids. *J. Clin. Invest.* **71:**565–571, 1983.

91. Hui, K. P., Conolly, M. E., and Tashkin, D. P. Reversal of human lymphocyte β-receptor desensitization by glucocorticoids. *Clin. Pharmacol. Ther.* **32:**566–571, 1982.

92. Barnes, P. J., Jacobs, M. M., and Roberts, J. M. Steroids selectively increase β-adrenoceptors in foetal alveoli: Autoradiographic evidence. *Clin. Sci.* **64:**10P (abstr.), 1983.

93. Fraser, C. M., and Venter, J. C. The synthesis of beta-adrenergic receptors in cultured human lung cells: Induction by glucorticoids. *Biochem. Biophys. Res. Commun.* **94:**390–397, 1980.

DISCUSSION

Tattersfield: Was the amount of exercise carried out by the asthmatic and normal subjects the same?

Dollery: The exercise loads in the two groups were the same.

Lichtenstein: I would like to address the question of whether beta-agonists block histamine release *in vivo*. There are several studies that differ from yours. Years ago Perper *et al.* (R. J. Perper, M. Sanda, and L. M. Lichtenstein, *Int. Arch. Allergy Appl. Immunol.* **43:**837, 1972) showed in monkeys that oral theophylline and beta-agonists blocked the ascaris skin test but not the histamine skin test. Antihistamines did the reverse. Dr. Zweiman in Philadelphia has shown in man that β-agonists block the appearance of plasma histamine and NCF after antigen challenge (G. L. Martin, P. C. Atkins, E. H. Dunsky, and B. Zweiman, *J. Allergy Clin. Immunol.* **66:**204, 1980). Dr. Ken Adams also has data that show that fenoterol blocks antigen-induced contraction of guinea pig trachea at concentrations 10- to 100-fold lower than those required to block contractions induced by exogenous histamine (G. K. Adams III, unpublished observation).

Dollery: Our experiments were undertaken in the expectation that we should be able to demonstrate beta-receptor modulation of mediator release. The fact that we have not been able to do so does not prove that such mechanisms are inoperative, but it casts some doubt upon their importance.

Adams: In guinea pig tracheal rings *in vitro* pretreatment with low concentrations of fenoterol ($<10^{-8}$ M) inhibited the antigen-induced contraction and tracheal histamine release without inhibiting the contractile response to histamine.

Kaliner: We studied and published analyses of beta-adrenergic responsivity in groups of atopics (M. Kaliner, J. H. Shelhamer, P. B. Davis, C. J. Smith, and J. C. Venter, *Ann. Intern. Med.* **96**:349, 1982) in order to assess this very question. The asthmatics were very mild, taking no medications, and they demonstrated impressive β-adrenergic hyporeactivity in regards to both cardiovascular and plasma cyclic AMP responses. Other atopics were similarly hyporeactive. Then, more recently, Marilyn Haloner has found that immunizing California rabbits neonatally with HRP results in the concurrent development of IgE antibodies and beta-adrenergic hyporesponsiveness (M. Haloner and M. Kaliner, *Int. J. Immunopharmacol.* in press). Thus, in both humans and animals, evidence exists indicating that beta-adrenergic hyporeactivity does exist and is unrelated to drug administration.

Dollery: The evidence for an autonomic abnormality independent of treatment is small. Our observation of a diminished rise in plasma adrenaline during exercise in asthmatics was a surprise. Adrenaline release in response to hypoglycaemia or histamine in asthmatics is normal. We have no explanation for the observation and it seems unlikely to be of much importance in asthma apart from a possible role in modifying exercise-induced asthma.

Barnes: There is little evidence to suggest that a basic defect in β-receptor function is the underlying cause of asthma, but it is still possible that there may be a secondary impairment in β-receptor function in the airways as a result of the disease. Dr. Tattersfield's finding that very mild asthmatics have no impairment in the airway β-receptor-mediated bronchodilator responses does not exclude the possibility that there be some such defect in more severe asthmatics. This is difficult to test *in vivo* and may only be possible to study *in vitro*.

Tattersfield: Our studies do not exclude the possibility that β-receptor dysfunction may occur as asthma deteriorates. However, our understanding of Szentivanyi's hypothesis is that β-receptor dysfunction is a basic abnormality in asthma. If this is the case, it should be present in patients with mild asthma, and we are confident that as far as the airways are concerned this does not occur.

Morley: While it is evident that exposure to β-adrenoceptor agonists can strongly desensitize lymphocyte reactivity to these drugs, this cannot wholly account for observations of defective reactivity in these cells, since we and others have observed this property in lymphocytes from atopics who did not receive such medication.

Dollery: I agree that there are small differences in beta-receptor function in lymphocytes derived from asthmatics. However, these changes are small compared with those induced by tachphylaxis and very small compared with the effect of therapeutic doses of propranolol. Thus, I accept the observation but do not believe it is important in the pathogenesis of asthma.

Holgate: Another explanation for your inability to find an inhibitory effect of a β-agonist on the skin wheal and flare response is that the skin mast cells may not contain $β_2$-adrenergic receptors. Mast cells in different anatomical sites may respond to pharmacological agents in different ways. Have you carried out any immunofluorescent β-receptor studies in human skin?

Dollery: We have been careful to make clear that our results apply only to skin mast cells. However, there is data from Dr. Basran at the Brompton Hospital that β-agonists and antagonists will modify the antigen wheal and flare response if they are injected together. Presumably the local concentrations achieved were much higher. Thus these mast cells may be able to respond but did not do so for systemic doses of salbutamol or propranolol.

Wasserman: The only direct data regarding β-adrenergic receptors on mast cells have been obtained by Dr. Diana Marquardt in our laboratory. Rat serosal mast cells possess 40,000 high-affinity β-receptors per cell, 90% of which are β_2 and 10% β_1. These receptors are linked to adenylcyclase as determined by cAMP increases induced by β-agonists, but these increases are short lived and do not alter mediator release in response to antigen.

Dollery: All I can do is to invoke species differences in mast cell responses.

Hargreave: Another effect of β-agonists in asthma is to reduce bronchial hyperresponsiveness. This is partly due to bronchodilation and partly to other effects (M. R. Hetzel, J. C. Batten, and T. J. H. Clark, *Br. J. Dis. Chest* **71**:109, 1977, P. M. O'Byrne, M. Morris, R. Roberts, and F. E. Hargreave, *Thorax* **37**:913, 1982).

Dollery: There are several possible actions of beta-agonists on the lung. β-Agonists might inhibit smooth muscle-mediated responses while leaving mucosal oedema and mucous plugging unaffected or even aggravated. There is an old story that excessive doses of β-agonists can lead, to a condition called "locked lung" in which the patients become unresponsive. A possible mechanism may be stimulation of mucous secretion and mucous plugging by chronic β-receptor stimulation.

Barnes: In response to Dr. Wasserman, with Drs. Phillips and Gold I have studied the autonomic receptors in cell-differentiated canine mastocytoma cells. There is a high density of β-receptors on these cells (approximately 30,000 per cell) and β-agonists inhibit antigen-induced histamine release. By contrast, there were no alpha-receptors or cholinergic receptors as assessed by binding studies or functionally.

Kaliner: There have been studies indicating that propranolol administered to subjects with atopic rhinitis makes them behave as asthmatics. Thus, increasing β blockade in this one population does affect their pulmonary responses.

Schleimer: To follow up on the discussions of Drs. Wasserman and Barnes, we have found that the purified human lung mast cells respond to submicromolar concentrations of the β-agonist fenoterol with reduced histamine release and two- to fourfold elevation of cyclic AMP.

Dollery: I do not doubt the ability of beta-agonists to modulate mast cell release. I was trying to answer a different question, namely the role of realistic doses of β-agonists and antagonists in a whole man. We were unable to demonstrate that these doses modified mediator release.

Nadel: Two animal research observations might be relevant to the use of β-adrenoceptor agonists: (1) β-Agonists appear to stimulate selectively mucous cells of the submucosal glands. (2) β-Agonists cause experimental gland hypertrophy, a phenomenon whose functional implications are unknown.

Dollery: Recently I had cause to reexamine the data obtained during the investigation of the epidemic of asthma deaths in the United Kingdom in the period 1960–1966. I was struck by two facts. First, that those who died had severe mucous plugging of bronchi, and second, that the admission rate for asthma rose during the period 1960–1966, before attention was focused on the problem. Putting these two pieces of information together leads me to the conclusion that stimulation of mucous secretion by the inhaled beta-agonists may be the missing link in the puzzle.

CHAPTER 22

Corticosteroid Resistance in Chronic Asthma

I. W. B. GRANT, A. H. WYLLIE, M. C. POZNANSKY, A. C. H. GORDON, and J. G. DOUGLAS

Respiratory Unit, Northern General Hospital
and Departments of Pathology and Medicine
University of Edinburgh
Edinburgh, Scotland, U.K.

INTRODUCTION

All physicians with experience of chronic asthma have seen patients who are resistant to systemic treatment with corticosteroids, even when given in very large doses. There is no doubt that these patients are asthmatics since a pronounced reduction in airflow obstruction always occurs after they inhale a bronchodilator aerosol. Nevertheless, because their asthma is resistant to oral and inhaled corticosteroids, and because in many cases it is refractory to other drugs including inhaled cromoglycate and oral methylxanthines, their chronic symptoms can seldom be adequately controlled. The asthma in such patients is usually severe: they are seriously disabled for long periods and at any time may develop acute attacks for which hospital treatment is urgently required. Although such patients are relatively few, they account for a high proportion of the total number of patients at most respiratory outpatient clinics. The clinical characteristics of corticosteroid-resistant chronic asthma are as follows:

1. Observed in 5 to 10% of patients with severe chronic asthma.
2. More common with long duration and family history.
3. Typically associated with good response to bronchodilator aerosols.
4. Nocturnal wheeze and morning "dip" in PEFR are common features.

ASTHMA: Physiology,
Immunopharmacology,
and Treatment
THIRD INTERNATIONAL SYMPOSIUM

359

The means by which this can be distinguished from corticosteroid sensitive asthma are shown in Table I.

There must be some reason why airflow obstruction is rapidly and completely relieved by a short course of oral prednisolone in some patients with asthma (Fig. 1), while in others corticosteroids administered in high dosage, either by mouth or by intravenous infusion, have little or no effect (Fig. 2). In seeking an explanation for this phenomenon, the proposition was first considered that "corticosteroid-resistant" and "corticosteroid-sensitive" asthmatics might be suffering from two aetiologically distinct forms of the disease, only one of which responded to treatment with corticosteroids. The alternative hypothesis, which we also decided to explore, was that corticosteroid resistance might result from disturbance of the "normal" mechanism by which corticosteroids can modify the cell-mediated response to antigenic stimuli.

A previously reported study (1) of 58 patients with corticosteroid resistant chronic asthma and an equal number of corticosteroid sensitive asthmatics, chosen at random from this series, showed only two differences in clinical status (Table II). The first was that corticosteroid-resistant chronic asthma was of longer duration, but this difference may have been biased by population selection whereby fewer corticosteroid-sensitive asthmatics with a long history were included in the study because many such patients had been discharged from observation with their asthma well controlled. The second difference, apparently genuine, was that a family history of asthma was significantly more common in the resistant cases. This raised the possibility that corticosteroid resistance might have a genetic basis, and HL-A typing is being undertaken to test this hypothesis.

TABLE I

Identification of Corticosteroid-Resistant and Corticosteroid-sensitive Chronic Asthma

Diagnostic preconditions
  Baseline FEV_1 <60% of predicted normal
  FEV_1 increases by >30% after bronchodilator aerosol

Corticosteroid-resistant
  FEV_1 increases by <15% after short-term systemic administration of corticosteroid in high dosage

Corticosteroid-sensitive
  FEV_1 increases by >30% after short-term systemic administration of corticosteroid in high dosage

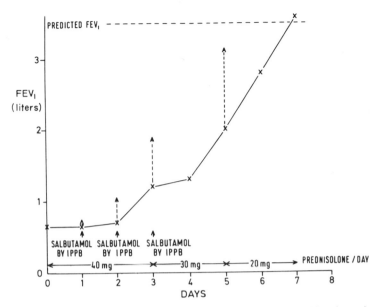

Fig. 1. Daily recordings of forced expiratory volume in 1 sec (FEV₁) in patient with corticosteroid-sensitive chronic asthma showing good response to oral prednisolone and an initially poor but a subsequent good response to salbutamol (5 mg) aerosol administered by intermittent positive-pressure breathing (bronchodilator aerosol).

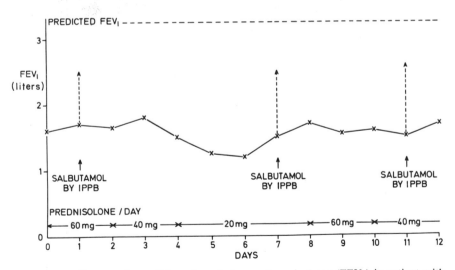

Fig. 2. Daily recordings of forced expiratory volume in 1 sec (FEV₁) in patient with corticosteroid-resistant chronic asthma showing no response to oral prednisolone but good response to salbutamol (bronchodilator) aerosol administered by intermittent positive-pressure breathing.

TABLE II
Clinical Status of Patients with Corticosteroid-Resistant and
Corticosteroid-sensitive Chronic Asthma

	Corticosteroid-resistant	Corticosteroid-sensitive
Number of patients	58	58
Male : female ratio	38 : 20	38 : 20
Average age (years)	42.8	43.5
Chronic asthma for >5 years (%)	60[a]	33[a]
Current smokers (%)	9	21
Family history of asthma (%)	62[b]	29[b]
Atopic on skin testing (%)	54	64

[a] $p < .01$.
[b] $p < .001$.

Bronchial reactivity to methacholine was tested by the method of Chai *et al.* (2) in 20 patients on similar maintenance doses of oral prednisolone, 10 from the resistant group and 10 from the sensitive group. As shown in Fig. 3, bronchial reactivity was significantly greater in the resistant group ($p < .001$), but in these patients the mean prechallenge forced expiratory volume in 1 sec (FEV_1) was lower, and this may have exaggerated the difference in bronchial reactivity between the two groups.

In Fig. 4A, the striking difference in terms of FEV_1 between the response of resistant and sensitive cases to the short-term administration of systemic corticosteroids in high dosage is illustrated. This contrasts

TABLE III
Laboratory Investigations in Corticosteroid-Resistant and
Corticosteroid-Sensitive Chronic Asthma

Blood	Sputum
Total white cell count	Cell counts: neutrophils,
Absolute eosinophil count	eosinophils, macrophages
IgG, IgA, IgM, IgE	Histamine
Complement C_4	SRS-A
Monocyte complement receptors (%)	Arylsulphatase
complement receptor enhancement	Immunoglobulins
Neutrophil superoxide radical production	
(HL-A typing)	

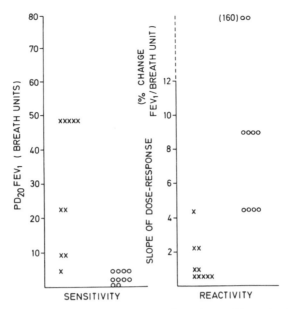

Fig. 3.   Results of methacholine challenge tests in patients with corticosteroid-resistant and corticosteroid-sensitive chronic asthma. One breath unit is equivalent to one inhalation of 1% methacholine. PD$_{20}$ is the cumulative number of breath units of methacholine that produces a 20% reduction in forced expiratory volume in 1 sec (FEV$_1$). O, corticosteroid-resistant; X, corticosteroid-sensitive.

sharply with the similar response in both groups to the inhalation of 5 mg of salbutamol as an aqueous aerosol.

A wide range of laboratory investigations have been undertaken in an attempt to identify factors that might be related to the response of chronic asthma to corticosteroids (Table III), but with one exception these failed to discriminate between resistant and sensitive populations. The exception was the measurement of monocyte complement receptors (MCR) and of their enhancement (CRE) by casein, a monocyte chemotactic factor. The formula used for this measurement is as follows:

$$\frac{\text{Patient's monocytes (\% rosettes) with diluent or casein}}{\text{Control's monocytes (\% rosettes) with diluent}} \times 100$$

This investigation (3) showed that monocyte complement receptors were enhanced by casein in cells obtained from both corticosteroid-resistant and -sensitive asthmatics provided they had not been treated with prednisolone or with any other systemically administered glucocorticoid drug. In patients who had been so treated, receptor enhancement was

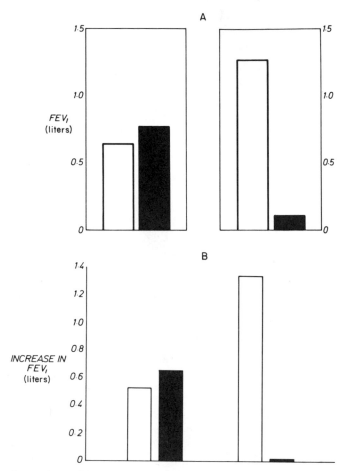

Fig. 4. Comparison of increase in forced expiratory volume in 1 sec (FEV$_1$) following inhalation of salbutamol (5 mg) aerosol (left; not significant) and short course of oral or intravenous (systemic) glucocorticoid (right; $p < .001$) in 58 patients with corticosteroid-sensitive (open bars) and 58 with corticosteroid-resistant (shaded bars) chronic asthma. B. Similar comparison of 30 chronic asthmatics (15 corticosteroid-sensitive and 15 cortico-steroid-resistant) included in an *in vitro* study. Left: after salbutamol aerosol (open bar, sensitive; shaded bar, resistant) (not significant). Right: after corticosteroid (open bar, sensitive; shaded, resistant) ($p < .001$).

unchanged in the resistant asthmatics but was diminished in the sensitive patients (Table IV). The results of this study prompted us to explore the possibility that abnormal responsiveness to glucocorticoid could be demonstrated in peripheral blood leucocytes of corticosteroid-resistant patients by *in vitro* tests.

TABLE IV
Effect of Corticosteroid Medication on Monocyte Complement
Receptors and Their Enhancement *In Vitro* by Casein
(2 mg/ml)[a]

Prednisolone	Asthma status	Mean % monocyte rosettes	
		Without casein	With casein
No	CR[b]	90.4	158.1
No	CS[b]	94.4[c]	186.9[c]
Yes	CR	100.7	165.4
Yes	CS	78.1[d]	122.7[d]

[a] Data from Kay *et al.* (3).
[b] CR, corticosteroid resistant; CS, corticosteroid sensitive.
[c] Not significant.
[d] $p < .005$.

PATIENTS

For the present study, peripheral blood leucocytes were obtained from 30 patients randomly selected from the 116 included in the original investigation of corticosteroid resistance in chronic asthma: 15 from the resistant and 15 from the sensitive group. Their response in terms of FEV_1 to the inhalation of bronchodilator aerosol and to systemic treatment with corticosteroids is illustrated in Fig. 4B. None of the 30 patients had taken an oral corticosteroid drug for 4 weeks prior to the study, but most were on regular treatment with a small dose (not exceeding 400 μg per day) of beclomethasone dipropionate by inhalation. Identical studies were also performed on 14 normal subjects within the same age range.

METHODS

Ficoll-Hypaque-separated peripheral blood mononuclear cells were cultured in soft agar, in the presence of phytohaemagglutinin (PHA) to permit growth of colonies (4,5) (Fig. 5). These colonies consist mostly of T cells bearing OKT4 (inducer) and OKT8 (cytotoxic-suppressor) immunophenotypes. Colony growth, however, is critically dependent on the presence of monocytes, and this requirement can also be met by soluble factors of monocyte origin. Colony growth is also dependent on

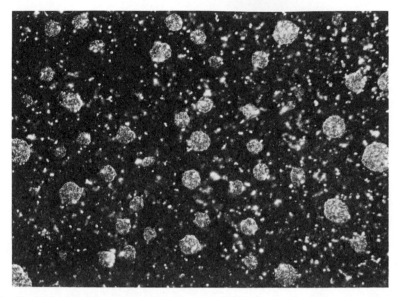

Fig. 5. Colonies of lymphocytes, predominantly T cells, developed from human peripheral blood mononuclear cells after 5 days culture in soft agar in the presence of PHA (×150).

other cell interactions in which soluble factors from T cells are generated. Hence, following other workers (6–8), we envisage that the colonies are the result of interleukin 1 (IL-1) production by monocytes, leading to production of interleukin 2 (IL-2; T-cell growth factor) by a subset of T cells, which then sustains the proliferation of T cells recognised as the colony. It is well known that IL-1 production is inhibited by glucocorticoids (6,9) and that these hormones also inhibit the capacity of T cells to respond to IL-1 by production of IL-2. This accounts for the marked sensitivity of colony growth to inhibition by glucocorticoids *in vitro*. Concentrations of methylprednisolone as low as 10^{-10} M are effective (4); this is within the normal range of the equivalent concentrations of physiological glucocorticoids in plasma and less than that required to saturate cytoplasmic glucocorticoid receptors in human lymphocytes (10,11).

RESULTS

We used colony growth *in vitro* to answer two questions about corticosteroid resistance in asthma: Can this phenomenon be demonstrated *in vitro?*—and if so, which cell type is responsible for such resistance?

TABLE V
Immunophenotype of Peripheral Blood Mononuclear
Cells of Controls and Asthmatic Patients

Phenotype	Mean % of mononuclear cells ($\pm$ SD)		
	Controls	Sensitive asthmatics	Resistant asthmatics
OKT3	47.2 $\pm$ 11.6	46.2 $\pm$ 7.0	45.1 $\pm$ 10.9
OKT4	30.9 $\pm$ 9.1	26.0 $\pm$ 7.1	27.2 $\pm$ 7.9
OKT8	16.3[a] $\pm$ 4.7	21.6[a] $\pm$ 6.3	17.8 $\pm$ 5.5
Ia231	12.9 $\pm$ 6.9	13.5 $\pm$ 4.9	13.8 $\pm$ 6.2
OKM1	29.3 $\pm$ 9.4	26.7 $\pm$ 7.4	29.0 $\pm$ 10.0

[a] $p < .01$ (t test).

Steroid Resistance Can Be Demonstrated *in Vitro*

The immunophenotypes of the mononuclear cells at the time of initiating the cultures were broadly similar: the proportion of OKT8 positive cells was slightly higher in corticosteroid-sensitive asthmatics than in controls, but there were no significant differences in phenotype between the corticosteroid resistant and sensitive patients (Table V).

In the absence of corticosteroid *in vitro*, peripheral blood mononuclear cells from all three groups generated similar numbers of colonies (Table VI). Addition of methylprednisolone (MP) at 10^{-8} M from the outset of culture strongly inhibited colony formation in the control and cortico-

TABLE VI
Effect of Glucocorticoid on Colony Formation by Peripheral Blood
Mononuclear Cells from Control and Asthmatic Patients

Culture conditions	Mean colony number ($\pm$ SD)		
	Controls	Sensitive asthmatics	Resistant asthmatics
No glucocorticoid	37.7 $\pm$ 5.2	38.3 $\pm$ 6.6	35.3 $\pm$ 9.5
Methylprednisolone 10^{-8} M[a]	14.7 $\pm$ 8.8	13.9 $\pm$ 7.3	31.8 $\pm$ 12.8

[a] The reduction in colony number with methylprednisolone is significant for controls and sensitive asthmatics ($p < .0001$) but not for resistant asthmatics.

steroid-sensitive groups but had little effect on the resistant group (Table VI). To facilitate comparison between individuals and normalise purely technical factors affecting "plating efficiency" in setting up the cultures, we expressed the colony number in the presence of 10^{-8} *M* MP as a percentage of the number obtained from the same patient, at the same time, in corticosteroid-free conditions (Fig. 6). It is clear that the sensitive and resistant patients differed markedly in the responsiveness of their peripheral blood mononuclear cells to glucocorticoid *in vitro*. All the experiments were performed without prior knowledge of the clinical status of the subjects from whom the cells were derived, and repeated tests on cells from patients and controls showed consistent responses.

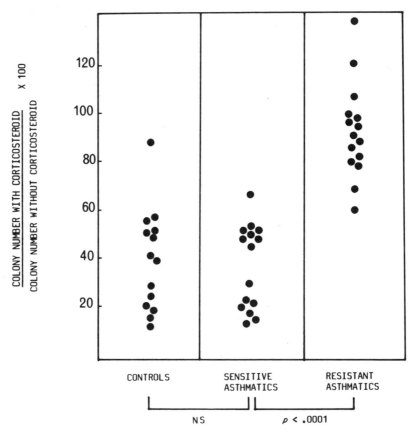

Fig. 6. Number of colonies from mononuclear cells developing in the presence of 10^{-8} *M* methylprednisolone expressed as a percentage of the number that developed in the absence of MP, using cells from the same subject. Each point derives from a different subject. NS, not significant.

Steroid Resistance Is a Property of Monocytes

The interleukin-mediated interactions between monocytes and T cells are not HLA restricted (12). Hence it was possible to conduct experiments in which monocytes from one patient were cocultured with lymphocytes from another. By combining monocytes from corticosteroid-resistant patients with lymphocytes from sensitive patients, and vice versa, we sought to establish whether resistance was determined principally by monocytes or lymphocytes.

Semipurified populations of lymphocytes were obtained by selected lysis of monocytes, using complement and the monocyte-specific monoclonal antibody OKM1. Similarly, cell populations enriched in monocytes were prepared by complement lysis in the presence of the T cell–specific antibody OKT3. When such "T cell" and "monocyte" populations were cultured in soft agar in various combinations, the subsequent yield of colonies made possible a number of conclusions (Table VII).

First, when monocytes and lymphocytes from the same patient were recombined, colonies grew well. Growth of colonies from the cells of corticosteroid-sensitive patients was strongly inhibited by MP at 10^{-8} M, whereas that from the cells of resistant patients was not inhibited. This demonstrated that the manipulations involved in preparing the cell populations had neither destroyed their capacity to interact and proliferate nor

TABLE VII

Colony Formation by Combinations of Mononuclear Cells from a Sensitive and a Resistant Asthmatic Patient

Source of cells		Number of colonies	
Lymphocytes	Monocytes	Without MP[a]	With MP
Sensitive	Sensitive	20	0
Resistant	Resistant	30	24
Sensitive	—	0	2
Resistant	—	4	0
—	Sensitive	2	0
—	Resistant	2	0
Sensitive (without PHA)	Resistant (without PHA)	0	0
Sensitive	Resistant	32	22
Resistant	Sensitive	18	0

[a] MP, methylprednisolone, applied at 10^{-8} M. Similar results were obtained from two additional pairs of patients.

altered their characteristic responses to glucocorticoid. Second, the semi-purified monocyte and lymphocyte populations cultured separately produced few or no colonies. This demonstrated that, however crude the purification procedure may have been, colony formation faithfully indicated interaction between the two populations. Third, mixtures of lymphocytes and monocytes from different patients in the absence of PHA did not generate colonies. This demonstrated that the colonies observed in these experiments were not the result of a mixed leucocyte reaction. Finally, the combination of corticosteroid-resistant monocytes with sensitive lymphocytes yielded colony growth that was not inhibited by MP at 10^{-8} M, whereas the combination of sensitive monocytes with resistant lymphocytes produced colony growth that was completely inhibited. This demonstrated that corticosteroid resistance is a property of monocytes rather than lymphocytes.

DISCUSSION

These studies show that steroid resistance in asthma is associated with a distinctive cellular abnormality: a defect in monocyte responsiveness to glucocorticoid *in vitro*. Although at present this is presumptive, we suggest that this monocyte defect accounts for the lack of response to corticosteroid *in vivo*.

There are two main routes whereby an effect of corticosteroid on monocytes might influence atopic reactions in sensitive patients: direct action of monocyte products on inflammatory mediators and indirect action via immunoregulatory cells (Fig. 7). Our assay has focused attention on the indirect route. We infer from our results that corticosteroid-resistant monocytes fail to shut off IL-1 production in response to glucocorticoids in the normal way. It is possible that *in vivo* this results in continuing interaction between, and proliferation of, T and B cells even in the presence of corticosteroids, with resultant continuing IgE production. Furthermore, IL-1 possesses interesting properties in its own right as an inducer of inflammatory mediators (13,14). It is equally probable, however, that in corticosteroid-resistant asthma there is a general defect in monocyte responsiveness to glucocorticoid. Indeed this is suggested by the data of Kay and his colleagues (3) who observed corticosteroid unresponsiveness in a monocyte function (complement receptor enhancement) entirely different from that studied here. Monocyte unresponsiveness to corticosteroid may lead to low lipomodulin production *in vivo*,

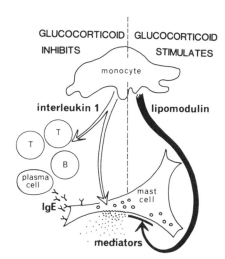

Fig. 7. Schematic representation of the role of the monocyte in corticosteroid-sensitive asthma. Although not shown, cells other than mast cells may be involved in mediator release in this context.

with resultant unrestrained synthesis of mast cell mediators. With assays for both the interleukins and lipomodulin becoming practicable, it should soon be possible to examine these alternatives directly.

It is of interest to inquire whether a monocyte defect of this type could account for the observed clinical differences between corticosteroid-resistant and -sensitive patients. If endogenous glucocorticoids play a role in aborting reactions to anaphylactic stimuli, the tendency of resistant patients to have more frequent attacks would be explained, since their monocyte resistance is evident at supraphysiological glucocorticoid concentrations *in vitro*. The association of a more prominent family history of asthma with glucocorticoid resistance may suggest that the monocyte defect is hereditary.

Study of corticosteroid-resistant asthmatic patients, coupled with analysis of the cellular site of the defect, may serve three purposes. First, it may lead to greater insight into the management of this difficult clinical problem. In particular, our cellular studies suggest that it may be possible to predict which patients are resistant and thus spare them the complications of corticosteroid medication. Second, the cell biology of the corticosteroid-resistant asthmatic directs attention to the major cellular targets of corticosteroid in the more common corticosteroid-sensitive patient. We have not positively excluded other cell types, but the results of this work suggest that the monocyte is this target cell. Finally, although our studies have been solely concerned with chronic asthma, they raise the possibility that corticosteroid-resistant individuals may exist within the general population. In that event, corticosteroid resistance with this cellular basis could give rise to poor therapeutic responses in other disorders for which corticosteroids are used as antiinflammatory or immunosuppressive agents.

SUMMARY

Corticosteroid resistance occurs in a small but significant proportion of asthmatics. It is associated with a defect in monocyte responsiveness to glucocorticoid *in vitro*. This observation emphasises the role of the monocyte as a target cell for corticosteroid action.

ACKNOWLEDGMENTS

AHW is supported by a Career Development Award from the Cancer Research Campaign. A grant from Upjohn Ltd. is gratefully acknowledged.

REFERENCES

1. Carmichael, J., Paterson, I. C., Diaz, P., Crompton, G. K., Kay, A. B., and Grant, I. W. B. Corticosteroid resistance in chronic asthma. *Br. Med. J.* **282:**1419–1422, 1981.
2. Chai, H., Farr, R. S., Froehlich, L. A., Mathison, D. A., McLean, J. A., Rosenthal, R. R., Sheffer, A. L., Spector, S. L., and Townley, R. G. Standardization of bronchial inhalation challenge procedures. *J. Allergy Clin. Immunol.* **56:**323–327, 1975.
3. Kay, A. B., Diaz, P., Carmichael, J., and Grant, I. W. B. Corticosteroid-resistant chronic asthma and monocyte complement receptors. *Clin. Exp. Immunol.* **44:**576–580, 1981.
4. Krajewski, A. S., and Wyllie, A. H. Inhibition of human T lymphocyte colony formation by methylprednisolone. *Clin. Exp. Immunol.* **46:**206–213, 1981.
5. Colledge, N. R., Krajewski, A. S., Smyth, J. F., and Wyllie, A. H. Action of deoxycoformycin on human T cell colonies *in vitro*. *Clin. Exp. Immunol.* **50:**115–122, 1982.
6. Smith, K. A., Lachman, L. B., Oppenheim, J. J., and Favata, M. F. The functional relationship of the interleukins. *J. Exp. Med.* **151:**1551–1556, 1980.
7. Gillis, S., and Watson, J. Interleukin 2 dependent culture of cytolytic T cell lines. *Immunol. Rev.* **54:**81–110, 1981.
8. Rosenszajn, L. A., Goldman, I., Kalechman, Y., Michlin, H., Sredni, B., Zeevi, A., and Shoham, D. T lymphocyte colony growth *in vitro:* Factors modulating clonal expansion. *Immunol. Rev.* **54:**157–186, 1981.
9. Smith, K. T-cell growth factor. *Immunol. Rev.* **51:**337–357, 1980.
10. Thomson, E. B., Norman, M. R., and Lippman, M. E. Steroid hormone action in tissue culture cells and cell hybrids—their relation to human malignancies. *Recent Prog. Horm. Res.* **33:**571–615, 1977.

11. Duval, D., Homo, F., and Thierry, C. Glucocorticoid sensitivity of normal lymphocyte populations. *Proc. Tenovus Workshop* **7**:143–154, 1979.
12. Palacios, R. Mechanism of T cell activation: Role and functional relationship of HLA-DR antigens and interleukins. *Immunol. Rev.* **63**:73–110, 1982.
13. Mizel, S. B., Dayer, J.-M., Krane, S. M., and Mergenhagen, S. E. Stimulation of rheumatoid synovial cell collagenase and prostaglandin production by partially purified lymphocyte activating factor (interleukin 1). *Proc. Natl. Acad. Sci. U.S.A.* **78**:2474–2477, 1981.
14. Dinarello, C. A., Marnoy, S. O., and Rosenwasser, L. J. Role of arachidonate metabolism in the immunoregulatory function of human leucocyte pyrogen/lymphocyte activating factor/interleukin 1. *J. Immunol.* **130**:890–895, 1983.

DISCUSSION

Schiffmann: Have you measured the corticosteroid receptor numbers in the resistant monocytes? If lipomodulin is a crucial entity in restoring sensitivity to steroids in resistant cells, then one might administer lipomodulin to the monocytes in your *in vitro* experiments. It is also conceivable that lipomodulin can be produced in the "resistant" monocytes but that it is inactivated by endogenous hypernormal phosphorylation.

Wyllie: Glucocorticoid receptor numbers in monocytes would provide interesting information but we do not have an assay sensitive enough to measure these at present.

Yes, we look forward to studying the effect of lipomodulin on cellular interactions in corticosteroid-resistant patients.

Morley: Human alveolar macrophages produce PGE_2 and TXA_2 that is sensitive to glucocorticosteroids at therapeutic concentrations. These cells (or more conveniently peripheral blood monocytes) could be tested for their capacity to produce PGE_2 as a relatively simple assay system. Has this been considered?

Wyllie: We have not yet done so, but hope to proceed to this.

Schleimer: You have presented an interesting hypothesis. I wonder if you plan to see, or have already directly tested, whether steroids inhibit IL-1 synthesis by the mononuclear cells?

With regards to the human lung mast cell, *in vitro* steroid treatment does not inhibit mediator release, while it does inhibit basophil histamine release. My recollection of the experiments of Dr. T. Ishizaka and collaborators is that exogenous lipomodulin does not inhibit histamine release. With regard to the potential role of lipomodulin as a hormone, both the Burroughs Wellcome group [R. J. Flower and G. J. Blackwell, *Nature (London)* **278**:456, 1979] and Dr. K. Ishizaka's group (T. Vede, F. Hirata, M. Hirashima, and K. Ishizaka, *J. Immunol.* **130**:878, 1983) have evidence that lipomodulin/macrocortin can exert effects on cells when presented exogenously.

Wyllie: Our current IL-1 assay is the conventional thymocyte proliferation bioassay. IL-1 measurement from monocyte populations is certainly relevant and we aim to measure this in the future, perhaps when a radioimmunoassay becomes available.

Hargreave: Were there any diurnal indices of bronchial inflammation in the resistant group after treatment with steroids? The diurnal features of the resistant group suggest that their bronchial responsiveness is severely increased.

Grant: We found no specific *clinical* indices in the corticosteroid-resistant asthmatics, but patients in that group showed a significantly greater degree of bronchial reactivity to methacholine challenge than patients in the sensitive group.

Wasserman: Your findings in asthma are somewhat reminiscent of the defective regulation of EB virus-induced B cell outgrowth in rheumatoid arthritis, a finding shown to be due to defective response to PGE_2. Have you examined PGE_2 levels on outgrowth or have you data on the effect of cyclooxygenase inhibition?

As triacetyloleandomycin (TAO) enhances the effect of steroids in some studies it would be of interest to know the clinical efficacy of this drug in your steroid-resistant patients.

Grant: It is conceivable, if the hypothesis put forward in this paper is correct, that it will be possible to identify patients with corticosteroid-resistant rheumatoid arthritis and other steroid treated disorders.

The possibility regarding TAO has not been explored.

Lewis: Since you have identified differences in peripheral monocyte responses to steroid in your populations, it might be useful to explore functional difference of pulmonary alveolar macrophages in the presence and absence of steroids in the two asthmatic sets (e.g., cyclooxygenase product generation and macrophage-derived growth factor).

Wyllie: A very attractive suggestion!

Kaplan: I would like to point out that in your diagram, a connection was drawn (apart from the lipomodulin effects) between the stimulated monocyte and the mast cell. Given that IL-1 regulation of IgE synthesis is an unlikely explanation of steroid responsiveness or resistance, I think that some sort of direct communication (a monokine, for instance) between the monocyte and mast cell is an interesting possibility.

Wyllie: Yes, I agree. IL-1 may be one such agent and there may well be others.

Platts-Mills: To what extent are the *in vitro* findings consistent, and can you say whether the *in vitro* phenomenon is secondary to the disease?

Grant: The *in vitro* phenomenon appear to be consistent as far as we have tested it: repeated assays on both sensitive and resistant patients have given consistent results. We think that corticosteroid resistance may be a primary phenomenon—at any rate it is not attributable to therapy, for in a small series of new asthmatics we have been able to predict the ultimate corticosteroid sensitivity or resistance from the *in vitro* responses. I appreciate this is not really definitive evidence that corticosteroid resistance is not caused by the asthma, but we do have one nonasthmatic control subject who was resistant to glucocorticoids *in vitro*.

Turner-Warwick: Could you describe for us in more detail the type of peak flow pattern over the weeks before and after the data you showed to illustrate the "steroid-sensitive" patients?

With regard to the steroid resistant group—you plotted the morning peak flow reading—were these "pure," "morning dippers," or were they unstable through the day?

Grant: Many of the corticosteroid-sensitive asthmatics had their symptoms adequately, although often not perfectly, controlled by steroid aerosols and required only occasional short courses of prednisolone by mouth.

Most of the corticosteroid-resistant asthmatics exhibited a marked degree of "morning dipping" in the PEFR, but this was not as prominent a feature in the corticosteroid-sensitive cases, in whom it was quickly reduced by prednisolone.

CHAPTER 23

Physiological and Pharmacological Control of the Respiratory Drive in Asthma

D. C. FLENLEY

Department of Respiratory Medicine
City Hospital
Edinburgh, Scotland, U.K.

HYPERVENTILATION AND ASTHMA

Asthmatics hyperventilate. This statement stems largely from the observation that the arterial P_{CO_2} is low in untreated patients suffering from an acute attack of clinical asthma; when they are breathing spontaneously (1–4) a high P_{CO_2} only rarely develops and then only in those with severe airflow limitation (Fig. 1). This low P_{CO_2} is usually accompanied by a respiratory alkalosis, at least in adults, whereas in children respiratory acidosis is not uncommon (5,6). Actual measurements of ventilation are rare in severe asthma, for clearly such patients will not tolerate the mouthpiece and nose clip (or even face mask) that are conventionally required for such measurements, and the newer noninvasive techniques [e.g., Respitrace (7)] are only just being applied to acute clinical problems at the bedside (Fig. 2). In unsedated asthmatic dogs (8) and monkeys (9), antigen challenge induces both bronchoconstriction and rapid shallow breathing. In an attack of clinical asthma in man, an increase in functional residual capacity (FRC) is characteristic (10), thus increasing the apparent stiffness of the lungs in the tidal volume range at this high FRC; this, coupled with the increased airways resistance and rapid breathing, must increase the metabolic cost of breathing, although this also has not been directly measured in the acute attack of asthma for the reasons given above. The low Pa_{CO_2} when combined with this increase in CO_2 produc-

ASTHMA: Physiology,
Immunopharmacology,
and Treatment
THIRD INTERNATIONAL SYMPOSIUM

375

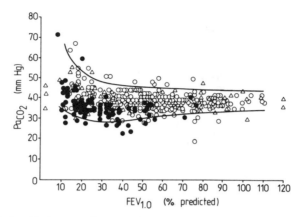

Fig. 1. Relationship between Pa_{CO_2}, and FEV_1 in asthma, as drawn from three studies of adult asthmatics. [Solid circles (2); open circles (Palmer and Kelman, 1973); open triangles (4).]

tion ($\dot{V}_{CO_2}$) must therefore imply that alveolar ventilation is increased. How does this come about?

Hypoxia

Despite hyperventilation, arterial hypoxaemia is usual in the asthmatic attack, largely from an increase in variance of the distribution of ventilation/perfusion ratios ($\dot{V}/\dot{Q}$) among the 3,000,000 alveoli of the lungs, as shown directly in asymptomatic asthma (11), but as such measurements are only valid in a steady state; they have not been used to confirm the $\dot{V}/\dot{Q}$ abnormalities in the acute clinical attack of asthma. The ventilatory response to progressive isocapnic hypoxia in normal subjects is a linear

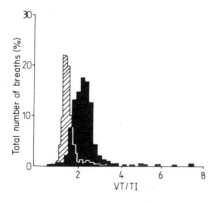

Fig. 2. Frequency histogram of chest wall circumference changes (V_t) divided by inspiratory time (T_i), giving the ratio V_t/T_i, before and after inhalation of a β_2-agonist, which caused an increase in peak expiratory flow rate in a moderately severe asthmatic during emergency hospital treatment. Note that the ventilatory drive, as assessed by V_t/T_i, is reduced as the β_2-agonist relieved airflow limitation [before β_2, PEFR = 200 liter/min (solid bars); after, PEFR = 320 liter/min (shaded bars)].

function of arterial oxygen saturation, with a mean value of 1.7 liter min^{-1} per 1% fall in Sa_{O_2} (12). Calculations based on these figures, with assumption of reasonable values for respiratory frequency, dead space, and $\dot{V}_{CO_2}$ in an asthmatic attack severe enough to lower Pa_{CO_2} to 30 mm Hg and Pa_{O_2} to 50 mm Hg, suggests that the fall in Pa_{CO_2} might result in part from such hypoxic stimulation of ventilation. However, these studies of hypoxic drive depend upon preservation of isocapnia.

Comparison with acute altitude exposure may be more appropriate. For 27 astronomers who motored in 24 hr from sea level to the Mauna Kea Observatory at 4200 m, where mean arterialised P_{O_2} was 42 mm Hg, hyperventilation lowered P_{CO_2} to 28 mm Hg on an average (13). Furthermore, in 10 men who ascended to nearly 4000 m over 4 days, mean Pa_{O_2} was then 46 mm Hg, but Pa_{CO_2} was 23 mm Hg (14). In comparison, in acute asthma (Fig. 3) hyperventilation to P_{CO_2} values of this order only occurred when arterial P_{O_2} values were ~10 mm Hg higher, implying that the hypoxic ventilatory drive alone probably did not account for this degree of hyperventilation (15–17). Correction of the hypoxaemia of the asthmatic by oxygen therapy does not restore Pa_{O_2} to normal values (18),

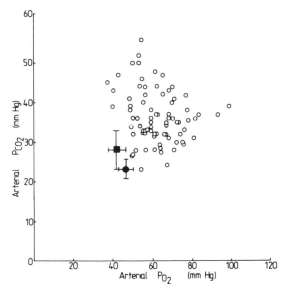

Fig. 3. O_2/CO_2 diagram in acute asthma and in acute altitude exposure. Note that in the asthmatics who have a similar P_{CO_2} to that seen in acute altitude exposure, the arterial P_{O_2} is higher in asthma, thus indicating that hyperventilation of the asthmatic does not arise from hypoxaemia alone. Acute asthma (air), ○. From Karetzkey (16); Rudolf *et al.* (15); Flenley and Warren (17). ■} High altitude (air). From Forster (13); Birmingham Medical Research Expeditionary Society (14).

again indicating that some other factor must therefore be stimulating ventilation. Again, at least some symptoms of acute mountain sickness, such as headache, nausea, anorexia, insomnia, dizziness, vomiting, lassitude, and ataxia occurred in up to 85% of 101 subjects (mean age, 31 years) who trekked to at least 4243 m in 4 days from 2800 m (19). However, such symptoms are not common in clinical asthma, where there is a similar severity of arterial hypoxaemia; as noted above, this will be associated with more hypocapnia in the altitude exposure.

Respiratory Neural Receptors

Stimulation of nasal receptors produces sneezing, apnoea, bronchodilatation, and possibly bronchoconstriction, so that such stimulation may be important in asthma; the receptors in the nose may be stimulated as a result of nasal deposition of the powerful antigen contained in the 20-μm diameter house mite faecal particles (20,21). Bronchopulmonary receptor fibres travelling in the vagus include those derived from irritant receptors in the epithelium of the trachea and bronchi, which are probably separated from airway lumen by tight intracellular junctions. These receptors are stimulated by histamine, probably both directly and as a consequence of the resultant bronchial smooth muscle contraction. Pulmonary stretch receptors also line the walls of the upper airways and are stimulated by distention of the lungs and airways and also by a fall in Pa_{CO_2} and the bronchoconstriction following on histamine inhalation (at least in guinea pigs). J receptors (with small diameter vagal fibres) were initially recognised by their response to intravascular injections of diphenylguanide but are also stimulated by microembolism, lung oedema, and irritant gases. Their stimulation results in rapid shallow breathing, pharyngeal constriction, and inhibition of spinal reflexes. Physiological evidence suggests that J receptors lie within the alveolar wall, but they are difficult to identify there by histological methods, including electron microscopy.

Vagal Afferents in Asthma

Clearly, all these bronchopulmonary receptors could be stimulated by some or all of the mediators that provoke asthmatic bronchoconstriction. However, direct recording from such single-fibre vagal afferents in experimental asthma in animals has not been reported. There is strong experimental evidence, nonetheless, that vagal afferents do play an important role in hyperventilation of the asthmatic attack. Thus, in four unsedated dogs during treadmill exercise, inhalation of *Ascaris suum* antigen aerosol consistently increased ventilation by increasing breathing rate, despite a fall in tidal volume, but only if the vagus nerves were functionally intact. However, when the vagi (exteriorised at a previous surgical procedure) were cooled to inhibit conduction, similar antigen challenge no longer influenced either ventilation, breathing rate, or tidal volume, although pulmonary resistance to airflow still increased as it did before cooling the vagi (8).

In unanaesthetised man, bilateral vagal block at the base of the skull also blocks the IX, X, and XI cranial nerves (22), including carotid chemoreceptors and baro-receptor fibres. In one mild chronic asthmatic physiologist in whom histamine inhalation (after atropine) provoked bronchoconstriction with tachypnoea and a fall in end tidal P_{CO_2}, the same stimulus of histamine inhalation (after atropine) after vagal block then produced no tachypnoea. In another two asthmatics, responses to vagal block during spontaneous breathing without histamine challenge were only trivial, however (23). The role of the vagus in causing the hyperventilation of the asthmatic attack in man is thus still unclear, but there is little enthusiasm today by patients, ethical committees, or investigators to resolve this problem by further direct experimentation in man.

Ventilatory Drive in Asthma

The ventilatory response to CO_2 is depressed in some (24) but not in all asthmatics [at least in children (25)]. The wide variability in the CO_2 response in normal subjects (26,27) also makes clear-cut interpretation of such measurements difficult. However, in 16 of 19 asthmatics the ventilatory response to CO_2 improved over several days as conventional treatment improved their FEV_1 from the initial acute airway obstruction; this did not occur in 3 of the 19 patients, but these persistently low responders could possibly still have responses within the normal range. In contrast, the central respiratory drive [as measured by $P_{0.1}$, the mouth occlusion pressure (28)], which must be transmuted into tidal volume by the inspiratory muscles and depends on the mechanical properties of the lungs and thorax, was in fact *higher* for any given P_{CO_2} during CO_2 rebreathing in asthmatics as compared to normal subjects; this implied that the central respiratory drive from CO_2 was increased in asthma (24), whereas the ventilatory response to CO_2 in these same subjects was reduced. This increase in $P_{0.1}$ in the asthmatic has been confirmed by Kelsen *et al.* (29), but in their studies the ventilatory response to CO_2 was normal in the asthmatics. Furthermore, the same authors also found that the response of the central drive ($P_{0.1}$) to an external flow-resistive load during CO_2

breathing was increased in asthma, and they attributed this effect to stimulation of sensory receptors in the airways (29). $P_{0.1}$ was also increased during spontaneous breathing at rest in 17 moderately severe adult asthmatics (FEV$_1$/VC, 46%; Pa_{O_2}, 65 mm Hg; Pa_{CO_2}, 31 mm Hg), but the mean $P_{0.1}$ was slightly reduced when oxygen therapy was used to raise the Pa_{O_2} of these patients to 114 mm Hg on an average, although the Pa_{CO_2} still remained low (18).

These same authors also found that the hypoxic drive to breathing was normal in asthmatics, when assessed by ventilatory responses, and this again has been confirmed in some asthmatic children (30) but not in others (31). Severe hypoxia and CO_2 retention in a 17-year-old asthmatic has been attributed to a possible hereditary absence of the hypoxic drive to breathing (32). We have also studied a 21-year-old male asthmatic who presented with cor pulmonale and persistent hypoxaemia that became much worse at night and during an asthmatic attack (33), and in this patient the ventilatory response to hypoxia also was absent.

Before the 1960s, bilateral carotid body resection began to be used for the treatment of asthma in Japan, and this controversial surgical procedure has also been carried out in California (34). The technique, which removes the carotid bodies alone yet preserves the baro-receptor responses intact, is believed by some to relieve bronchospasm; this is based upon animal studies (35) that showed that hypoxic stimuli mediated through the carotid bodies could provoke bronchoconstriction. However, many physicians fear that bilateral carotid body resection may render the patient particularly liable to fatal hypoxaemia during an asthmatic attack. Nonetheless, it must be admitted that the role of bilateral carotid body resection in the treatment of bronchial asthma has never been tested by a controlled clinical trial.

Respiratory Muscles

Although the very large increases in total lung capacity (TLC) previously described in acute asthma (36) are now recognised to be an artefact [swings in mouth pressure during panting in the body plethysmograph are less than oesophageal pressure swings when airways obstruction is severe (37)], it still seems that the FRC is considerably increased in asthma (10). This hyperinflation will thus impose severe burdens on inspiratory muscles of respiration (yet assist the expiratory muscles) whereas the increase in airflow resistance (38) will increase the demands on both. Thus shortening the resting length of the inspiratory muscles will reduce the tension which they can develop for a given stimulus; the low flat diaphragm must geometrically reduce its ability to generate a negative intrapleural pressure [by the Laplace relationship (39)]; and the static pressure volume curve of the thorax becomes flatter at high lung volumes (40). The hyperinflation seems to result from sustained contraction of the respiratory muscles throughout the breathing cycle, as shown by both mechanical (41) and electromyographic (42) measurements. This sustained activity will also impair blood flow into the respiratory muscles, yet at the same time the metabolic demands on these muscles is very great, as shown by the great increase in the work of breathing (43). The scene thus seems set for a Micawber-like catastrophe, which must end in respiratory muscle failure, CO_2 retention, lactacidosis, and ultimately death, unless the airways obstruction that initiates this sequence is reversed either spontaneously or in response to treatment. It is possible that less severe degrees of hypoxia in the respiratory muscles may generate some of the excess respiratory drive in the asthmatic by stimulation of small diameter muscle afferents during hypoxic exercise (44), as has been suggested in other skeletal muscles.

Summary

It seems probable that the undoubted hyperventilation of the asthmatic attack results from considerable increase in the intensity of central ventilatory drive, which in turn probably arises largely from stimulation of bronchopulmonary afferents running in the vagus nerves, with also a potential minor component arising from the hypoxaemia that results from the variation in ventilation/perfusion balance within the asthmatic lungs. These bronchopulmonary receptors may be stimulated by histamine, or possibly by the more potent mediators including leukotrines that are released as a consequence of the antigen/antibody response, which is responsible for the bronchospasm of asthma; at this time, however, this mechanism of stimulation must be regarded as purely speculative.

DRUGS AND THE VENTILATORY DRIVE IN ASTHMA

Pharmacological modification of the respiratory drive in asthma has rarely been a primary aim of therapy, and indeed such treatment could carry hazards. Reduction of the excessive respiratory drive in the asthmatic would obviously increase hypoxaemia, from the arithmetic dictates of the alveolar air equation (45). The potential danger of catastrophic respiratory muscle fatigue (see above) would then be increased by further arterial hypoxaemia (46), and unless the hyperinflation and airway narrowing were also reduced, any reduction in inspiratory work from the reduced ventilatory demand may thus be offset by this even greater danger. This reasoning may underly the traditional clinician's view that "Morphia is dangerous, and may be deadly" in asthma (47). Similar arguments would apply to other ventilatory depressants [morphine analogues, short-acting barbiturates, and even benzodiazepimes (48)]. Thus, at least in the acute asthmatic, even modest sedation is safe only if accompanied by relief of airway obstruction, and even then the effects of the sedative should be carefully monitored (unless of course the patient is mechanically ventilated).

β_2-Agonists and theophyllines are used primarily to relieve airways obstruction, but they also have important effects on ventilatory control, at least in normal subjects. Thus, in seven healthy men, 10 μg/min of iv salbutamol infusion significantly increased the ventilatory response to inhaled CO_2, in both hypoxia and hyperoxia, implying a central effect. The infusion also increased heart rate, particularly when hypoxia was combined with hypercapnia, and reduced the serum potassium on an average from 4.0 to 3.1 mM/liter, presumably as the result of an increase in both plasma glucose and serum insulin, which cause potassium to move into the intracellular fluid (49). Extrapolating to the asthmatic (which may not be justified), one may conclude that β_2-agonist therapy, at least in this dose, may further increase hyperventilation, particularly if hypoxia is allowed to persist. Hypokalaemia, which could impair function of respiratory muscles as well as induce cardiac irregularities, is also clearly important in the practical management of the asthmatic attack, as β_2-agonists, at least by nebuliser (either by metered dose or wet nebulisation), are widely regarded as the first-line treatment of choice in the acute attack of asthma (50).

Theophyllines (51), given either intravenously in the treatment of the acute attack (52) or by mouth (now often used in prevention of asthma when given as a slow-release preparation) were also found to lower resting end tidal P_{CO_2} from 38 to 34 mm Hg when the average theophylline serum level was 13.2 mg/ml in seven healthy men following iv infusion, with similar but smaller effects when serum levels were somewhat lower following oral dosage. Furthermore, theophylline also increased the hypoxic ventilatory drive in these subjects when this was measured at constant end tidal P_{CO_2} (53), confirming earlier observations (54).

Aubier *et al.* (55) has found that aminophylline increased the transdiaphragmatic pressure generated for a given integrated electromyographic activity in the diaphragm in eight men; in four of these subjects aminophylline increased the transdiaphragmatic pressure generated at a given level of stimulation of the phrenic nerve, as compared to control studies in the same subjects without aminophylline. All of these responses were obtained when serum theophylline levels were in the therapeutic range, suggesting that a direct action of the drug on muscle may be important in treatment of asthma, as well as in chronic bronchitis and emphysema. However, Green and Moxham (56) have found that aminophylline did not affect either the twitch tension, frequency force curve, or low frequency fatigue of the human adductor pollices muscle, nor was the amplitude of the transdiaphragmatic twitch pressure that resulted from stimulation of the phrenic nerve in normal men affected by intravenous infusion of aminophylline. More studies are clearly needed to resolve these experimental conflicts, for this could have important indications for understanding the full role of theophylline in the treatment of human asthma.

Isoprenaline [isoproterenol (57)] and intravenous aminophylline (58) are both well recognised to cause a minor fall in arterial P_{O_2} in the asthmatic despite relieving airflow limitation, an effect that appears to result from change in $\dot{V}/\dot{Q}$ distribution between alveoli in the asthmatic following drugs. In contrast, prednisolone appears to increase Pa_{O_2} as well as relieving airflow limitation, as has been clearly documented in longstanding chronic asthmatics in which 40 mg of prednisolone by mouth increased PEF and Pa_{O_2} within 9 hr of administration (59).

BREATHING AND VENTILATORY CONTROL IN NOCTURNAL ASTHMA

Although nocturnal asthma was clearly described in 1698 (60), recognition that FEV_1 (61) or the PEF (62) could vary throughout 24 hr in asthmatics has led to the recognition that the "early morning dip" (62) of PEF is common in many asthmatics. This dip usually occurs around 2 to 4 AM, and although a circadian effect is important (63) a recent study in paired adult asthmatics, both of whom were woken to measure PEF when one of the pair entered rapid eye movement (REM) sleep, has also shown that some airflow limitation is associated with REM sleep (64). Modest hypoxaemia and irregular breathing during sleep are also both more common in stable asthmatics than in age-matched control subjects (65,66). The mechanism of this nocturnal airflow limitation, which may be subclinical but is more commonly recognised when it awakens the patients with wheeze, is not yet understood. The relationship to REM sleep may be important. Breathing is characteristically erratic in REM sleep, and this is particu-

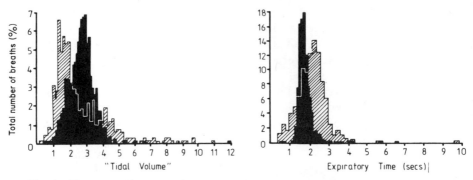

Fig. 4. Frequency histogram of the changes in chest wall diameter ("tidal volume") and expiratory time during nonrapid eye movement sleep (NREM) when oxygenation was stable at a high level, and during rapid eye movement sleep (REM) when arterial oxygen saturation fell during nocturnal sleep in a patient with atopic asthma. Note that in REM sleep breathing is more irregular, and that tidal volume tends to be reduced and expiratory time prolonged, which is compatible with the occurrence of bronchoconstriction at this time. NREM, stable Sa_{O_2} (solid bars); REM, hypoxaemic episodes (shaded bars). From Catterall *et al.* (65).

larly true in hypoxic REM sleep of the asthmatic (Fig. 4), when this is compared with either wakefulness or non-REM sleep, and both the CO_2 and hypoxic drives to breathing are now known to be reduced in REM sleep in man (67). Thus an asthmatic attack that triggered hypoxaemia (by whatever mechanism) may give less ventilatory stimulation if this occurred during REM sleep.

Although Clark and Hetzel (68) suggested that allergy plays little part in nocturnal asthma, the discovery that the house mite faecal pellet contains a very potent antigen (21), and that prolonged avoidance of such allergen will reduce bronchial hyperreactivity in house mite-sensitive asthmatics (69), might imply a role for such a mechanism. House mites often live in the mattress, and it seems very probable that the faecal pellets (20 μm in diameter) may therefore be inhaled during the night. If they deposit in the nose, which aerodynamic theory would predict for such a particle size (70), it seems possible that an allergic reaction at this site could cause occlusion of the nasal airway (71), known to interfere with breathing during sleep (72).

Furthermore, Sullivan *et al.* (73) found that in four trained dogs tracheal calibre (which they assessed by variation of the pressure in the cuff of an endotrachael tube inserted through a previously fashioned tracheostomy) fluctuated erratically during REM sleep, whereas this tracheal muscle tone was stable in non-REM sleep. However, the fluctuations in tracheal tone during REM sleep were abolished (although resting tone was not) when both vagus nerves (previously exteriorised in skin loops) were cooled, implying that muscular contraction of the central airways depended upon vagally mediated influences. It thus seems possible that the bronchoconstriction, which we believe to be a relatively common feature of REM sleep in asthmatics, may be mediated by a similar neural mechanism although clearly this proposal will require much further study to establish.

It will be obvious that much remains to be learned as to the mechanisms of nocturnal asthma. However, this also remains a challenge therapeutically; the commonly used β_2-agonists, given by metered-dose inhaler, rarely persist long enough to provide protection throughout the night, and this may be a specific area where slow-release theophyllines (74) or even ketotifen (75) could provide

> A bower quiet for us, and a sleep
> full of sweet dreams and health, and quiet
> breathing
>
> (John Keats, *Endyminon*)

for the asthmatic.

REFERENCES

1. Tai, E., and Read, J. Blood-gas tensions in bronchial asthma. *Lancet* 1:444–446, 1967.
2. McFadden, E. R., and Lyons, H. A. Arterial blood-gas tension in asthma. *N. Engl. J. Med.* 278:1027–1032, 1968.
3. Rees, H. A., Millar, J. S., and Donald, K. W. A study of the clinical course and arterial blood gas tensions of patients with status asthmaticus. *Q. J. Med.* 37:541–561, 1968.
4. Miyamoto, T., Mizuno, K., and Furuya, K. Arterial blood gases in bronchial asthma. *J. Allergy* 45:248–254, 1970.
5. Simons, F. E. R., Pierson, W. E., and Bierman, C. W. Respiratory failure in childhood status asthmaticus. *Am. J. Dis. Child.* 131:1097–1101, 1977.
6. Simpson, H., Forfar, J. O., and Grubb, D. J. Arterial blood gas tensions and pH in acute asthma in childhood. *Br. Med. J.* 3:460–464, 1968.
7. Duffty, P., Spriet, L., Bryan, M. H., and Bryan, A. C. Respiratory induction plethysmography (Respitrace TM): Evaluation of its use in the infant. *Am. Rev. Respir. Dis.* 123:542–546, 1980.
8. Cotton, D. J., Bleecker, E. R., Fischer, S. P., Graf, P. D., Gold, W. M., and Nadel J. A. Rapid shallow breathing after *Ascaris suum* antigen inhalation: Role of vagus nerves. *J. Appl. Physiol.* 42:101–106, 1977.
9. Pare, P. D., Michoud, M. C., and Hogg, J. C. Lung mechanics following antigen challenge of *Ascaris suum*–sensitive rhesus monkeys. *J. Appl. Physiol.* 41:668–676, 1976.
10. McFadden, E. R., and Lyons, H. A. Serial studies of factors influencing airway dynamics during recovery from acute asthma attacks. *J. Appl. Physiol.* 27:452–459, 1969.
11. Wagner, P. D., Dantzker, D. R., Iacovoni, V. E., Tomlin, W. C., and West, J. B. Ventilation–perfusion inequality in asymptomatic asthma. *Am. Rev. Respir. Dis.* 118:511–524, 1978.

12. Rebuck, A. S., and Slutsky, A. S. Measurement of ventilatory responses to hypercapnia and hypoxia. *Lung Biol. Health Dis.* **17:**745–772, 1981.
13. Forster, P. J. G. Work at high altitude: A study at the United Kingdom infra red telescope, Mauna Kea, Hawaii, 1983 (personal communication).
14. Birmingham Medical Research Expeditionary Society Mountain Sickness Study Group. Acetazolamide in control of acute mountain sickness. *Lancet* **1:**180–183, 1981.
15. Rudolf, M., Riordan, J. F., Grant, B. J. B., Maberly, D. J., and Saunders, K. B. Arterial blood gas tensions in acute severe asthma. *Eur. J. Clin. Invest.* **10:**55–62, 1980.
16. Karetzky, M. S. Blood studies in untreated patients with acute asthma. *Am. Rev. Respir. Dis.* **112:**607–613, 1975.
17. Flenley, D. C., and Warren, P. M. Personal series (1983).
18. Kassabian, J., Miller, K. D., and Lavietes, M. H. Respiratory center output and ventilatory timing in patients with acute airway (asthma) and alveolar (pneumonia) disease. *Chest* **81:**536–543, 1982.
19. Hackett, P. H., Rennie, D., and Levine, H. D. The incidence, importance, and prophylaxis of acute mountain sickness. *Lancet* **2:**1149–1154, 1976.
20. Widdicombe, J. G. Nervous receptors in the respiratory tract and lungs. *Lung Biol. Health Dis.* **17:**429–472, 1981.
21. Tovey, E. R., Chapman, M. D., and Platts-Mills, T. A. E. Mite faeces are a major source of house dust allergens. *Nature (London)* **289:**592–593, 1981.
22. Guz, A., Nobel, M. I. M., Eisele, J. H., and Trenchard, D. The role of vagal inflation reflexes in man and other animals. *In* "Breathing: Hering-Breuer Centenary Symposium," pp. 17–40. Churchill, London, 1970.
23. Eisele, J. H., and Jain, S. K. Circulatory and respiratory changes during unilateral and bilateral cranial nerve IX and X block in two asthmatics. *Clin. Sci.* **40:**117–125, 1971.
24. Zackon, H., Despas, P. J., and Anthonisen, N. R. Occlusion pressure responses in asthma and chronic obstructive pulmonary disease. *Am. Rev. Respir. Dis.* **114:**917–927, 1976.
25. Hutchison, A. A., and Okinsky, A. Hypoxic and hypercapnic response in asthmatic subjects with previous respiratory failure. *Thorax* **36:**759–763, 1981.
26. Rebuck, A. S., and Read, J. Patterns of ventilatory response to carbon dioxide during recovery from severe asthma. *Clin. Sci.* **41:**13–21, 1971.
27. Saunders, N. A., Leeder, S. R., and Rebuck, A. S. Ventilatory response to carbon dioxide in young athletes: A family study. *Am. Rev. Respir. Dis.* **113:**497–502, 1976.
28. Whitelaw, W. A., Derenne, J. P., and Milic-Emili, J. Occlusion pressure as a measure of respiratory centre output in conscious man. *Respir. Physiol.* **23:**181–199, 1975.
29. Kelsen, S. G., Fleegler, B., and Altose, M. D. The respiratory neuromuscular response to hypoxia, hypocapnia, and obstruction to airflow in asthma. *Am. Rev. Respir. Dis.* **120:**517–527, 1979.
30. Morrill, C. G., Dickey, D. W., and Cropp, G. J. A. Ventilatory response and drive of asthmatic children to alveolar hypoxia. *Pediatr. Res.* **15:**1520–1524, 1981.
31. Smith, T. F., and Hudgel, D. W. Decreased ventilation in response to hypoxia in children with asthma. *J. Pediatr. (St. Louis)* **97:**736–741, 1980.
32. Hudgel, D. W., and Weil, J. V. Asthma associated with decreased hypoxic ventilatory drive. *Ann. Intern. Med.* **80:**622–625, 1974.
33. Catterall, J. R., Calverley, P. M. A., MacNee, W., and Flenley, D. C. Unpublished data.
34. Winter, B. J. Carotid body resection. Controversy—confusion—conflict. *Ann. Thorac. Surg.* **16:**648–659, 1973.

35. Nadel, J. A., and Widdicombe, J. G. Reflex control of airway size. *Ann. N. Y. Acad. Sci.* **109:**712–722, 1963.
36. Woolcock, A. J., Rebuck, A. S., Cade, J. F., and Read, J. Lung volume changes in asthma measured concurrently by two methods. *Am. Rev. Respir. Dis.* **104:**703–709, 1971.
37. Rodenstein, D. O., and Stanescu, D. C. Frequency dependence of plethysmographic volume in healthy and asthmatic subjects. *J. Appl. Physiol.* **54:**159–165, 1983.
38. McFadden, E. R., Kiser, R., and deGroot, W. J. Acute bronchial asthma. Relations between clinical and physiologic manifestations. *N. Engl. J. Med.* **288:**221–225, 1973.
39. Marshall, R. Relationships between stimulus and work of breathing at different lung volumes. *J. Appl. Physiol.* **17:**917–921, 1962.
40. Flenley, D. C., Pengelly, L. D., and Milic-Emili, J. Immediate effects of positive-pressure breathing on the ventilatory response to CO_2. *J. Appl. Physiol.* **30:**7–11, 1971.
41. Martin, J., Powell, E., Shore, S., Emrich, J., and Engel, L. A. The role of respiratory muscles in the hyperinflation of bronchial asthma. *Am. Rev. Respir. Dis.* **121:**441–447, 1980.
42. Muller, N., Bryan, A. C., and Zamel, N. Tonic inspiratory muscle activity as a cause of hyperinflation in asthma. *J. Appl. Physiol.* **50:**279–282, 1981.
43. Roussos, C. Lecture at International Congress of Chest Disease, Toronto, Canada, 1982.
44. Flenley, D. C., Brash, H., Clancy, L., Cooke, N. J., Leitch, A. G., Middleton, W., and Wraith, P. K. Ventilatory response to steady-state exercise in hypoxia in humans. *J. Appl. Physiol.* **46:**438–446, 1979.
45. Otis, A. B. Quantitative relationships in steady state gas exchange. *In* "Handbook of Physiology" (W. O. Fenn and H. Rahn, eds.), Sect. 3, Vol. I, pp. 681–698. Am. Physiol. Soc., Washington, D.C., 1964.
46. Roussos, C. S., and Macklem, P. T. Diaphragmatic fatigue in man. *J. Appl. Physiol.* **43:**189–197, 1977.
47. Coope, R. "Diseases of the Chest." Livingstone, Edinburgh, 1948.
48. Hickey, R. F., and Severinghaus, J. W. Regulation of breathing: drug effects. *Lung Biol. Health Dis.* **17:**1251–1312, 1981.
49. Leitch, A. G., Clancy, L. J., Costello, J. F., and Flenley, D. C. Effect of intravenous infusion of salbutamol on ventilatory response to carbon dioxide and hypoxia and on heart rate and plasma potassium in normal men. *Br. Med. J.* **1:**365–367, 1976.
50. Flenley, D. C. New drugs in respiratory medicine. *Br. Med. J.* **286:**871–875, 1983.
51. Weinberger, M., and Hendeles, L. Theophyllines. *In* "Recent Advances in Respiratory Medicine" (D. C. Flenley and T. L. Petty, eds.), Vol. 3. Churchill-Livingstone, Edinburgh and London, pp. 63–77, 1983.
52. Jenne, J. W. Pharmacology of the airways. *In* "Pulmonary Disease Reviews" (R. C. Bone, ed.), Vol. 2, pp. 295–318. Wiley, New York, 1981.
53. Sanders, J. S., Berman, T. M., Bartlett, M. M., and Kronenberg, R. S. Increased hypoxic ventilatory drive due to administration of aminophylline in normal men. *Chest* **78:**279–282, 1980.
54. Lakshminarayan, S., Sahn, S. A., and Weil, J. V. Effect of aminophylline on ventilatory responses in normal man. *Am. Rev. Respir. Dis.* **117:**33–38, 1978.
55. Aubier, M., De Troyer, A., Sampson, M., Macklem, P. T., and Roussos, C. Aminophylline improves diaphragmatic contractility. *N. Engl. J. Med.* **305:**249–252, 1981.
56. Green, M., and Moxham, J. Respiratory muscles. *In* "Recent Advance in Respiratory Medicine" (D. C. Flenley and T. L. Petty, eds.), Vol. 3. Churchill-Livingstone, Edinburgh and London, pp. 1–20, 1983.

57. Knudson, R. J., and Constantine, H. P. An effect of isoprotenerol on ventilation-perfusion in asthmatic versus normal subjects. *J. Appl. Physiol.* **22**:402–406, 1967.
58. Rees, H. A., Borthwick, R. C., Millar, J. S., and Donald, K. W. Aminophylline in bronchial asthma. *Lancet* **2**:1167–1169, 1967.
59. Ellul-Micallef, R., Borthwick, R. C., and McHardy, G. J. R. The effect of oral prednisolone on gas exchange in chronic bronchial asthma. *Br. J. Clin. Pharmacol.* **9**:479–482, 1980.
60. Floyer, J. A. "A Treatise of the Asthma." Wilkin, London, 1698.
61. Lewinsohn, H. C., Capel, L. H., and Smart, J. Changes in forced expiratory volumes throughout the day. *Br. Med. J.* **1**:462–464, 1960.
62. Turner-Warwick, M. On observing patterns of airflow obstruction in chronic asthma. *Br. J. Dis. Chest* **71**:73–86, 1977.
63. Hetzel, M. R., and Clark, T. J. H. Does sleep cause nocturnal asthma? *Thorax* **34**:749–754, 1979.
64. Shapiro, C., Montgomery, I., and Catterall, J. R. Breathing, bronchoconstriction, and sleep stage in nocturnal asthma. *Thorax* **37**:238 (abstr.), 1982.
65. Catterall, J. R., Douglas, N. J., Calverley, P. M. A. *et al.* Irregular breathing and hypoxaemia during sleep in chronic stable asthma. *Lancet* **1**:301–304, 1982.
66. Montplaisir, J., Walsh, J., and Malo, J. L. Nocturnal asthma: Features of attacks, sleep and breathing patterns. *Am. Rev. Respir. Dis.* **125**:18–22, 1982.
67. Douglas, N. J., White, D. P., Weil, J. V. *et al.* Hypoxic ventilatory response decreases during sleep in normal men. *Am. Rev. Respir. Dis.* **125**:286–289, 1982.
68. Clark, T. J. H., and Hetzel, M. R. Diurnal variation of asthma. *Br. J. Dis. Chest* **71**:87–92, 1977.
69. Platts-Mills, T. A. E., Tovey, E. R., Mitchell, E. B., Moszoro, H., Nock, P., and Wilkins, S. Reducation of bronchial hyperreactivity during prolonged allergen avoidance. *Lancet* **2**:675–678, 1982.
70. Morrow, P. E. Clearance kinetics of inhaled particles. *Lung Biol. Health Dis.* **5**:491–543, 1977.
71. McNicholas, W. T., Tarlo, S., Cole, P. *et al.* Obstructive apneas during sleep in patients with seasonal allergic rhinitis. *Am. Rev. Respir. Dis.* **126**:625–628, 1982.
72. Zwillich, C. W., Pickett, C., Hanson, F. N., and Weil, J. V. Disturbed sleep and prolonged apnea during nasal obstruction in men. *Am. Rev. Respir. Dis.* **124**:158–160, 1981.
73. Sullivan, C. E., Zamel, N., Kozar, L. F., Murphy, E., and Phillipson, E. A. Regulation of airway smooth muscle tone in sleeping dogs. *Am. Rev. Respir. Dis.* **119**:87–99, 1979.
74. Barnes, P. J., Greening, A. P., Neville, L., Timmers, J., and Poole, G. W. Single-dose slow-release aminophylline at night prevents nocturnal asthma. *Lancet* **1**:299–301, 1982.
75. Catterall, J. R., Calverley, P. M. A., Wraith, P. K. *et al.* The role of ketotifen in nocturnal asthma. *Res. Clin. Forums* **4**:21–26, 1982.

DISCUSSION

Leitch: Can you tell whether the P_{O_2} falls further during sleep in asthmatics compared with normals? The data given were Sa_{O_2} values, and both groups presumably start at different points on the O_2 dissociation curve.

Flenley: In normal (older) subjects, asthmatics and bronchitics, *on average,* the P_{O_2} falls by about 10 mg in REM sleep, and the saturation fall thus depends upon where the P_{O_2} is at the time of starting the REM sleep. However, the *absolute* level of P_{O_2} achieved is lower in asthmatics than normals, and I believe it is this absolute level of P_{O_2} that produces the physiological effects such as pulmonary hypertension, altered cardiac output, arrythmias, etc.

McFadden: Could the effect of histamine that you are describing be caused by (a) direct or (b) reflex effects on the glottis?

Flenley: I do not know what histamine inhalation does to the glottis or what happens to the glottis in sleep. Obstructive sleep apnoea was not common in our studies.

Pride: I am concerned you are suggesting another potentially unfavourable effect of β-agonists in asthma, that is, a reduction in respiratory drive. But when you have improved airway mechanics, I do not believe you can use changes in V_t/T_i to assess respiratory drive.

Flenley: I agree that the measurement of drive from V_t/T_i by the "Respitrace" is not ideal, as it depends on lung volume (which will change as airways dilate) and on the mechanical changes in the lungs, which will themselves change the relationship between phrenic nerve activity (the true drive) and the V_t/T_i, but we cannot make better measurements of drive, such as $P_{0.1}$, in severely sick asthmatics. The results *suggest* that drive *might* decline with relief of bronchospasm but cannot prove it.

McFadden: Could you comment on the effects of oxygen administration on respiratory drive in patients with airway obstruction?

Flenley: That is a very large subject. In brief, in acute exacerebations of CO_2 retention in COPD, oxygen *sometimes* causes a further rise in P_{CO_2} but by no means in all, despite the predictions of classical theory [P. M. Warren, D. C. Flenley, J. S. Millar, and A. Avery, *Lancet* 1:467, 1980; P. M. Warren, A. Jeffrey, C. Haslett, R. A. Wilkie, and D. C. Flenley, *Clin. Sci.* 63:53p (45 abstr.), 1982]. In those without CO_2 retention initially, (as in most asthmatics) oxygen almost never causes P_{CO_2} to rise to a clinical level of significance.

Grant: Is there sound evidence that selective β-agonists are any less liable to reduce the PO_2 than isoprenaline or aminophylline? Is there any risk that salbutamol inhaled last thing at night will aggravate the periodic hypoxaemia that occurs during sleep in some patients with asthma?

Flenley: No, I feel that the problem with β-agonist by inhalation last thing at night (on retiring) is that it will not last long enough (only ~3 to 4 hr) and that this may be a specific indication for slow-release theophylline, as suggested by a study by Barnes *et al.* (P. J. Barnes, A. P. Greening, L. Neville, J. Timmers, and E. W. Poole, *Lancet* 1:229, 1982).

Grant: In 1981–1982, 6000 asthmatic patients in New Zealand privately purchased nebulizers for inhalation of bronchodilator aerosols (mainly salbutamol in a dose of 5–10 mg several times per day). By any standards, the dose of drug actually inhaled was up to 50 times that obtained from pressurized inhalers in the usual recommended dose. This is now being investigated as one possible cause of the recent increase in asthma deaths in New Zealand.

Nadel: Are pollens and other inhaled antigens retained in the nose for significant periods in asthmatics? Could they be aspirated at night and trigger attacks?

Platts-Mills: I think it is unlikely that pollen is present in the air of the bedroom at night in sufficient concentrations to contribute directly to nasal or bronchial nocturnal symptoms. The size of pollen grains is about 20 nm in diameter, and these settle rapidly in undisturbed rooms.

Clark: A number of factors are associated with the abnormal circadian rhythm in asthma. These include gastro-oesophageal reflux, inhalation of mites, and changes in plasma adrenaline and histamine. None of these factors produces asthma in healthy subjects, and in asthma the common denominator appears to be bronchial hyperreactivity.

McFadden: If one were to consume an entire cannister of salbutamol at one time, how much drug would one get?

Tattersfield: If you give the same dose of terbutaline by nebulizer and by metered-dose inhaler, blood levels are lower after the nebulizer. The dose of β-agonist given by nebulizer can be up to 50 times higher than the dose recommended by metered-dose inhaler, for example, 5–10 mg salbutamol by nebulizer compared to 200 mcg by metered-dose inhaler. Studies in Southampton (R. A. Lewis, M. J. Cushley, J. S. Fleming, and A. E. Tattersfield, *Am. Rev. Respir. Dis.* **25**:94, 1982; M. J. Cushley, R. A. Lewis, D. J. B. Cragg, I. L. Jackson, and A. E. Tattersfield, *Thorax* **36**:714, 1981) suggested that roughly the same proportion of the dose from a nebulizer enters the lung as from a metered-dose inhaler, that is, ~10%.

Flenley: I am worried about the possibility that large doses of β-agonist, which can be given by nebulization using inhaler solution, could induce further severe and potentially fatal hypoxia in a hypoxic severe asthmatic. This needs study, in my view, because the nebulizer may be driven by air and not O_2 in the patient's home.

CHAPTER 24

Pharmacological Modulation of Airway Calibre and Mediator Release in Human Models of Bronchial Asthma

STEPHEN T. HOLGATE, MARTIN K. CHURCH, MICHAEL J. CUSHLEY, CLIVE ROBINSON, JONATHAN S. MANN, and PETER H. HOWARTH

*Faculty of Medicine, University of Southampton
and Department of Clinical Pharmacology
Southampton General Hospital
Southampton, U.K.*

INTRODUCTION

Bronchial asthma is a disease that can be characterized clinically by reversible airways obstruction, physiologically by increased bronchial reactivity to specific and/or nonspecific stimuli, and pathologically by airway inflammation (1). The pathological features of asthma are well defined and include destruction of the bronchial epithelium and mucosal oedema, hypersecretion of mucus, infiltration of the airway wall with eosinophils and neutrophils, thickening of the basement membrane, and hypertrophy of airway smooth muscle (2,3). Most of these pathological features can be accounted for by the release of mast cell and mast cell-associated inflammatory mediators (4,5).

In contrast, the mechanism(s) of airway hyperreactivity are not defined, although they may be linked to airway inflammation. It has been suggested that release of inflammatory mediators from bronchial mucosal mast cells opens up epithelial tight junctions allowing penetration of inflammatory mediators to afferent vagal receptors and the bronchial smooth muscle (6). This may occur acutely in seasonal allergic asthma or chronically in perennial asthma in which permanent disruption of the epithelial barrier may be an important factor in maintaining enhanced

ASTHMA: Physiology,
Immunopharmacology,
and Treatment
THIRD INTERNATIONAL SYMPOSIUM

391

airway reactivity (3). An alteration in airway epithelial permeability may coexist with other mechanisms contributing to hyperreactivity such as an acquired or genetic defect of airway smooth muscle (7) and enhanced bronchoconstrictor neural reflex pathways (8,9).

In an attempt to define the role of the mast cell in airway hyperreactivity, parallel measurement of airway and plasma mediator responses have been undertaken with specific and nonspecific bronchial provocation in patients with mild asthma. These *in vivo* studies have been compared to *in vitro* modulation of mediator release from dispersed human lung mast cells.

MAST CELLS OF HUMAN LUNG AND THEIR ACTIVATION

Human lung tissue contains 0.01–0.1% mast cells (5), of which at least 80% are situated in the airways where they comprise 0.12–0.42% of the bronchial epithelial cells (10). These mast cells are mostly located beneath the respiratory epithelium, although a number are also found adjacent to the bronchial lumen (10,11) which, with alveolar mast cells, account for the 0.1–0.4% of histamine-containing cells found in bronchoalveolar lavage fluid (12,13). Because of their position, luminal mast cells assume particular importance in the initial airway response to inhaled allergen (6). Mast cells from the gastrointestinal tract of the rat (14,15) and possibly of the human (16) differ from mesenchymal mast cells in their cell of origin, mechanism of differentiation, content of mediators, and mechanisms of activation. Comparable studies have not been reported for mast cells of human airways, although the lysozomal granules of intraepithelial mast cells (10) have a crystalline ultrastructure similar to mast cells enzymatically dispersed from lung parenchyma (17).

Since exposure to a number of nonspecific proteases may alter the response of mast cells to immunological activation (18), initial studies to characterize human lung mast cells were carried out with cells dispersed mechanically or with collagenase alone. These cells may be activated to release mediators by specific antigen, antihuman IgE, the ionophores A23187 and ionomycin, and concanavalin A, but in contrast to rat serosal mast cells, they are not activated by compound 48/80, basic polyamines (polyarginine, polylysine, ACTH 1-24, and the bee venom peptide 401), or dextran (19,20). Mechanically dispersed mast cells have on their cell surface in excess of 1.5×10^5 free high-affinity (K_A, $10^8 \ M^{-1}$) binding sites for the Fc C4 domain of IgE (21). Following the bridging of IgE-Fc receptors, histamine secretion begins after 10 to 15 sec, and proceeds rapidly to

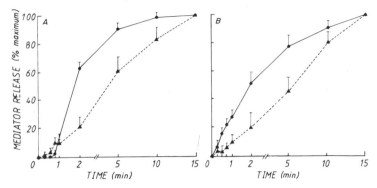

Fig. 1. Time course of histamine (●) and prostaglandin D_2 (▲) release from dispersed human lung mast cells challenged with 1/10 antihuman IgE (A) and ionophore A23187, 2.5 μM (B). Each point represents the mean ± 1 SEM of eight observations for anti-IgE and five for A23187.

reach completion by 5 to 10 min. Both IgE- and ionophore-dependent histamine release are totally dependent on extracellular calcium and an intact glycolytic pathway (20). Furthermore, in individual mast cell preparations a positive correlation between immunologically induced and A23187-induced histamine release suggests that "mediator releasability" is a property of human lung mast cells that is independent of the type or strength of secretory stimulus.

The early bronchoconstrictor response observed with antigen challenge in asthma results from mediator release from mast cells. Human lung tissue is a rich source of the bronchoconstrictor mediator histamine that is present, preformed, in mast cell lysozomal granules, along with exoglycosidases, chemotactic peptides, neutral proteases, and heparin (22). In addition to releasing preformed mediators, activation of human lung mast cells with antihuman IgE and A23187 generates prostaglandin D_2 (PGD_2) (50–100 ng/10^6 mast cells) at a slower rate than histamine release (Fig. 1). A number of studies have now confirmed that PGD_2 is by far the most prominent cyclooxygenase product of arachidonic acid generated by human mast cells (23,24). In contrast, immunological stimulation of human lung fragments or enzymatically dispersed human lung cells enriched with 1–5% mast cells also releases significant amounts of the cyclooxygenase products; thromboxane (Tx) A_2 (measured as TxB_2), PGI_2 (measured as 6-keto-$PGF_{1\alpha}$), $PGF_{2\alpha}$, and PGE_2 (25,26). While human lung mast cells alone may generate small amounts of these prostanoids (24), we have recently provided evidence that other inflammatory cells respond to IgE-dependent stimulation with prostanoid synthesis both directly and indi-

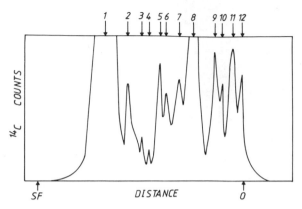

Fig. 2. Thin-layer chromatogram of ^{14}C-labelled products, released from dispersed human lung cells 20 min after challenge with antihuman IgE and [^{14}C]arachidonic acid. O, origin; SF, solvent front. Solvent, toluene : dioxane : acetic acid 65 : 34 : 1.5. The peaks are identified as (1) arachidonic acid, (2–4) monoHETES, (5) HHT, (6) 5-HETE, (7) 5,12-diHETE, (8) PGD$_2$, (9) TxB$_2$, (10) PGE$_2$, (11) PGF$_{2\alpha}$, (12) polar peak ? LTC$_4$.

rectly through an interaction with released mast cell mediators (26). Some of the secondary prostanoid generation by lung fragments may arise *inter alia* from the contractile actions of mast cell mediators on airway smooth muscle (25,27). The recognition of a mast cell-dependent prostaglandin-generating factor of anaphylaxis (PGF-A), may be of particular relevance since this newly generated oligopeptide has the capacity to stimulate synthesis of TxA$_2$ and PGF$_{2\alpha}$ by lung tissue in the absence of antigen challenge (28,29).

To further study the way in which dispersed human lung cells containing 5–9% mast cells respond to IgE-dependent or ionophore A23187 stimulation, we have pulsed cells with [^{14}C]arachidonic acid at the time of challenge. Twenty minutes after challenge the ^{14}C-labelled products released were extracted by C-18 reverse-phase partition and separated by thin layer chromotography (TLC). The individually labelled compounds were quantified by computer-assisted radiochromatogram scanning using a linear analyser (Fig. 2). Prostaglandin D$_2$ accounted for 60% of the released radiolabelled lipid, but significant amounts of the cyclooxygenase products PGF$_{2\alpha}$ and PGE$_2$, the TxA$_2$ hydrolysis product TxB$_2$, and (12 S)-12-hydroxy-5,8,10-heptadecatrienoic acid (HHT) were also detected (15%). Immunological activation also stimulated the release of the lipoxygenase products 5-(S)-hydroxy-6,8,11,14-eicosatetraenoic acid (5-HETE) (8%), other monoHETES (8%), 5,12-dihydroxy-6,8,10,14 eicosatetraenoic acid (5,12-diHETE) (5%), and a polar peak tentatively identified as sulfidopeptide leukotrienes (9%). The chemical characteristics and cells of origin of these mediators require further definition, but these studies confirm that IgE-dependent activation of human lung cells releases an array of highly active inflammatory mediators, which almost certainly are pertinent to the pathophysiology of allergic asthma.

PHARMACOLOGICAL MODULATION OF MEDIATOR RELEASE *IN VITRO*

From the foregoing discussion, the pharmacological modulation of mast cell-associated mediator release should have profound effects on the airway inflammatory response of bronchial asthma. From a theoretical standpoint, this control may be achieved by inhibiting crucial enzymes required for the coupling of mast cell activation to secretion or by activating the intrinsic down regulation of mast cells. Table I illustrates that many of the pharmacological agents that inhibit activation–secretion coupling of rat peritoneal mast cells and human basophils are also potent at inhibiting IgE-dependent mediator release from human dispersed lung mast cells. The ability of these agents to inhibit immunological mediator release in rat mast cells (30,31) and human basophils (32–34) has been used as an argument for the participation of certain biochemical pathways in activation–secretion coupling, but all too frequently their specificity for inhibiting particular enzymes in inflammatory cells has not been proven.

An alternative approach to pharmacological interference of the mast cell secretory process is by stimulating cell-surface receptors that recruit endogenous inhibitory mechanisms. Both rat peritoneal (35) and human lung mast cells (36) have on their cell surface β_2-adrenergic receptors whose stimulation by drugs such as isoprenaline and salbutamol stimulate adenylate cyclase to increase cellular levels of $3'5'$-cyclic adenosine monophosphate (cAMP). However, in rat mast cells both β_2-agonists and PGD_2, which stimulate adenylate cyclase, are notably ineffective at inhibiting mediator release despite increasing cAMP levels (37). This lack of effect probably results from ineffective coupling of intracellular cAMP to the activation of cAMP-dependent protein kinase (38,39). Prostaglandin D_2 is also ineffective in inhibiting mediator release from dispersed human mast cells, whereas β_2-agonists such as salbutamol and rimiterol are highly effective (36,40) (Fig. 3). These observations suggest that in mast cells of different species there exist separate pools of cAMP only some of which are linked to the inhibitory mechanism of mediator secretion (41).

TABLE I

Comparative Effects of Inhibitors of Phospholipid Metabolism on IgE-Dependent Histamine Release

Pharmacological agent	Enzyme(s) inhibited	Metabolic pathway	IC_{50}		
			Human mast cell (M)	Rat mast cell (M)	Human basophil (M)
3-deazaadenosine + homocysteine thiolactone	Methyltransferase I	Methylation	3.3×10^{-5}	3.3×10^{-5} [a]	—
Eicosatetraynoic acid (ETYA)	Cyclooxygenase = lipoxygenase	Arachidonic acid oxidation	2×10^{-5}	6.5×10^{-5} [a]	2×10^{-4} [b]
BW 755C	Lipoxygenase > cyclooxygenase	Arachidonic acid oxidation	3×10^{-4}	—	3×10^{-5} [b]
Nordihydroguaierteric acid (NDGA)	Lipoxygenase > cyclooxygenase	Arachidonic acid oxidation	5×10^{-5}	—	1×10^{-5} [b]
p-Bromphenacylbromide	Phospholipase A_2	Phospholipid cleavage	2×10^{-6}	—	1×10^{-6} [b]
Mepacrine	Phospholipase A_2	Phospholipid cleavage	2×10^{-6}	—	$3-10 \times 10^{-5}$ [b]

[a] Data from Ishizaka et al. (30) and Sullivan and Parker (31).
[b] Data from Magro (32), Marone et al. (33), and Marone et al. (34).

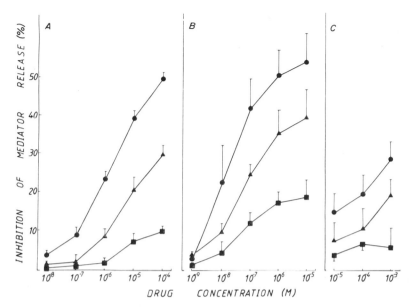

Fig. 3. Concentration-related inhibitory effects of (A) adenosine, (B) salbutamol, and (C) sodium cromoglycate on histamine release from dispersed human lung mast cells challenged with antihuman IgE at 1/10 (■), 1/100 (▲), and 1/300 (●) final dilution. Each point represents the mean ± 1 SEM for six to nine experiments.

The cellular role of cAMP in regulating mediator secretion may depend not only on intracellular compartmentalization of the nucleotide but also on other biochemical events of mast cell activation. Evidence for this is derived from observations with the purine nucleoside adenosine, which when added to rat mast cells enhances both ionophore (42) and IgE-dependent (43) mediator secretion through a cAMP-dependent mechanism. Adenosine is formed by the 5'-nucleotidase cleavage of 5'-adenosine monophosphate (AMP) and is an important substrate for many intracellular biochemical events (e.g., transmethylation and energy metabolism). In addition to its intracellular function, adenosine serves as an extracellular mediator by stimulating specific cell-surface receptors linked to adenylate cyclase to increase (R_A or A_2 receptor) or decrease (R_I or A_1 receptor) cellular levels of cAMP (44).

Preincubation of human basophils (45) or dispersed human lung mast cells (40,46) with adenosine inhibits IgE-dependent mediator release, whereas addition of the nucleoside immediately following immunological stimulation enhances mediator release (46) (Fig. 4). Both effects of adenosine are competitively antagonised ($pA_2 \simeq 5$) by concentrations of theophylline which have no effect on cAMP phosphodiesterase (PDE),

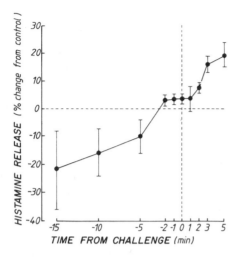

Fig. 4. Effect of 10^{-5} M adenosine on IgE-dependent histamine release from dispersed human lung mast cells when added at intervals before (left) or after (right) challenge with 1/100 antihuman IgE. Net histamine release in the absence of adenosine was $28 \pm 3\%$. Each point represents the mean $\pm$ 1 SEM for four experiments.

suggesting that they are mediated by stimulation of cell-surface adenosine receptors (47). More pronounced inhibition and potentiation of immunological mediator release occurs with N-ethylcarboxamideadenosine (NECA), which preferentially stimulates A_2 receptors, whereas L-N^6-phenylisoproplyadenosine (L-PIA), which is more selective for A_1 receptors, is less effective than adenosine (44–46). Stimulation of A_2 receptors in all cells tested including human basophils (48) activates adenylate cyclase to increase cellular cAMP levels. Thus for the human mast cell, adenosine's effect in increasing intracellular cAMP levels depends upon biochemical events of mast cell activation (41). Preincubation of mast cells with adenosine or NECA before immunological challenge reduces the rate of histamine release; addition of the nucleosides after challenge prolongs the rapid phase of mediator secretion. Both in rat and human lung mast cells, IgE-dependent activation stimulates adenylate cyclase causing an early rise in cAMP (49) and activation of cAMP-dependent protein kinase (50) before the onset of mediator secretion. If this early rise in cAMP had the effects of enhancing rather than inhibiting mediator release, then our results with adenosine could be explained. Stimulation of A_2 receptors to increase cAMP before immunological challenge would cause a premature activation of cAMP-dependent protein kinase and depletion of activatable protein kinase available at the time of challenge, therefore reducing mediator secretion. Stimulation of A_2 receptors after challenge would enhance the IgE-dependent increase in cAMP, causing greater protein kinase activation and therefore enhanced mediator secretion.

Sodium cromoglycate (SCG) and other related compounds have been investigated as mast cell-stabilizing agents for use in the treatment of a variety of allergic diseases including asthma (51). Sodium cromoglycate is highly effective at inhibiting IgE-dependent mediator release from rat mast cells *in vitro* possibly by the cyclic guanosine monophosphate-dependent phosphorylation of a 78,000-dalton inhibitory protein (52,53). In contrast to β_2-adrenergic agonists, SCG is markedly less effective at inhibiting anaphylactic histamine release from fragments (54) or dispersed cells (36) of human lung (Fig. 3). The strength of mast cell stimulation for mediator release is an important factor in interpreting efficacy of drugs that act on mast cell receptors compared to those agents that directly inhibit enzymes involved in the secretory process. For the three receptor agonists we have recently investigated (adenosine, salbutamol, and SCG), inhibition of mediator release was inversely proportional to the strength of immunological stimulation (36, Fig. 3). Thus for 3–5% mediator release from mast cells, which is reported to occur *in vivo*, drugs such as SCG may be more effective than is apparent from *in vitro* observations. Furthermore, if mucosal mast cells in the airways are important in initiating antigen-induced bronchoconstriction as is currently proposed (6), then high concentrations of drugs such as SCG on the surface of the airway may be highly efficacious in preventing propagation of the ensuing inflammatory response with antigen challenge.

AIRWAY AND MEDIATOR RESPONSES TO BRONCHIAL PROVOCATION IN ASTHMA

One of the major problems that has hindered understanding of the pathophysiology of bronchial asthma is the lack of satisfactory animal models for the disease. While progress is being made in this area, it must be recognized that asthma is a disease unique to man. In asthma, bronchial provocation with antigen challenge is associated with immediate (12–15 min) and late (6–12 hr) bronchoconstrictor responses. Since late asthmatic reactions depend upon events that occur in the airways immediately following antigen exposure, we and other investigators have focused attention on the immediate effects of agents that provoke bronchoconstriction.

To investigate the possible contribution of mast cells to the bronchoconstrictor response of specific and nonspecific challenge, a group of mild atopic asthmatic subjects (mean FEV_1, 94% predicted) underwent bronchial provocation with exercise, isocapnic hyperventilation (ICH), methacholine, and antigen. The airway responses were measured by body ple-

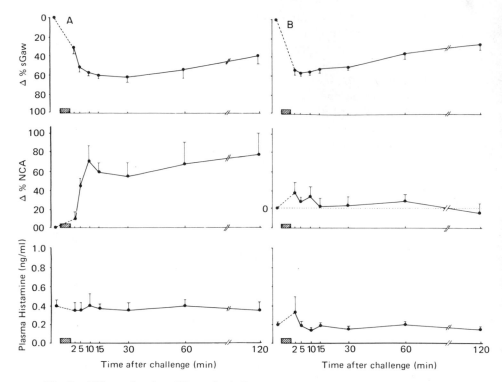

Fig. 5. Effects of antigen (A), methacholine (B), exercise (C), and isocapnic hyperventilation (D) in asthma on specific airways conductance (sGaw), serum neutrophil chemotactic activity (NCA), and plasma levels of histamine. Each point is the mean ± 1 SEM for eight subjects.

thysmography as airway resistance and computed to specific airway conductance (sGaw) by an on-line microprocessor. The challenges in each individual were adjusted to produce approximately a 60% fall in sGaw. The exercise and ICH challenges were matched minute by minute to achieve the same respiratory heat exchange. Before and at regular time points after challenge, venous blood was taken for plasma histamine levels [measured by a sensitive microenzymatic radiotransfer assay (55)] and serum neutrophil chemotactic activity (NCA) (assayed by the Boyden chamber technique in Prof. A. B. Kay's laboratory at the Cardiothoracic Institute, Brompton Hospital).

The time course of bronchoconstriction induced by each of the challenges differed. Methacholine, exercise, and ICH all produced rapid falls in sGaw that reached maximum 2–5 min postchallenge, whereas broncho-

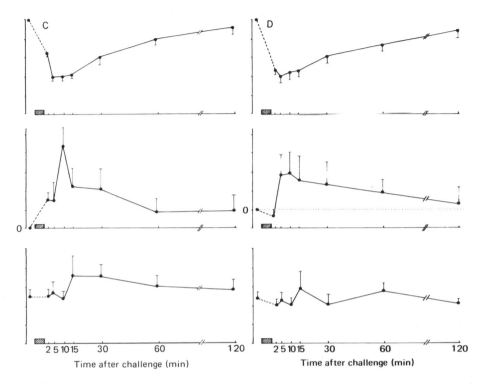

Fig. 5. (*continued*)

constriction induced by antigen was slower in onset, reaching maximum after 15–30 min (Fig. 5). Resting plasma histamine levels were higher in the asthmatic (0.52 ± 0.04 ng/ml, mean ± SEM) than in a matched group of normal subjects (0.31 ± 0.07 ng/ml, $p < .05$). These values are similar to reported plasma levels determined by radioenzymatic methods in which a TLC step was used to separate methylhistamine from other methylated products (56–58). In both the asthmatic and normal subjects there was a highly significant correlation between plasma and total blood histamine levels ($p < .01$). More than 99% of total blood histamine is contained in basophils, and therefore a significant component of histamine measured in plasma may be basophil derived. The spontaneous *in vitro* release of histamine from basophils from asthmatic subjects was higher than that of the normal subjects (13.4%; cf. 6.5%, ($p < .005$). This finding is consistent with previous reports of enhanced basophil ''releasability'' in asthma (59–61) and could account for the increased plasma levels of histamine observed in this disease.

We were unable to demonstrate any significant increase in plasma histamine levels following any of the four bronchial provocations (Fig. 5). Considerable care was taken during the sampling and handling of blood. It is possible that the changes in plasma histamine reported following exercise, but not ICH, (62) may be accounted for by the basophilia of exercise, which does not occur with ICH. In contrast to histamine, we observed significant increases in serum NCA following exercise, ICH, and antigen challenge, although not with methacholine challenge in asthma or with exercise in normal subjects. The rise in NCA after ICH differs from a previous report (63) but is entirely consistent with the correlation of NCA changes with respiratory heat exchange discussed by Dr. Lee. The discrepancy between NCA and histamine with the various forms of challenge may reflect rapid clearance of histamine (64) or separate origins of the two mediators.

One reason why increases in plasma histamine with antigen challenge have been found by some investigators (57) but not by others (65, Fig. 5) could lie in the characteristics of the patients chosen for study. We have recently confirmed the observation of Cockroft *et al.* (66) that the airway response to inhaled antigen is a function of two interracting components, nonspecific airway reactivity and mast cell sensitivity to inhaled antigen. In the previous study (Fig. 5) the asthmatic subjects had mean baseline FEV_1 values of 94% of their predicted, but they also had hyperreactive airways as indicated by a geometric mean concentration of inhaled methacholine (MC), which produced a 20% fall in FEV_1 (PC_{20} MC) of 0.09 mg/ml.

A similar challenge study was therefore undertaken in a separate group of 6 mild allergic asthmatics whose mean baseline FEV_1 value was 113% of predicted, and who had less reactive airways, as indicated by a geometric mean PC_{20} MC of 1.89 mg/ml. In contrast to the previous study (Fig. 5), we were able to detect an increase in plasma histamine from 0.17 ± 0.04 ng/ml to a peak at 5 min of 0.44 ± 0.01 ng/ml ($p < .05$) in parallel with the onset of bronchoconstriction. Thus, whether an increment in plasma histamine can be detected with antigen challenge in asthma is highly dependent upon the relative contributions of mast cell degranulation and airway reactivity to the ensuing airway response. Variations in these factors may also be important in determining individual responses to anti-asthmatic drugs, particularly those which are reported to inhibit mediator secretion.

PHARMACOLOGICAL MODULATION OF AIRWAY CALIBRE AND MEDIATOR RELEASE *IN VIVO*

From a theoretical standpoint, drugs that are useful in the treatment of asthma may exert their effects by inhibiting mast cell mediator release, by blocking the effects of mediators on target cells (pharmacological antagonism), or by relaxing airway smooth muscle (functional antagonism). The mechanisms of action proposed for many antiasthmatic drugs have been largely derived from observations in animals; as has been discussed, studies in animals may not be relevant to asthma in man. Therefore, we carried out a study to investigate the comparative effects of drugs on airway and mediator responses to antigen provocation in asthma. A patient group was chosen with high mast cell sensitivity and low airway reactivity, because in this patient group antigen bronchial provocation stimulated a reproducible two- to fourfold increase in plasma histamine levels paralleled by a 20–40% fall in FEV_1 and a 40–60% fall in sGaw (Figs. 6 and 7). Grass pollen-sensitive subjects were given a control challenge with inhaled grass pollen extract. The same challenge was then repeated on separate days, at least 1 week apart, each challenge being preceded by nebulised aerosol inhalations of saline (placebo), SCG (20 mg), salbutamol (200 μg), ipratropium bromide (1 mg), and 2 weeks of oral treatment with the selective histamine H_1-antagonist, astemizole (10 mg/day), which was sufficient to abolish the intradermal skin reaction to 50 μg/ml histamine. Measurements of FEV_1 and sGaw were made before and after drug treatment and at regular intervals following antigen challenge. Blood was taken at the same time points for measurement of plasma histamine.

Figure 6 illustrates the mean FEV_1 and sGaw responses to challenge in six asthmatic subjects. Inhalation of saline placebo had a small but insignificant effect on antigen-induced bronchoconstriction. Sodium cromoglycate inhibited the FEV_1 response to antigen by 75%, while it had only a partial inhibitory effect on sGaw. Astemizole partially but significantly attenuated antigen-induced bronchoconstriction. Previous studies on the effects of H_1-antagonists on antigen-induced bronchoconstriction have used drugs that have at least some local anaesthetic, antiserotonin, and anticholinergic effects. Astemizole is reported to be free of such actions (67), and yet it still produced significant inhibition of antigen-induced bronchoconstriction. This indicates that histamine has at least some role in the immediate airway response to antigen, although other mast cell derived-mediators such as those illustrated in Fig. 2 are likely to be more important. In principle, antagonism of a single bronchoconstric-

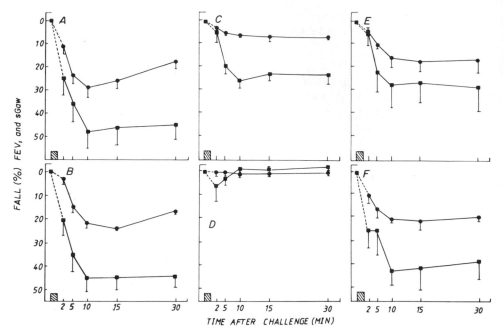

Fig. 6. Specific airways conductance, sGaw (■), and FEV₁ (●) responses to antigen bronchial challenge in asthma before (A, control) and after treatment with inhaled saline (B, placebo), sodium cromoglycate (20 mg) (C), salbutamol (200 μg) (D), oral astemizole (10 mg daily for 2 weeks) (E), and ipratropium bromide (1 mg) (F). Each point is the mean ± 1 SEM for six subjects.

tor mediator is unlikely to have much impact on a disease in which many inflammatory mediators are released and interacting with each other.

Salbutamol and ipratropium bromide were the only drugs used in this study that caused bronchodilatation. Neither drug had any effect on FEV₁, but this would be expected since baseline FEV₁ measurements were within the predicted normal range. Both salbutamol and ipratropium bromide increased mean values for sGaw, by 51.2% and 45.5%, respectively. The doses of ipratropium bromide and salbutamol were chosen from previous concentration–response studies in mild asthmatic subjects to produce comparable bronchodilatation. However, in contrast to their common bronchodilator action, salbutamol and ipratropium bromide differed profoundly in their effects on the airway response to antigen challenge. Salbutamol totally inhibited the FEV₁ and sGaw bronchoconstriction, while ipratropium bromide was no more effective than a placebo (Fig. 6). Thus, the protective effect of salbutamol on antigen-induced

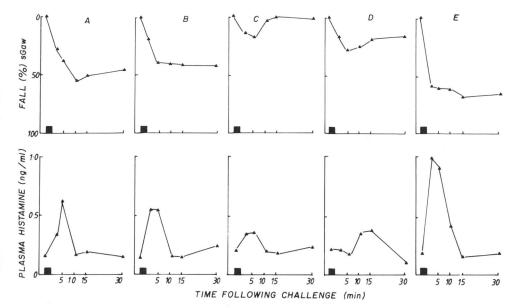

Fig. 7. Specific airways conductance (sGaw) and plasma histamine responses to antigen bronchial provocation in a single subject before (control) and after treatment with inhaled saline (placebo), salbutamol (200 μg), sodium cromoglycate (20 mg), and ipratropium bromide (1 mg). ■, time following challenge in minutes. A. Control; B. Placebo; C. Salbutamol; D. Cromoglycate; E. Iprotropium.

bronchoconstriction could not be due to the bronchodilator effect of the drug alone. The difference observed between the two drugs could be that stimulation of β_2-adrenergic receptors to increase smooth muscle levels of cAMP fundamentally alters the response of the airways to bronchoconstrictor stimuli, while ipratropium bromide, a muscarinic cholinergic antagonist, only has the capacity to remove extrinsic parasympathetic tone of the airways (68). In addition, salbutamol directly inhibits IgE-dependent mediator release from mast cells *in vitro* (Fig. 3), which would also appear to be a mechanism of action *in vivo* (Fig. 7).

For the group of stable mild asthmatic patients studied, resting levels of plasma histamine on each of the study days were reproducible (Fig. 7). Following inhalation of saline placebo, antigen bronchial provocation produced an almost identical increase in plasma histamine to that observed with the control challenge. Both SCG and salbutamol inhibited the antigen-induced increase in plasma histamine by >50%. In contrast, ipratropium bromide either had little effect or enhanced the antigen-induced increase in plasma histamine consistent with its lack of provocation produced an almost identical increase in plasma histamine to that observed with the control challenge. Both inhaled SCG (20 mg) and salbutamol (200 μg) inhibited the antigen-induced increase in plasma histamine, with salbutamol appearing to be more effective than SCG. In contrast, inhaled ipratropium bromide (1 mg), which produced equivalent bronchodilatation as achieved with salbutamol, had little effect on the antigen-induced increase in plasma histamine, consistent with its lack of effect on antigen-induced bronchoconstriction (Figs. 6 and 7). Astemizole, which had a partial inhibitory effect on the immediate airway response to challenge, had no significant effect on antigen-induced plasma histamine levels, indicating that its predominant pharmacological effect is antagonism of H_1-receptors and not mast-cell stabilization.

MECHANISM OF ACTION OF METHYLXANTHINES IN ASTHMA

Methylxanthines such as theophylline and its diethylamine salt aminophylline are used widely as effective therapeutic agents in asthma. Following from the discovery that β-adrenergic agonists directly relax airway smooth muscle and also inhibit mast cell mediator release by stimulating adenylate cyclase to increase cellular levels of cAMP, it was soon realised that methylxanthines also increase cAMP levels by inhibiting cyclic nucleotide phosphodiesterase (PDE), and that this might be their mechanism of action in asthma. However, a number of *in vitro* studies have shown that levels of theophylline achieved therapeutically in asthma (10-20 mcg/ml) are too low to effectively inhibit human airway smooth muscle PDE *in vitro* (69). Theophylline and related methylxanthines also inhibit the receptor-mediated effects of adenosine at concentrations 50- to 100-fold lower than required for PDE inhibition (47).

Since we had previously shown that adenosine potentiates on-going IgE-dependent mediator release from human lung mast cells (Fig. 4), it is possible that at least some of the effect of theophylline in asthma might result from antagonism of released adenosine. We have recently shown that adenosine by inhalation is a potent bronchoconstrictor in both allergic and nonallergic asthmatic subjects, with a time course similar to that of inhaled methacholine (70). Specificity of the response was suggested by showing that AMP, which can be metabolised to adenosine, was almost equipotent with adenosine in causing bronchoconstriction. By contrast, inosine, the major metabolite of adenosine and guanosine (a related nucleoside) were without effect (70,71). Adenosine and AMP in concentrations up to 400 times those producing bronchoconstriction in asthma had no significant effect on normal airways.

To examine the effects of methylxanthines on adenosine-induced bronchoconstriction, a group of asthmatic subjects were challenged on separate days with increasing concentrations of saline, adenosine, or histamine, each inhalation being preceded by either inhaled saline (control) or theophylline (5 mg/ml; total cumulative dose, 35 mg). When nebulised saline was followed by histamine or adenosine, dose-dependent bronchoconstriction occurred in all subjects with adenosine being about one-third as potent as histamine. Inhalation of theophylline followed by saline produced a small but significant bronchodilatation (2% increase in FEV_1, $p <$ .05). Theophylline also had a small effect in displacing the FEV_1 and sGaw histamine concentration–response curves to the right, as indicated by an increase in the geometric mean PC_{20} values by 90% when airway calibre was measured as FEV_1. Theophylline had a far greater effect in antagonising adenosine-induced bronchoconstriction, as reflected in a 515% increase in the geometric mean PC_{20} value (72). That theophylline was more effective in antagonising bronchoconstriction induced by adenosine when compared to histamine strongly suggests an effect mediated through adenosine receptors.

In a separate study, the bronchoconstrictor effect of adenosine but not histamine was also inhibited by inhaled SCG (20 mg/ml) (73); this might suggest that adenosine is mediating its effect by enhancing mast cell mediator release (Fig. 3). However, SCG also inhibits bronchoconstriction induced by agents that are not thought to activate mast cells, such as sulphur dioxide, propranolol, sodium salicylate, ICH, and inhaled water vapour, suggesting that this drug has pharmacological activities other than mast cell stabilization. Other possible mechanisms for adenosine's bronchoconstrictor effect include presynaptic inhibition of catecholamine release (74), stimulation of neural reflex pathways (75), or a direct effect on airway smooth muscle. What is particularly intriguing is that adenosine causes bronchoconstriction in asthma, whereas it relaxes smooth muscle in isolated animal airway preparations (76) and it has no effect on normal human airways. It is tempting to speculate that adenosine's bronchoconstrictor effect in asthma results from an altered response fundamental to the pathophysiology of the disease.

For adenosine antagonism to be a significant effect of theophylline's action in asthma, the nucleoside must be released endogenously within the lung. In animal experiments, increased release of adenosine and its metabolites inosine and hypoxanthine from the lung have been reported with hypoxia (77) and antigen challenge (78), two conditions that occur in asthma. We have recently carried out a study in a group of mild asthmatic subjects to determine whether adenosine is released into the circulation following antigen bronchial provocation. Before and at regular intervals after antigen challenge, FEV_1 was measured and blood taken for measurement of adenosine and inosine levels. After separating the plasma at 4°C, it was deproteinised and the supernatants applied to phenylboronate–acrylamide affinity gel to selectively retain *cis*-diols (79). The eluted purine nucleosides were separated by high performance liquid chromatography, and adenosine and inosine were quantified by UV absorbance at 254 nm. By carrying through an internal radiolabelled standard, the overall recovery of adenosine was >90%. Antigen challenge resulted in a maximum 25% fall in FEV_1 at 15 min, which was accompanied by significant increases in plasma adenosine levels from 5.0 ± 0.8 to 7.9 ± 1.3 ng/ml at 2 min and 15.0 ± 2.8 ng/ml at 45 min. Plasma levels of inosine were higher than those of adenosine (26.5 ± 2.8 ng/ml), but no significant increase occurred following antigen challenge. Adenosine may therefore be a hitherto unrecognized bronchoconstrictor mediator in asthma whose pharmacological and functional antagonism by theophylline and SCG, respectively, might account for at least some of the therapeutic effects of these drugs in this disease.

Methylxanthines may exert a more indirect effect in increasing airway calibre. Intravenous aminophylline (80) and oral theophylline (unpublished data) cause bronchodilatation in normal subjects, accompanied by a parallel fall in postural systolic blood pressure and reflex tachycardia. Since ~50% of these responses could be blocked by prior administration of propranolol, it is likely that theophylline and aminophylline stimulate the release of catecholamines, which in themselves exert a bronchodilator effect. This has been confirmed more directly by showing that aminophylline increases the urinary excretion of catecholamine metabolites (81); in two recent studies theophylline-based drugs have been shown to stimulate significant increases in plasma adrenaline and noradrenaline levels (82,83). Theophylline has several other effects, some of which may be relevant to its action in asthma; it causes a redistribution of calcium within airway smooth muscle at concentrations that do not effect cAMP levels, decreases pulmonary hypertension, increases the contractility of the diaphragm under conditions of fatigue, and improves mucociliary clearance.

REFERENCES

1. Holgate, S. T. The human lung mast cell; Morphology biochemistry and role in allergic asthma. *Adv. Med.* **19:**287–306, 1983.

2. Hogg, J. C., Pare, P. D., Boucher, R., Michoud, M. C., Guerzon, G., and Moroz, L. Pathologic abnormalities in asthma. *In* "Asthma: Physiology, Immunopharmacology, and Treatment" (L. M. Lichtenstein, K. F. Austen, and A. S. Simon, eds.), Vol. 2, pp. 1–14. Academic Press, New York, 1977.

3. Laitinen, L. A., Kava, T., and Heino, M. Ultrastructure of the airways and bronchial reactivity in asthma. *In* "International Conference on Bronchial Hyperreactivity" (J. A. Nadel and R. Pauwels, eds.), p. 71. Medicine Publ. Found., Oxford, 1982.

4. Austen, K. F. Biological implications of the structural and functional characteristics of the chemical mediators of immediate hypersensitivity. *Harvey Lect.* **73**:93–161, 1979.

5. Kaliner, M. A. Mast cell derived mediators and bronchial asthma. *In* "Airway Reactivity, Mechanisms and Clinical Relevance" (F. E. Hargreave, ed.), pp. 175–187. Astra, Ontario, 1980.

6. Hogg, J. C. Bronchial mucosal permeability and its relationship to airways hyperreactivity. *J. Allergy Clin. Immunol.* **67**:421–425, 1981.

7. Antonissen, L. A., Michell, R. W., Kroeger, E. A., Kepron, K., Tse, K. S., and Stephens, N. L. Mechanical alterations of airway smooth muscle in a canine asthmatic model. *J. Appl. Physiol.* **46**:681–687, 1979.

8. Empey, D. W., Laitinen, L. A., Jacobs, L., Gold, W. M., and Nadel, J. A. Mechanisms of bronchial hyperreactivity in normal subjects after upper respiratory tract infection. *Am. Rev. Respir. Dis.* **113**:131–139, 1976.

9. Holtzman, M. J., Sheller, J. R., Dimeo, M., Nadel, J. A., and Boushey, H. A. Effect of ganglionic blockade on bronchial reactivity in atopic subjects. *Am. Rev. Respir. Dis.* **122**:17–25, 1980.

10. Lamb, D., and Lumsden, A. Intraepithelial mast cells in human airway epithelium: Evidence for smoking-induced changes in their frequency. *Thorax* **37**:334–342, 1982.

11. Guerzon, G. M., Parb, P. D., Michoud, M. C., and Hogg, J. C. The number and distribution of mast cells in monkey lungs. *Am. Rev. Respir. Dis.* **119**:59–66, 1979.

12. Patterson, R., McKenna, J. M., Suszko, I. M., Solliday, N. H., Pruzansky, J. J., Roberts, M., and Kehol, T. J. Living histamine containing cells from the bronchial lumen of humans. *J. Clin. Invest.* **59**:217–225, 1977.

13. Fox, B., Bull, T. B., and Guz, A. Mast cells in the human alveolar wall: An electronmicroscopic study. *J. Clin. Pathol.* **34**:1333–1342, 1981.

14. Miller, H. R. P. The structure and function of mucosal mast cells. *Biol. Cell.* **39**:229–234, 1980.

15. Haig, D., McKee, T., Jarrett, E. E. E., Woodbury, R. G., and Miller, H. R. P. Generation of mucosal mast cells is stimulated *in vitro* by factors derived from T cells of helminth-infected rats. *Nature (London)* **300**:188–193, 1982.

16. Strobel, S., Miller, H. R. P., and Ferguson, A. Human intestinal mucosal mast cells: Evaluation of fixation and staining technique. *J. Clin. Pathol.* **34**:851–858, 1981.

17. Caulfield, J. P., Lewis, R. A., Hein, A., and Austen, K. F. Secretion in dissociated human pulmonary mast cells. Evidence for solubilization of granule contents before discharge. *J. Cell Biol.* **85**:299–311, 1980.

18. Church, M. K., Mageed, R. A. K., and Holgate, S. T. Human tonsilar mast cells: Characteristics of histamine secretions and methods of dispersion. *Int. Arch. Allergy, Appl. Immunol.* **72**:188–190, 1983.

19. Ennis, M. Histamine release from human pulmonary mast cells. *Agents Actions* **12**:60–63, 1982.

20. Church, M. K., Pao, G. J.-K., and Holgate, S. T. Characterization of histamine secretion from mechanically dispersed human lung mast cells: Effects of anti-IgE, calcium

ionophore A23187, compound 48/80 and basic polypeptides. *J. Immunol.* **129:**2116–2121, 1982.

21. Coleman, J. W., and Godfrey, R. C. The number and affinity of IgE receptors on dispersed human lung mast cells. *Immunology* **44:**859–863, 1981.

22. Schwartz, L. B., Lewis, R. A., Seldin, D., and Austen, K. F. Acid hydrolases and tryptase from secretory granules of dispersed human lung mast cells. *J. Immunol.* **126:**1290–1294, 1981.

23. Lewis, R. A., Soter, N. A., Diamond, P. T., Austen, K. F., Oates, J. A., and Roberts, J. L., II. Prostaglandin D$_2$ generation after activation of rat and human mast cells with anti-IgE. *J. Immunol.* **129:**1627–1631, 1982.

24. Schleimer, R. P., MacGlashan, D. W., Jr., Schulman, E. S., Peters, S. P., Adkinson, N. F., Newball, H. H., Adams, G. K., and Lichtenstein, L. M. Effects of glucocorticoids on mediator release from human basophils and mast cells. *Fed. Proc., Fed. Am. Soc. Exp. Biol.* **41:**487a, 1982.

25. Schulman, E. S., Newball, H. H., Demers, L. M., Fitzpatrick, F. A., and Adkinson, F. A., Jr. Anaphylactic release of thromboxane A$_2$, prostaglandin D$_2$ and prostacyclin from human lung parenchyma. *Am. Rev. Respir. Dis.* **124:**402–406, 1981.

26. Holgate, S. T., Burns, G. B., Robinson, C., and Church, M. K. Anaphylactic- and calcium-dependent generation of prostaglandin D$_2$(PGD$_2$), thromboxane B$_2$ and other cyclooxygenase products of arachidonic acid by dispersed human lung cells and relationship to histamine release. *J. Immunol.* (in press).

27. Platshon, L. F., and Kaliner, M. A. The effects of the immunologic release of histamine upon human lung cyclic nucleotide levels and prostaglandin synthesis. *J. Clin. Invest.* **62:**1113–1121, 1978.

28. Steel, L. K., and Kaliner, M. A. Prostaglandin generating factor of anaphylaxis: Identification and isolation. *J. Biol. Chem.* **256:**12692–12698, 1981.

29. Steel, L. K., Bach, D., and Kaliner, M. A. Prostaglandin generating factor of anaphylaxis. II Characterisation of Activity. *J. Immunol.* **129:**1233–1238, 1982.

30. Ishizaka, T., Hirata, F., Ishizaka, K., and Axelrod, J. Transmission and regulation of triggering signals induced by bridging of IgE receptors on rat mast cells. *In* "Biochemistry of the Acute Allergic Reactions" (E. L. Becker, A. S. Simon, and K. F. Austen, eds.), pp. 213–227. Alan R. Liss, Inc., New York, 1981.

31. Sullivan, T., and Parker, C. W. Possible role of arachidonic acid and its metabolites in mediator release from rat mast cells. *J. Immunol.* **122:**431–436, 1979.

32. Magro, A. M. Effects of inhibitors of arachidonic acid metabolism upon IgE- and non-IgE-mediated histamine release. *Int. J. Immunopharmacol.* **4:**15–20, 1982.

33. Marone, G., Kagey-Sobotka, A., and Lichtenstein, L. M. Effects of arachidonic acid and its metabolites on antigen-induced histamine release from human basophils *in vitro*. *J. Immunol.* **123:**1669–1677, 1979.

34. Marone, G., Kagey-Sobotka, A., and Lichtenstein, L. M. Possible role of phospholipase A$_2$ in triggering histamine secretion from human basophils *in vitro*. *Clin. Immunol. Immunopathol.* **20:**231–239, 1981.

35. Marquardt, D. L., and Wasserman, S. I. Characterization of the rat mast cell beta-adrenergic receptor in resting and stimulated cells by radioligand binding. *J. Immunol.* **129:**2122–2126, 1982.

36. Church, M. K., Holgate, S. T., and Pao, G. J.-K. Histamine release from mechanically and enzymatically dispersed human lung mast cells: Inhibition by salbutamol and cromoglycate. *Br. J. Pharmacol.* **79** Suppl: 374P, 1983.

37. Holgate, S. T., Lewis, R. A., Maguire, J. F., Roberts, J. L., II, Oates, J. A., and Austen, K. F. Effects of prostaglandin D$_2$ on rat serosal mast cells: Discordance be-

tween immunologic mediator release and cyclic AMP levels. *J. Immunol.* **125:**1367–1373, 1980.

38. Holgate, S. T., Winslow, C. M., Lewis, R. A., and Austen, K. F. Effects of prostaglandin D_2 and theophylline on rat serosal mast cells: Discordance between increased cellular levels of cyclic AMP and activation of cyclic AMP-dependent protein kinase. *J. Immunol.* **127:**1530–1533, 1981.

39. Lewis, R. A., Holgate, S. T., Roberts, J. L., II, Oates, J. A., and Austen, K. F. Preferential generation of prostaglandin D_2 by rat and human mast cells. *In* "Biochemistry of the Acute Allergic Reactions" (E. L. Becker, A. J. Simon, and K. F. Austen, eds.), pp. 239–254. Alan R. Liss, Inc., New York, 1981.

40. Peters, S. P., Schulman, E. S., Schleimer, R. P., MacGlashan, D. W., Newball, H. H., and Lichtenstein, L. M. Dispersed human lung mast cells. Pharmacologic aspects and comparison with human lung tissue fragments. *Am. Rev. Respir. Dis.* **126:**1034–1039, 1982.

41. Holgate, S. T., Lewis, R. A., and Austen, K. F. Role of cyclic nucleotides in mast cell activation and secretion. *Prog. Immunol.* **4:**486–492, 1980.

42. Marquardt, D. L., Parker, C. W., and Sullivan, T. J. Potentiation of mast cell mediator release by adenosine. *J. Immunol.* **120:**871–878, 1978.

43. Holgate, S. T., Lewis, R. A., and Austen, K. F. The role of adenylate cyclase in the immunologic release of mediators from rat mast cells: Agonists and antagonist effects of purine- and ribose-modified adenosine analogs. *Proc. Natl. Acad. Sci. U.S.A.* **77:**6800–6804, 1980.

44. Daly, J. W. Adenosine receptors: Targets for future drugs. *J. Med. Chem.* **25:**197–206, 1982.

45. Church, M. K., Holgate, S. T., and Hughes, P. J. Adenosine inhibits and potentiates IgE-dependent histamine release from human basophils by an A_2-receptor mediated mechanism. *Br. J. Pharmacol.* **80:**719–726, 1983.

46. Church, M. K., Hughes, P. J., and Holgate, S. T. Adenosine modulation of histamine release from human basophils and mast cells. *Fed. Proc., Fed. Am. Soc. Exp. Biol.* (in press).

47. Fredholm, B. B. Theophylline actions on adenosine receptors. *Eur. J. Respir. Dis.* **61**(Suppl. 109):29–36, 1980.

48. Hughes, P. J., Holgate, S. T., and Church, M. K. Relationship between cyclic AMP changes and histamine release from basophil-rich human leucocytes. *Biochem. Pharmacol.* **32:**2557–2563, 1983.

49. Lewis, R. A., Holgate, S. T., Roberts, J. L., II, Maguire, J. F., Oates, J. A., and Austen, K. F. Effects of indomethacin on cyclic nucleotide levels and histamine release from rat serosal mast cells. *J. Immunol.* **123:**1663–1668, 1979.

50. Holgate, S. T., Lewis, R. A., and Austen, K. F. Rat serosal mast cell 3'5'-cyclic adenosine monophosphate-dependent protein kinase and its immunologic activation. *J. Immunol.* **124:**2093–2099, 1980.

51. Church, M. K. Cromoglycate-like anti-allergic drugs: A review. *Drugs Today* **14:**282–341, 1978.

52. Sieghart, W., Theoharides, T. C., Douglas, W. W., and Greengard, P. Phosphorylation of a single mast cell protein that inhibits secretion. *Biochem. Pharmacol.* **30:**2737–2738, 1981.

53. Wells, E., and Mann, J. Phosphorylation of a mast cell protein in response to treatment with anti-allergic compounds. Implication for the mode of action of sodium cromoglycate. *Biochem. Pharmacol.* **32:**837–842, 1983.

54. Church, M. K., and Young, K. D. The characteristics of inhibition of histamine release

from human lung fragments by sodium cromoglycate, salbutamol and chlorpromazine. *Br. J. Pharmacol.* **78:**671–879, 1983.

55. Howarth, P. H., Pao, G. J.-K., Church, M. K., and Holgate, S. T. Exercise- and isocapnic hyperventilation-induced bronchoconstriction in asthma. *J. Allergy Clin. Immunol.* **73:**391–399, 1984.

56. Brown, M. J., Ind, P. W., Barnes, P. J., Jenner, D. A., and Dollery, C. T. A sensitive and specific radiometric method for the measurement of plasma histamine in normal individuals. *Anal. Biochem.* **109:**142–146, 1980.

57. Brown, M. J., Ind, P. W., Causon, R., and Lee, T. H. A novel double-isotope technique for the enzymatic assay of plasma histamine, application to estimation of mast cell activation assessed by antigen challenge in asthmatics. *J. Allergy Clin. Immunol.* **69:**20–24, 1982.

58. Dyer, J., Warren, K., Merlin, S., Metcalf, D., and Kaliner, M. A. Measurement of plasma histamine: Description of an improved method and normal values. *J. Allergy Clin. Immunol.* **70:**82–87, 1982.

59. Neijens, H. J., Raatgeep, H. C., Degenhart, H. J., and Kerrebijn, K. F. Release of histamine from leucocytes and its determinants *in vitro* in relation to bronchial responsiveness to inhaled histamine and exercise *in vivo*. *Clin. Allergy* **12:**577–586, 1982.

60. Findlay, S. R., and Lichtenstein, L. M. Basophil releasability in patients with asthma. *Am. Rev. Respir. Dis.* **122:**53–59, 1980.

61. Neijens, H. J., Duiverman, E. J., Raatgeep, H. C., Degenhart, H. J., and Kerrebija, K. F. Altered responses of leucocytes *in vitro* in relation to the presence of asthma and bronchial hyperreactivity. *In* "International Conference on Bronchial Hyperreactivity" (J. A. Nadel and R. Pauwels, eds.), pp. 42–43. Medicine Publ. Found., Oxford, 1982.

62. Barnes, P. J., and Brown, M. J. Venous plasma histamine in exercise- and hyperventilation-induced asthma in man. *Clin. Sci.* **61:**159–162, 1981.

63. Deal, E. C., Wasserman, S. I., Soter, N. A., Ingram, R. H., and McFadden, E. R. Evaluation of role played by mediators of immediate hypersensitivity in exercise-induced asthma. *J. Clin. Invest.* **65:**659–665, 1980.

64. Ind, P. W., Brown, M. J., L'hoste, F. J. M., Macquin, I., and Dollery, C. T. Determination of histamine and its metabolites: Concentration effect relationship of infused histamine in normal volunteers. *Agents Actions* **12:**12–16, 1982.

65. Moodley, I., Morgan, D. J. R., and Davies, R. J. The measurement of histamine during allergen-induced asthma. *Clin. Sci.* **64:**12P, 1983.

66. Cockcroft, D. W., Ruffin, R. E., Frith, P. A., Cartier, A., Juniper, E. F., Dolovich, J., and Hargreave, F. E. Determinants of allergen-induced asthma: Dose of allergen, circulating IgE antibody concentrations and bronchial responsiveness to inhaled histamine. *Am. Rev. Respir. Dis.* **120:**1053–1058, 1979.

67. Emanuel, M. B., and Young, G. A. The pharmacology of astemizole, a novel H_1-antagonist. *Int. Congr. Allergol. Clin. Immunol., 11th, 1982* Abstracts, p. 61, 1983.

68. Tattersfield, A. E. Measurement of bronchial reactivity—a question of interpretation. *Thorax* **36:**561–565, 1982.

69. Fredholm, B. B. Are methylxanthines effects due to antagonism of endogenous adenosine? *Trends Pharmacol. Sci.* **1:**129–132, 1980.

70. Cushley, M. J., Tattersfield, A. E., and Holgate, S. T. Inhaled adenosine and guanosine in normal and asthmatic subjects. *Br. J. Clin. Pharmacol.* **15:**161–165, 1983.

71. Cushley, M. J., and Holgate, S. T. Adenosine-induced bronchoconstriction in asthma: Specificity and relationship to airway reactivity. *Thorax* **38:**705, 1983.

72. Cushley, M. J., Tattersfield, A. E., and Holgate, S. T. Adenosine antagonism as an

alternative mechanism of action of methylxanthines in asthma. *In* "Pharmacology of Asthma" (J. Morley and K. D. Rainsford, eds.), pp. 109–113. Birkhaeuser, Berlin, 1983.

73. Cushley, M. J., Church, M. K., Pao, G. J.-K., and Holgate, S. T. Adenosine-induced bronchoconstriction is not caused by enhanced immunological release of mast cell mediators. *Br. J. Clin. Pharmacol.* **14:**607P, 1982.

74. Fredholm, B. B., and Hedqvist, P. Modulation of neurotransmission by purine nucleotides and nucleosides. *Biochem. Pharmacol.* **29:**1635–1643, 1980.

75. Bleehan, T., and Keele, C. A. Observations on the algogenic action of adenosine compounds on the human blister base preparation. *Pain* **3:**367–377, 1977.

76. Brown, C. M., and Collis, M. G. Evidence for an A_2/R_A adenosine receptor in the guinea pig trachea. *Br. J. Pharmacol.* **76:**381–387, 1982.

77. Mentzer, M. R., Rubio, R., and Bern, R. M. Release of adenosine by hypoxic canine lung tissue and its possible role in pulmonary circulation. *Am. J. Physiol.* **229:**1625–1631, 1975.

78. Fredhom, B. B. Release of adenosine from rat lung by antigen and compound 48/80. *Acta Physiol. Scand.* **111:**507–508, 1981.

79. Gehrke, C. W., Kuo, K. C., Davis, G. E., and Suits, R. D. Quantitative high performance chromatography of nucleosides in biological materials. *J. Chromatogr.* **150:**455–476, 1978.

80. MacKay, A. D., Baldwin, C. J., and Tattersfield, A. E. Action of intravenously administered aminophylline on normal airways. *Am. Rev. Respir. Dis.* **127:**609–613, 1983.

81. Atuk, N. O., Blades, M. C., Westervelt, F. B., and Wood, E. J. Effect of aminophylline on urinary excretion of epinephrine and norepinephrine in man. *Circulation* **35:**745–750, 1967.

82. Higbee, M. D., Kumar, M., and Galant, S. P. Stimulation of endogenous catecholamine release by theophylline: A proposed additional mechanism of action for theophylline effects. *J. Allergy Clin. Immunol.* **70:**377–382, 1982.

83. Warren, J. B., Turner, C., Dalton, N., Thompson, A., Cochrane, G. M., and Clark, T. J. H. Effect of posture on the sympathoadrenal response to theophylline infusion. *Thorax* **38:**239, 1983.

DISCUSSION

McFadden: Would you care to give us your view of the role of mediators in the various types of challenge situations you used?

Holgate: This is a highly relevant question but unfortunately our knowledge on the cellular origin of many on the already defined mediators and their interactions with each other on target tissues have yet to be defined before this question can be answered.

Lichtenstein: Where is the adenosine coming from?

Lewis: If you do a methacholine challenge can you find adenosine in the peripheral blood? This is particularly relevant if you think adenosine is deriving from smooth muscle.

Holgate: We have just completed a study in which adenosine levels were being measured following exercise and methacholine induced bronchoconstriction, but the analyses are not yet completed.

Kay: It is possible that NCA is mast cell granule-associated but that its release is retarded compared to histamine. This might explain the fact that NCA was detectable in patients with hyperresponsive airways and high baseline histamine values; that is, it was easier, in this situation, for the NCA to leak out.

Holgate: Yes, this is indeed a possibility although I know of no data that would help answer this question.

Piper: The dose–response curves for the bronchoconstrictor effects of PGD_2 and $PGF_{2\alpha}$ were not parallel, clearly showing that PGD_2 has an action of its own that is not due to conversion to $PGF_{2\alpha}$. How does the duration of bronchoconstriction to PGD_2 compare with that to $PGF_{2\alpha}$? Do you have any information on the metabolism of PGD_2 in the circulation?

Holgate: In time course studies PGD_2 had a more prolonged effect compared to $PGF_{2\alpha}$. Preliminary studies suggested that PGD_2 is degraded in human whole blood and plasma to a as yet unidentified metabolite which is not $PGF_{2\alpha}$ or 13, 14-dihydro-15-keto $PGF_{2\alpha}$. Since similar degradation occurs in aqueous buffer containing human serum albumin, it is likely to be nonenzymatic.

Schwartz: Do adenosine deaminase-deficient patients, who have high plasma levels of adenosine, also have hyperreactive airways?

Holgate: As far as I am aware there have been no reported studies of pulmonary function or airways reactivity in these patients. Adenosine does not have any effect on normal airways.

Dollery: I should like to comment on the action of PGD_2 in man. We have infused the compound intravenously in a dose that caused flushing and fall in diastolic blood pressure. Only one subject has a significant fall in peak expiratory flow rate. PGD_2 plasma concentrations were measured by a gas chromatography/mass spectroscopy method (a GC-MS NICF) and reliably measurable concentrations were found.

Holgate: Prostaglandins are likely to act in the airways as local mediators. Dr. Newball has reported a study comparing intravenous with inhaled $PGF_{2\alpha}$ in asthma in which bronchoconstriction was only produced when the prostanoid was inhaled (H. H. Newball, H. R. Keiser, and C. Lenfant, *Respir. Physiol.* 41:183, 1980). We also need to know more about the metabolism of PGD_2 when given intravenously.

Morley: Persson and his colleagues [C. G. A. Persson, in "Pharmacology of Asthma" (J. Morley and K. D. Rainsford, eds.), p. 115. Birkhaueser, Basel, 1983] undertook a structure–activity study of theophylline and dissociated bronchodilator effects from adenosine antagonism. They developed a compound, enprophylline (3-propylxanthine), which has been shown to be more a potent bronchodilator than theophylline in man despite lacking significant adenosine antagonism. I do not think that it is reasonable to attribute the bronchodilator effect of theophylline to adenosine antagonism.

Holgate: The compound enprophylline was reported to be a cyclic AMP phosphodiesterase inhibitor and to be free from adenosine antagonism. However, in a recent study it was shown, at least in one assay system, that enprophylline was in fact a potent adenosine A_2 antagonist (B. B. Fredholm and C. G. A. Persson, *Eur. J. Pharmacol.* 812:673, 1982). Furthermore, its reported lack of adenosine antagonism was based on its inability to inhibit adenosine-induced *relaxation* of animal airway preparation *in vitro* (J. A. Karlsson, G. Kjellin, and C. G. A. Persson, *J. Pharm. Pharmacol.* 34:788, 1982). In asthma, adenosine causes *bronchoconstriction,* not bronchodilation, and therefore the animal test model was inappropriate.

Lewis: Have you begun looking at synergism between PGD_2 and adenosine on airways dysfunction, since both would presumably work through their effects on activating adenylate cyclases (although the adenosine would presumably be less selective for its spectrum of adenylate cyclase targets)?

Holgate: Having defined a bronchoconstrictor effect of PGD_2, we intend to proceed with interactive studies.

Lichtenstein: It looked as if DSCG did not block histamine release into the plasma following antigen bronchial challenge but merely delayed it; is that correct?

Holgate: This is true. I have no good explanation for this at the present time.

Schiffmann: Inhibition of adenosine deaminase is associated with depressed leucocyte chemotaxis. If, in the asthmatic patient during an attack, adenosine is present in greater than normal amounts, this might tend to reduce leucocyte activation. Does this line of evidence minimize the role of the PMN in the asthmatic response?

Holgate: I do not know. Certainly drugs that inhibit adenosine deaminase *in vitro,* such as *erythro*-9-(2-hydroxy-3-nonyl)adenine (EHNA) have not been given to man.

Schleimer: Are you considering adenosine to be a stimulus selective for asthmatics or is this a case of another mediator that is much more potent in asthmatics than normals? Also, have you considered the platelet as a possible source of adenosine, either in the lungs, or during blood collection, following antigen challenge?

Holgate: Adenosine monophosphate (AMP) (from which adenosine is derived) also causes bronchoconstriction, whereas inosine, the adenosine deaminase metabolite, is without effect on airway calibre. A dose of AMP 400-fold that which caused bronchoconstriction in asthmatics was without effect in normals. Furthermore, the airway response to adenosine correlates with nonspecific airway reactivity as assessed by histamine provocation testing.

It is possible that adenosine is platelet derived, possibly through the activation of platelets, which has been shown to occur following antigen bronchial provocation (K. A. Knauer, L. M. Lichtenstein, N. F. Adkinson, Jr. *et al., N. Engl. J. Med.* **304:**1404, 1981). In controls with the cannula *in situ* but with no antigen challenge, there was a much smaller late rise in adenosine.

CHAPTER 25

Summing Up*

MARGARET TURNER-WARWICK

Department of Medicine (Thoracic Medicine)
Cardiothoracic Institute, Brompton Hospital
London, U.K.

I would like to do three things in this summing-up session: first, remind you of some of the topics we have attempted to cover; second, emphasize other aspects that we have not covered; and third, make some general comments of my own regarding areas where I personally would like to see more activity. I have tried to illustrate many of these points with diagrams (see Figs. 1 and 2). Some of you might object to the liberties I have taken with this form of précis, but I hope you will question anything that you feel is inappropriate or inaccurate.

We started by considering some of the different characteristics of the mast cell and the basophil, and the differing spectra of mediators they produce. Mast cell heterogeneity in the mouse was considered, and the point emphasized that we do not know whether the same is true in man. This is a critical area because many of us who are interested in chronic inflammation have been struck by the prominence of mast cells in connective tissue. Perhaps these cells operate quite independently from the mast cells in atopic diseases. It would be a good theory if, as proposed by Frank Austen, the connective tissue mast cells were monitoring the microenvironment, and contrasted with the T cell–dependent mucosal cells thought to be of more importance to us in relation to diseases of the airways. In this regard, T-cell mediators might stimulate mast cells independent of antigen, and we heard of fascinating studies of basophils or basophil-like cells developing from cord blood in mononuclear cell cul-

*Edited transcript. Illustrations in this chapter are used with permission of the copyright holder, the Cardiothoracic Institute.

ASTHMA: Physiology,
Immunopharmacology,
and Treatment
THIRD INTERNATIONAL SYMPOSIUM

417

tures. We had an interesting description of mastocytosis, and during the course of that discussion the heterogeneity of that clinical population was emphasized. In some individuals the disease was exacerbated by aspirin, whereas in others the drug protected. Presumably we still have much to learn about the cyclooxygenase and lipoxygenase pathways, their enzymes, and the agents that control them.

We discussed at length mediators derived from a wide range of cell types, particularly highly purified mast cells from various species. The need to invoke the participation of "other cells" to explain some of the findings seemed to lurk in a nebulous way, and requires more specification. Clearly we must reckon with the macrophage, bearing in mind that, although it has IgE receptors of low affinity, it can be stimulated to release leukotrienes by IgE complexes. Nevertheless, the macrophage presents a problem because, although these cells may be *in* the airways, one could expect more "peripheral" lung disease if they were of importance in asthma. We should not forget that in clinical asthma the acinar parts of the lung are characteristically preserved, both clinically and histologically even after 30 to 40 years of severe asthma in atopic individuals. Therefore, I think we have to find a reason why alveolar macrophages exposed in their normal site to a variety of antigens do not seem to cause more problems.

Although there were elegant studies on the diversity of mediators produced by various cell types, with regard to asthma we must be very clear not only about species differences but also about the wide spectrum of mediators derived from various cells.

I was intrigued by the possible role of tryptase in asthma because it links complement activation and the various suggestions that have been put forward over the years regarding immune complex–mediated asthma and the Arthus reaction. This seems to provide a plausible explanation as to how complement activation might occur in this disease and perhaps "gets us off the hook" with the Arthus reaction, which seems to be out of fashion at present.

You will note that in my diagrams I have deliberately avoided putting the mediators too close to any one of the cell types, because we do not have sufficiently detailed information, especially in humans, to be more precise than this.

There were some interesting presentations about the neutrophil chemotactic factor, concerning both its capacity to attract neutrophils under certain circumstances and to activate them (that is why in the diagram the arrow goes in both directions). The possible relationship between neutrophils and the development of hyperreactivity is also of considerable interest. We were informed about some elegant studies applying mediators directly to isolated smooth muscle strips both in animals and humans. In

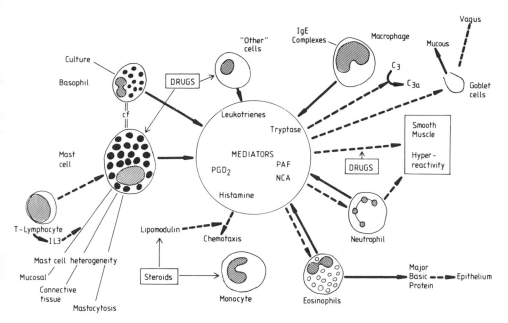

Fig. 1. The scope of the areas covered in this volume. Solid boldface arrows, generation of mediators; dashed arrows, actions of mediators; solid light arrows, modulating actions of drugs, etc.

these situations the effects of drugs could also be studied, but *in vitro* systems have the possible disadvantage of eliminating any control feedback mechanisms that might be important.

There was a splendid paper on the eosinophil; it was unfortunate that discussion of the eosinophil did not arise more frequently during the course of these three days. We are now beginning to understand the importance of the major basic protein and some of its effects on the epithelium and its location within the tissues in asthma. Is this study a lead-in to a better way of studying asthma? I hope that techniques for identifying mediators in the bronchial tissue will become more commonplace, because mediators identified in the circulation are quite distant from their origin. The paper on major basic protein supported a way toward more information on local tissue, if we could only get the material.

That is how we spent our time over the first one and one-half days of the meeting, and anything approaching bronchial asthma was wedged, properly, in one corner (Fig. 1).

We then proceeded to the second 36 hr, and the mast cell became a little "smaller" (figuratively speaking). We discussed bronchial challenge procedures in animals and humans and the circulating mediators that we were able to identify in the blood of humans, in relation to both the immediate

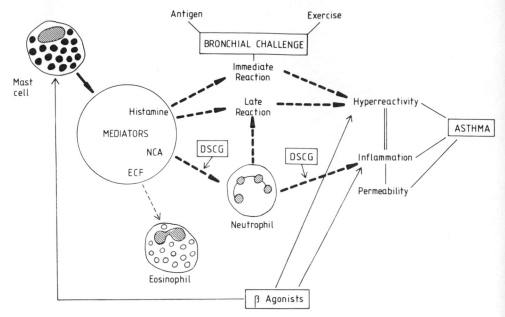

Fig. 2. The scope of the areas covered in this volume (continued).

and late reactions. In this respect, it is unfortunate that the number of mediators in the circle on my second diagram (Fig. 2) have now diminished. Nevertheless, those of you who are working on better assays for leukotrienes, prostaglandins, and other mediators have shown the need to apply these in relationship to bronchial challenge studies and, of course, in real clinical asthma. The importance of the different responses to various forms of challenge in humans, that is, antigen inhalation and exercise challenge, was emphasized many times. The general feeling seems to be that the many forms of challenge tests distinguish asthmatics from non-asthmatics on the basis of hyperreactivity rather than by any direct mechanism upon otherwise normal muscle. It is, therefore, very surprising that we have heard nothing about muscle studies during the last three days. I wonder whether you share my view that many of the chemicals, hormones, and mediators that we have considered are also likely to influence smooth muscle, which might in turn lead to altered responsiveness rather than being primarily involved in an asthma attack.

There was much discussion of whether those individuals expressing a late reaction were those whose late response had a close interrelationship with the development of hyperreactivity. Some of you were almost tempted to say that if we knew the immunopathogenesis of the late response, we could explain hyperreactivity. I am sure this is worth more discussion, and perhaps we should consider whether it is the neutrophil influx that determines the changed muscle properties. This leads me to consider the manner in which we are going to study bronchial smooth muscle in asthma. Even if we were able to obtain asthmatic material and study it *in vitro,* this might not give us the whole answer, because other factors vital for the expression of hyperreactivity might be eliminated. I cannot believe that it is beyond our ability to devise techniques for looking at muscle contractility, either by use of a bronchoscope or an implant of some kind. Ingenuity in other areas has been so extreme that I would like to suggest that some of you put your time into a study on intact muscle in asthmatic humans.

You remember the discussion we had on nonmuscle components of the asthmatic response: the relationship between inflammation and permeability and the sad observation that hyperreactivity did not seem to move closely with permeability of the bronchial epithelium. There may be some technical problems involved with these forms of study. Another point that was only discussed superficially was the mode of actions of drugs in asthma. Again, this was perhaps understandable because the meeting is primarily concerned with dissecting the asthmatic response. Drugs can help us, in part, to understand these mechanisms, although we had to resist the temptation of generating too much clinical discussion about drugs and patients. Nevertheless, there was an important discussion on β-agonists and muscle, their antiinflammatory possibilities, and their action on mucus as well as the mast cell. Equally important, while on the topic of drugs, we had a fascinating contribution on corticosteroids. We should dissect this problem further and look, not so much at antiinflammatory properties, but at precisely how cells vary in their abilities to handle corticosteroids. This may be fundamental in determining whether the asthmatic patient will respond or not.

There were also a few studies that unrepentantly related to asthma, and one considered, for instance, what happens to patients with this disease at night. There is still great value in talking deliberately about asthma as we really see it (as opposed to tidy *in vitro* models), so perhaps we should have more of this at our next meeting.

Now a few more general points. The meeting was essentially divided into two populations: scientists and physicians (although with considerable overlap). I noticed that during the first half of the meeting, the scientists tended to sit in the front rows and the physicians in the back rows. I did sense a slight transatlantic divergence of approach to the problem, but thankfully this became much less apparent as the meeting progressed. By the end of the day, the distribution of physicians and scientists achieved the proper blend and became what Barry Kay and his colleagues had originally intended. Clearly as a physician, I think that we have to thank the scientists for giving us this opportunity to see how they have tried to unpick a singularly difficult field. Also speaking as a physician, I think we must be very careful with what we do with the pickings. There are many difficulties, particularly methodological ones, not the least being the extrapolations from animal to man, which may not necessarily be sufficiently accurate to be useful. Ideas derived from animal experiments, presented in a fairly light-hearted manner, may go a long way, but any sort of rigid translation from an experimental model to real asthma will be fraught with disaster.

Throughout the meeting, I have been very impressed by the continual re-emphasis of the heterogeneity of almost every population of cells that has been considered, a point that I have emphasized on the diagrams. The heterogeneity of the mast cells has obviously taken some time to become apparent, but I think we are all aware of the potential importance of this area of research. The studies on the eosinophil also tended toward the view that there is possibly some functional heterogeneity, even though the evidence for morphological subtypes still seems to be lacking. If that is true, I think it is highly probable that there will be functional heterogeneity of neutrophils. In any study one must be aware of the fact that cells can be performing in a variety of ways at different times with varying results as to the types of mediators they are releasing under the various circumstances or the biological job they are trying to do.

While on the subject of heterogeneity, one point that has not emerged very much is the heterogeneity of the asthmatic population itself. I don't know what an asthmatic is, but I do know that the asthmatic population can be subdivided and that descriptions of these subgroups have to be more precise. For example, bronchial challenge tests are only undertaken on relatively mild asthmatics because it would be unethical to carry out these procedures on patients with more severe cases. If we extrapolate from many of the results of these studies to our more severe chronic patients, this might lead to erroneous conclusions. One elegant example of that was illustrated by the study from Dr. Holgate and his colleagues in which two populations of asthmatics were identified who showed a different balance between reactivity and mast cell degranulation. What other subgroups of asthma should we be alerted to? Ian Grant emphasized the importance of corticosteroid unresponsive asthma, which he defined in terms of patterns of physiological variations. There are other subgroups of asthma including those with a very substantial irreversible component. There has been little or no discussion about the possible immunopathogenesis of the irreversible component in asthma. We might be able to prevent these serious irreversible consequences, which are very common and very important, if we knew more about the pathogenesis at an earlier stage and adjusted our therapy accordingly. What about the group of asthmatics that is highly unstable all the time, very reversible, but impossible to stabilize? What message is that giving us, as opposed to that from the patients who maintain a steady level of normal airflow for long periods of time and then suddenly get a devastating attack of asthma from an apparently trivial exposure? Surely if we try and eliminate some of the heterogeneity, we can dissect our subpopulations more precisely, and in this way we may arrive at some answers more quickly and avoid the dangers of lumping patients together. I am not necessarily accusing you of overlooking this point, since the meeting has not considered the asthmatic patient in a major way.

Where can the bridge be built more firmly between scientists and clinicians? As soon as we have good blood measurements for all of the mediators this will surely open a substantial door, but we must not forget the problems that have been discussed throughout the meeting about the limitation of using blood samples to identify agents when they are taken far from the site of the disease. On the other hand, if this approach has been valuable with NCA and histamine, I do not see why it could not also yield useful information for some of the other mediators.

Another question to consider is how much these bronchial challenge procedures, eliciting either immediate or late reactions, have anything to do with natural asthma; specifically, either atopic asthma resulting from natural exposure or asthma in general, in which no specifiable extrinsic agent can be identified. I know there are many who favour the idea that we are very close to the real thing by analysing the late reaction, but other data suggested that this might not necessarily be the case. Perhaps no form of bronchial challenge really tells us everything about asthma. The point was often made that there is a correlation between the profiles of various parameters, either between cells and mediators or, in the broader context, among the disciplines such as physiology, immunology, and pharmacology. Study of these interrelationships may be the most productive means of moving ahead when the scientists have the tools and the physicians have the patients. The question of the real pathology of asthma, other than lethal disease, has been raised several times. Have we really worked over the histopathology of autopsy material from "incidental" asthmatics thoroughly? Have we looked critically at different parts of the airways? Have we used the right staining techniques? I imagine that some form of international collaboration in these areas would be very valuable. Anybody who has an asthmatic death might put a substantial amount of deep frozen material aside as well as tissue for electron microscopy, and these might be exchanged.

Linked with this was the question of whether or not lavage was going to give us any information. I think the general feeling is that people should properly consider the risk of inducing severe asthma, especially when such a study is being undertaken for pure research purposes. There has been some reservation for purely ethical reasons, as a result of either our own experiences or those of others, of inducing bronchospasm and other complications. However, as we have heard, the French have apparently overcome the problems, having now lavaged several hundred patients, with suitable and careful preparation (for instance, by giving bronchodilators as the fiberoptic bronchoscope goes through the cords), and they do not appear to have had significant problems. If this is true, then I think I should be more open minded. The procedure may be safe if it is supervised very carefully in centres that really do appreciate the problems, and if it is controlled meticulously. Just supposing we can do it and that the problem of bronchospasm is solved, what is it going to tell us? Again, I am sure any cells obtained from the lungs are going to be of interest, but we will have to devise ways of getting cells from the airways, as opposed to cells from the alveolar parts, which would be of less interest. In the meantime, we clearly have to go on quizzing our scientific colleagues about their models of asthma, because models are obviously useful for many reasons, but they must be valid with respect to the particular question being asked. If not, they could be highly misleading.

I suppose we will still be left with the hard core of our continuing asthmatic patients, that is those who have their asthma to a greater or lesser degree at all times. Is this due to persisting allergen? Is there enough allergen around to make this possible? How are the airways controlled in the moderate to severe cases? Is the mechanism pharmacological, neurological, or something completely different? I suspect that this will be a major area for work for "Asthma IV."

What are the laboratory and clinical people going to do next? I would like to have a more clearly defined statement on the control of mediator release. The question of cell control was raised many times and this exciting area clearly has a long way to go.

Technical methodology for mediator measurements as suitable for clinicians is a more mundane feature, but a very useful one. I have mentioned this endless question—What is hyperreactivity? On the clinical side, how are we going to explore further the component of inflammation, and would it not be possible to use noninvasive tools as is being done in the study of inflammation in many other disorders, perhaps with radioisotopes? I think, in particular for clinicians, the interdisciplinary studies become absolutely essential, provided we give our scientific colleagues the right sort of patients. Have I posed enough questions to safeguard the need for Asthma IV?

GENERAL DISCUSSION

Austen: Your summing up was so elegant that there is almost nothing more for us to add. Nevertheless, I would like to make the suggestion that perhaps asthma is no more than physical allergy of the mast cells of the lung. For those of you who are familiar with physical allergy, you can consider that either obvious, outrageous, or irrelevant. The reason I am willing to make the speculation is based on two points. First, there seems to be a similarity between antigen challenge and exercise challenge as regards the identification of the mediators released and the recognition of the delayed reaction. The other relates to the current understanding of physical allergy, which is known to involve mediator release from cutaneous mast cells by various eliciting agents. Patients with solar urticaria react to certain light wave lengths, whereas cold and cholinergic urticaria are elicited by extremes of temperature.

In each instance the same chemical mediators of mast cell origin can be shown as well as mast cell degranulation on biopsy of their urticarial eruptions. Finally, there is a newly recognized form of physical allergy related to exercise, in which individuals with exercise developed erythema, conventional hives, angiooedema, and vascular collapse, but no pulmonary manifestations or response to an elevated core temperature. So, from the cutaneous viewpoint there are a variety of examples of obviously nonantigenic external factors which will activate the mast cells and in which there are one or more different clinical presentations. The only thing not yet described in physical allergy is a late reaction. I suspect that we have to be resourceful to find a late reaction. If it is possible that the diverse physical allergies that we see in the skin, which are clearly mast cell mediated, can be shown to give us a late reaction, then the similarities to the pulmonary problem would increase. Airway hyperirritability could be either a late secondary event of mast cell activation or independent. Nonetheless, I am curious to hear whether my old protagonists would agree if I were to suggest that asthma is in fact a physical allergy of the mast cells in the pulmonary tissues.

Gleich: The suggestion that asthma (that is, the common form that we all recognize but have difficulty agreeing what to call) has as its basis the mast cell needs further evidence. This hypothesis nicely explains certain of the features of asthma due to allergy where there are acute bouts related to allergen exposure and associated with late-phase reactions. However, when one turns to chronic asthma (intrinsic, or perhaps better, idiopathic), the mast cell hypothesis lacks the cornerstone of the IgE–allergen relationship. In order to improve our ability to discriminate among models, I believe we need a modern description of the pathology of asthma using methods to analyse tissue in such a manner that the number of inflammatory cells, namely basophils, mast cells, eosinophils, and neutrophils, can be determined and their location and relationships described. Another approach to the same question may come through analysis of bronchial lavage fluids. French workers (P. Godard, J. Chaintreuil, M. Damon, M. Coupe, O. Flandre, A. Crastes de Paulet and F. B. Michel, *J. Allergy Clin. Immunol.* **70:**88, 1982) already have information about the kinds of cells recovered, and it seems clear that there are a large number of eosinophils in these fluids. One must also keep in mind that the pathology of the cutaneous late-phase reaction is characterized by a prominent neutrophil infiltration. If the infiltration in the late asthmatic reaction also is characterized by neutrophils, it then becomes difficult to equate chronic asthma with an ongoing persistent late reaction because it appears that neutrophils are not prominent in the pathology of asthma. In the last analysis our hypotheses must explain the striking eosinophil infiltration in asthma, and I am not sure that they do so adequately at the present time.

Kay: We (T. H. Lee, B. K. Assoufi and A. B. Kay, *Lancet,* 1:520, 1983) and others (P. J. Barnes, P. W. Ind and M. J. Brown, *Clin. Sci.,* **62:**661, 1982) previously suggested that in asthma, mast cells are intermittently "leaky." A situation is envisaged in which mast cells or other mediator cells release pharmacological agents as a result of a variety of specific or nonspecific stimuli. The "leakiness" can be intermittent (episodic asthma) or continuous (chronic asthma) with the degree of putative membrane permeability reflecting the severity of the disease. Thus many of the features of asthma such as hyporesponsiveness to β-adrenergic agents, bronchial hyperreactivity, and bronchial inflammation might be secondary to this primary mast cell defect.

Turner-Warwick: Dr. Austen, do you really think that in "physical allergy" the mast cell is the only abnormal cell, performing in isolation?

Kaplan: I would like to comment about possible analogies between physically induced hives and nonallergic stimuli that trigger asthma. The analogy is perhaps best demonstrated by cholinergic urticaria since many patients with cold urticaria or dermatographism, or type I solar urticaria are IgE mediated. But in cholinergic urticaria there is no antibody involved, and by exercising and inducing sweating and muscle movement, generalized urticaria occurs. Skin biopsies show no infiltrate, but mast cell degranulation and oedema formation are seen. With a more sensitive assay, we find elevated venous histamine levels during attacks in all such patients. Further, injection of methacholine into the skin of many such patients causes localized hive formation that reproduces their lesions, hence the term *cholinergic*. This is an example of abnormal histamine release from cutaneous mast cells as a result of release of an otherwise normal neurohormone. We know from Dr. McFadden's work that when these patients are placed in heat retaining suits so as to raise cell temperature, they have bronchoconstriction even though most are not otherwise asthmatic. This is as close as possible to linking a physical form of hives with lung disease, but it may well be a model of nonimmune autosensitivity of mast cells and could have a relationship to exercise-induced asthma or perhaps "intrinsic" asthma.

I agree with Dr. Austen that desensitization of leucocytes, due to severe episodes of mediator release, could prevent a late phase infiltrate, but remember that a small "X" placed on the skin of a dermatographic does not yield a delayed reaction nor does an ice cube test in an cold-insensitive urticaria patient. Here one usually cannot measure any mediator in the circulation. I believe there is some other reason for absence of late reactions in physically-induced skin reactions, perhaps absence of antigen over time, or intrinsic differences between cell recruitment in the lung as compared to the skin.

Wasserman: It is important as we consider Dr. Austen's hypothesis that it need not explain everything in every patient. It is obvious that some of the controversies regarding mediator measurement in exercise bronchospasm reflect the fact that physical activation of lung mast cells is but one of many mechanisms responsible for asthma.

Nadel: In response to Dr. Austen's request to comment on our perception of asthma and how this has changed since "Asthma II," I would say (a) scientists and clinicians now recognize the importance of increased airway responsiveness in asthma—the *mechanisms* must now be identified; (b) the input signals to mast cells are now recognized to be broader than IgE; exploration of physical and chemical signals to discharge mast cells will be important; and (c) the recognition of the possible importance of inflammation for the pathogenesis of asthma has suddenly budded! We must recognize that inflammation and repair of tissues vary under different conditions. We cannot expect all "inflammatory responses" to have the same effects on airways or on other tissues.

Kay: The inflammatory response is particularly intriguing, but what are the signals for the infiltrations of inflammatory cells? Mast cell- or macrophage-derived mediators are obviously implicated, but the signal may be derived from other cells—possibly epithelial cells. Also, why do some people have this putative "leakiness" of mediator cells and others not? Perhaps there may be too much extrapolation from isolated human lung mast cells, since these may not be the cells that have the primary defect.

Lichtenstein: I have approximately the same model in my mind as Dr. Austen suggested, that most asthma results (in the simplest sense) from the nonimmune release of mediators. I would differ in that I would extend the list of appropriate stimuli to more than the physical— to things like hyperosmolarity, polyamines, anaphylatoxins, etc. A major lack is that we do not have stimuli that release *in vitro* which we know are relevant *in vivo*. Recall that the mechanism of release by anaphylatoxin, hyperosmolarity, etc., is different from antigen, and in particular different drugs inhibit different stimuli. It may well be that we will have to find drugs that inhibit the nonimmune stimuli before we make a big impact on the clinical disease.

Kay: To define the triggers and drugs that inhibit release it may be necessary to work with asthmatic mediator/mast cells.

Lewis: I would extend Barry Kay's comment. Since the human pulmonary mast cells we obtain are derived from lungs of pulmonary carcinoma patients, and not from asthmatics, we should expect them to teach us something, but not everything, about pulmonary mast cells in asthmatics. Likewise, we accept that whereas measuring mast cell mediators in systemic arterial or venous blood may tell us something about their generation in asthma, the site of sampling is far enough away from the critical site of local action as to have limited relevance to pathobiology of the disease. These reservations should be added to those readily voiced over *in vivo* and *in vitro* animal models, which (as pointed out by Margaret Turner-Warwick) should be used to ask specific rather than global questions.

Hogg: While we might all agree that asthma is an inflammatory disease of the airway, it is also true that many cases of acute and chronic airways inflammation do not display airways hyperreactivity and reversible bronchoconstriction. It thus seems possible that the hyperreactivity and bronchoconstriction relate to some factor other than inflammation, such as the nervous control of the smooth muscle or the smooth muscle itself.

Flenley: Inflammation of the airways, which it seems we are being told is the feature of asthma, is also seen in chronic bronchitis—yet by definition these patients do not have spontaneously variable airflow—or possibly excessive bronchial reactivity. If inflammation is the common cause, why is there this difference?

Also, why can a patient have a nearly fatal wheeze today, and yet not yesterday? Is this a sudden exposure to a physical or biological allergen today and not yesterday? That seems to be unlikely, in view of the clinical history often obtained in such patients.

Hargreave: The possibility that leaky mast (or other) cells are responsible for the type of inflammation that initiates and characterizes asthma is supported by some of our recent work. Dr. Helen Ramsdale, working with our group, has observed in chronic airflow obstruction associated with chronic bronchitis that there is a linear correlation between reduced FEV_1 and reduced PC_{20} methacholine and a lack of correlation between responsiveness to methacholine and responsiveness to respiratory heat loss (E. H. Ramsdale, M. M. Morris, R. S. Roberts and F. E. Hargreave, *Thorax*, in press). The patients were hyperresponsive to methacholine but not to respiratory heat loss. We think these results suggest that the increased methacholine responsiveness might be due to reduced airway calibre and that the lack of response to respiratory heat loss was due to the absence of release of appropriate mediators.

Schiffmann: It is conceivable that mediators may be released in the bronchi (perhaps from the mast cell) when challenged with a stimulus which can cause contractile events in smooth muscle cells. For example, it has been demonstrated that platelet-derived growth factor is a potent inducer of spreading and chemotaxis in vascular smooth muscle cells.

Clark; In response to the present role of the mast cell, as proposed by Frank Austen, I would make the following comments. First, mast cells are present in healthy man and therefore some other factor must be involved. Even in patients with abnormal mast cells such as those with urticaria, rhinitis or skin test hypersensitivity only a minority have asthma. The waxing and waning of asthma also requires an explanation for a change in behaviour of the mast cells. Another source of doubt is the failure to find suitable therapeutic agents for asthma based on animal work which has produced drugs that can block mast cell degranulation. These comments make me hesitate to accept the mast cell theory for asthma.

Bach: I would like to stress a point that has not been considered at these meetings, namely the possibility of genetic predisposition. Animal models of genetically defined hyperreactivity have now been described. To be sure, it is not a single genetic determinant that predisposes to asthma. Rather than accounting for asthma as the overlap of two circles, as was done at the beginning of this meeting, we might consider the partial overlap of 10 or more circles. A careful identification of the genetic inheritance of the recognizable components may ultimately aid in the definition of the multiple ramifications of disease.

I am struck by the fact that no single mediator is acting in isolation nor, in the real world, are they only acting acutely. I believe that much can be learned of the aetiology of hyperreactivity if we could study the effects of chronic administration of agonists or neurohormones singly or in combination.

Oates: To use a drug as evidence against the participation of the mast cell, there must be data indicating that the drug reaches sufficient concentration in biologic fluids in man and that it does indeed affect the putative pharmacologic action on the human mast cell.

Kay: Following on from Tim Clark's point, during the course of this meeting the origin of various mediators has been raised several times and there is the probability that many (of importance in asthma) might be derived from non–mast cell sources. Therefore arguments for or against the participation of mast cells are not necessarily all that apposite when considering mediators as a whole.

On a further point, it seems to me that the general field of the relationship between mediators and bronchial smooth muscle hyperreactivity needs more attention.

Nadel: In contrast to *vascular* tissue, few studies demonstrating changes in contractility of airway smooth muscle exist. This area of research urgently needs to be explored.

Lessof: I would like to suggest one area for further work. It has been suggested that the measurements of mediator release and other techniques that have been applied to asthma should now be applied to other diseases. One disease that cries out for that kind of study is chronic bronchitis. David Flenley said that you do not get bronchial hyperreactivity in chronic bronchitis, but that depends on how you define chronic bronchitis. Bronchial hyperreactivity is certainly observed in this poorly delineated condition, and more detailed studies would show how different patients in this group compare and contrast with bronchial asthma. Major basic protein measurements in sputum might also help to define the areas of overlap between asthma and cases of wheezy bronchitis at different ages.

Hargreave: Dr. Nadel's comment about the absence of any demonstrated *in vitro* abnormality of muscle emphasizes the need to study the muscle from people who have had definite clinical asthma.

Holgate: One factor that may be relevant to the finding of normal reactivity of asthmatic airway smooth muscle *in vitro* is disconnection from the nervous system. Furthermore, human airways contain a large number of neural ganglia which contain a variety of peptides and possibly purine neurotransmitters. It is possible that changes in these, with effects on airway tone, may be an important determinant of airway hyperreactivity *in vivo*.

Barnes: There are several regulatory peptides within the airways that may have important effects on smooth muscle either directly or by neuromodulation. Whether there is an abnormality in the peptides will be difficult to study until specific antagonists are available, but is an area of great interest.

Gleich: Dr. Hogg and I are developing plans to conduct a study of the pathology of asthma, but these are in a rather preliminary form at the present time. Perhaps by the time "Asthma IV" is held we will have the necessary information.

Index of Participants

Subject Index

A

Acetylcholine, 145
Acute severe asthma, 348–349
Adenosine, 178–180, 192, 397–398, 406, 413–415
Adenosine receptors, 398, 407
β-Adrenoceptors, airway, 339–358, 395
  dysfunction in asthma, 345–347
  effect of corticosteroids, 350
  function, 339–342
  localisation, 339–342
  regulation, 343–345
  tolerance, 349–350
Aerosol
  generation, 264–265
  inhalation, 264–265
AGEPC, see Platelet-activating factor
α-Agonists, 139–140
β-Agonists, 144–145, 261, 280, 339–358, 395, 420–421
  effect
    on gland secretions, 139–140
    on late-phase reactions, 253–254, 257
    on respiratory drive, 382, 385, 389–390
  tolerance, 349–350
  in treatment of asthma, 347–349
Airway resistance, 400–401
Airways
  in asthma, 129–130
  cooling, see Heat exchange, respiratory
  inflammation, see Inflammation
  mucosal inflammation, 325–338
  mucosal permeability, 329–338
  mucosal reactivity, 331–332, 337–338
  neural receptors, 378
  response
    to bronchial provocation, 399–402
    to leukotrienes, 71, 85–99

  responsiveness, 129–155
  secretions, see Mucus; Secretions
  smooth muscle, see Smooth muscle, airway
Allergen-inhalation challenge, 212–213
Allergens, see also specific allergens
  airborne, 297–314
    particle size, 303–308, 312–313
  avoidance, 297–314
  and bronchial reactivity, 305–306
Allergic asthma, 10–12, 93, 157–171, 195, 215–216, 265–266
Alternaria tenuis, 247–257, 260–261
Altitude exposure, 377–378
Aminophylline, 382–383, 389, 408
Anaphylaxis, 61, 117
Angina, 117, 122–123, 126
β-Antagonists, 343–345
Antigen inhalation, 214
  delayed response to, 130–131
Antigen P_1, 299, 300–303, 306–308
Antihistamine, tricyclic, 10
Arachidonic acid
  metabolism and airway smooth muscle, 101–112
  release
    from basophils, 47–49
    from mast cells, 42–43
Aspergillosis, allergic bronchopulmonary, 259–260
Aspirin, 57–62, 98, 102–104, 418
Aspirin-evoked asthma, 58–62
Aspirin-evoked mastocytosis, 57–62
Astemizole, 403–406
Asthma, see also Allergic asthma; Bronchial asthma; Chronic asthma; Exercise-induced asthma; Intrinsic asthma; Nocturnal asthma; Occupational asthma; Seasonal asthma
  mucociliary abnormalities, 138, 146